DATE DUE

DEC 0 1 2009	

EXAMINING YOUR DOCTOR

EXAMINING YOUR DOCTOR

A PATIENT'S GUIDE TO AVOIDING HARMFUL MEDICAL CARE

Timothy B. McCall, M.D.

A BIRCH LANE PRESS BOOK
Published by Carol Publishing Group

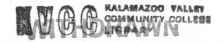

A Birch Lane Press Book
Published by Carol Publishing Group
Birch Lane Press is a registered trademark of Carol Communications,
    Inc.
Editorial Offices: 600 Madison Avenue, New York, N.Y. 10022
Sales & Distribution Offices: 120 Enterprise Avenue, Secaucus,
    N.J. 07094
In Canada: Canadian Manda Group, One Atlantic Avenue, Suite 105,
    Toronto, Ontario M6K 3E7
Queries regarding rights and permissions should be addressed to
Carol Publishing Group, 600 Madison Avenue, New York, N.Y. 10022

Carol Publishing Group books are available at special discounts for
bulk purchases, sales promotions, fund-raising, or educational
purposes. Special editions can be created to specifications. For
details, contact: Special Sales Department, Carol Publishing
Group, 120 Enterprise Avenue, Secaucus, N.J. 07094

Manufactured in the United States of America
10 9 8 7 6 5 4 3 2 1

Library of Congress Cataloging-in-Publication Data

McCall, Timothy, B.
    Examining your doctor : a patient's guide to avoiding harmful
medical care / by Timothy B. McCall.
        p.   cm.
    "A Birch Lane Press book."
    ISBN 1-55972-282-7
    1. Physician and patient.   2. Medical care—Evaluation.
3. Patient education.   I. Title.
R727.3.M394   1995
610.69'6—dc20   94-25244
                                                         CIP

In memory of my father, Raymond J. McCall,
who first showed me the beauty
and the power of the words.

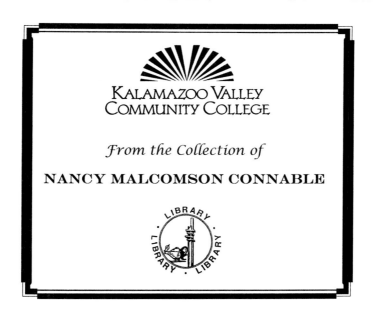

I observe the physician with the same diligence as the disease.
—JOHN DONNE

CONTENTS

FOREWORD

MY FIRST EXPERIENCES TAKING CARE OF PATIENTS AS A MEDICAL student changed forever the way I viewed doctors. I was appalled. In the university hospital where I was assigned, we treated one patient after another transferred from hospitals where they'd received medical care that nearly killed them. We managed to save some of them, though many of those we saved wound up disabled. We didn't tell these patients or their families that they'd been victims of poor medical care; we intentionally misled them.

Covering up malpractice is just one example of the systematic way that doctors withhold information from their patients. Rather than providing patients with enough information to make truly informed decisions, doctors, if anything, have encouraged attitudes of helplessness. Most act as if medicine is just too completed for the average person to understand. They seem to be saying, We wouldn't want to trouble you with all this information. It would probably just make you more anxious. If, as the saying goes, knowledge is power, then the power in doctor-patient relationships is distinctly one-sided. Even most bright and generally well informed people have little idea how to tell good medical care from bad—sometimes until it's too late.

In the fifteen years since I started medical school, I've seen thousands of examples of bad care ranging from the insensitive and mildly incompetent to outright malpractice. I've worked in major medical centers in Boston, private hospitals in small Wisconsin towns, welfare clinics deep in rural Alabama. I've worked in emergency rooms, walk-in clinics, community health centers, and private doctors' offices. Besides the unnecessary deaths and suffering, I've seen many patients become disillusioned and alienated by doctors in general. And I've seen a profession that not only doesn't admit its shortcomings but actively attempts to sweep them from sight.

Since every one of us is a medical consumer, we're all potentially vulnerable. My knowledge has allowed me to escape poor care so far, but I've had to watch my loved ones be victimized. I've seen friends misdiagnosed, treated like chattel, forced to undergo painful surgeries they never should have needed. Despite my best efforts, in the last few years of his life my father, living a thousand miles away, saw one second-rate physician after another. I could sometimes only intervene after the damage was done. Again and again the medical care he received lowered the quality of his life and probably cut it short as well.

My initial response was anger, but realized there is a more constructive path. I could help alter the lopsided power equation between doctors and patients by teaching people how to be smarter, more assertive medical consumers. I could give them the kind of inside information—vital to getting good medical care—that is rarely available to them.

A dozen years ago I began advising my friends and family on how to interact with their doctors. We talked about how to find good doctors, how to scrutinize their performance, how to demand more information, how to tell if you really need a drug or a test—in short, how to get the right medical care. More recently I wrote this book.

In fact, the hundreds of discussions I've had with friends and family members over the years were the seeds from which this book grew. If there is one overarching principle that came out of those discussions it is this: If you want to get consistently good medical care, you should begin by examining your doctor.

ACKNOWLEDGMENTS

THIS BOOK WOULD NOT HAVE BEEN POSSIBLE WITHOUT THE HELP, love and support of many people.

Thanks most of all to my friends and to my mother and the rest of my family for their unflagging help, interest and encouragement. I am grateful to Steve Nadis and Andy Chaikin who have believed in the book since the idea was first hatched eight years ago. Thanks, too, to Ann Dwyer, Theresa Murphy, Phyllis Segal, Ivan Mimica and Lisa Clark.

My brother Tony and my friends Tom Birch and Mark Pearlmutter, all physicians, read the manuscript and offered helpful suggestions. Two friends, Mike Eastman and Neal Burnham, solved computer disasters and, given the connection between stress and health, probably added years onto my life.

Fellow members of the National Writers Union aided me at every stage along the way. Christine Ammer, Barbara Beckwith, Ann Bernays, and especially Archie Brodsky took time from their hectic schedules to help me fing an agent, negotiate a contract and deal with other problems as they arose. Every writer should join this wonderful organization.

Several people have helped me become a better writer. They include my sister-in-law Madelyn Wessel, Mopsy Strange Kennedy and Ottone Riccio (a.k.a. Ricky). Martín Espada has been a friend, teacher, expert editor and tireless supporter.

Thanks to my editor at Birch Lane Press, Kevin McDonough, for his thoughtful, "less invasive" approach to his work. My friend Tom Begner, formally of Viking Press, introduced me to my agent Angela Miller who worked hard for the book *and* answered my phone calls.

Two people deserve special thanks. My brother Ray stayed with me the final week before the manuscript was due, read every word, and debated structure, syntax and punctuation with me, sometimes into the wee hours. I'm waiting for him to write his book so I can return the favor. Sibley Fleming spent long hours on the phone helping shape the manuscript. Her sharp eye made the book stronger and me a better writer in more ways than I can name.

Finally, I'd like to thank the people who let me tell their stories in these pages and the thousands of other patients who over the years have taught me a lot about medicine and more about life.

DISCLAIMER

Every effort has been made to ensure that the information contained in this book is accurate and up-to-date. Due to the constant evolution of medical knowledge and individual variation in symptoms, diseases, and responses to therapy, however, it is prudent to consult a competent physician before making medical decisions based on the information in these pages.

EXAMINING YOUR DOCTOR

I

ARE YOU SEEING
THE RIGHT DOCTOR?

MOST PEOPLE PASSIVELY FOLLOW THE DICTATES OF THEIR DOCTORS.
People who wouldn't buy a toaster without consulting *Consumer Reports* become meek and deferential in the presence of a stethoscope and a long white coat. They find themselves reduced to muttering, "Whatever you say. You're the doctor."

Probably the most important lesson I learned in medical school was that if you want to avoid a medical disaster, you've got to abandon this passive "you're the doctor" mentality and learn to take control of your medical care. You need to scrutinize the quality of your doctor and actively participate in the medical decisions that affect you. The quality of doctors varies enormously, and the quality of the doctor is the primary determinant of the quality of medical care. Blind faith in physicians is like Russian roulette.

American consumers *can* obtain the finest medical care in the world. We lead the world in medical technology and research. You have more to gain from medicine today than at any time in history. But because the quality of medical care is also more uneven today than at any time in history, you have more to lose by not choosing your doctor wisely. Consider the case of one of the first patients I cared for as a medical student.

Case History: Licensed to Kill

Bill Carlson,* a retired naval officer from a small farming community, came to the Veterans Administration Hospital be-

---

* The case histories in this book are true. Some names and personal characteristics have been changed to protect privacy.

cause of severe chest pain. He said he felt as if someone were sitting on his chest. An electrocardiogram (EKG) done in the emergency room revealed that he was in the process of having a heart attack, so he was rushed upstairs to the coronary care unit (CCU) where I'd been assigned as a third-year student. Medical students spend their first two years attending lectures, doing lab work, and burying their noses in books. They rarely see patients. It is only in the third year that they don their white coats and begin to learn the ways of the hospital, where they will spend the remainder of their training.

When I entered Bill's room, he was propped up in bed, wearing only a pair of blue pajama bottoms. He was thick-chested, like a bulldog, partly from boyhood work on his father's dairy farm and a career in the military. When I introduced myself, Bill was still experiencing chest pain from his heart attack, but he wasn't going to give into it. "How are you, kiddo," he said, smiling, and squeezed my hand hard enough to make it ache.

Under the direction of the medical resident, Dr. John Layton, the nurses gave Bill nitroglycerin tablets under the tongue and, when they proved ineffective, small injections of morphine to relieve his pain. I didn't understand everything going on around me, but I did my best to be helpful.

After Bill's condition stabilized and Dr. Layton had completed his evaluation, I was allowed to interview and examine Bill in detail. He told me that although he wasn't the type to go to the doctor much, he went to his physician, Dr. Charles Piper, within the first few hours of developing the pain in his chest. Dr. Piper had done an EKG, but it had looked okay to him. He couldn't figure out what was causing Bill's pain, so he suggested Bill drive to the VA, more than an hour away, to get it checked out.

As I'd rehearsed in my first two years of medical school, I asked Bill about his past medical problems, his allergies, and whether he'd ever had surgery. I examined his eyes and ears, listened to his chest with my stethoscope, prodded his abdomen, and tapped on his knees. After completing the exam, I went to discuss the case with Dr. Layton. We went over the EKG Dr. Piper had sent along, John pointing out the changes in the shapes of the waves that showed that Bill had already been suffering a heart *attack while he was in Dr. Piper's office. It was pretty obvious, but Piper had missed it. John snickered and shot a glance toward the tiled ceiling. "Dr. Piper," he said, "wouldn't recognize a heart attack if it bit him in the ass."*

John leaned back in his chair and began to talk about Dr. Piper. It seemed he regularly referred patients whom he had misdiagnosed or whom he'd been treating with medicines that had become outmoded years earlier. One guy had a cyst on the back of his hand which Dr. Piper had treated with a splint, a treatment about as likely to be effective as a pair of crutches for appendicitis. John told me the medical interns and residents, with typical black humor, referred to Dr. Piper as a "double O doc," because—like Secret Agent 007, James Bond—he was "licensed to kill." Everyone, John told me, knew Dr. Piper was dangerous.

Everyone, it turned out, except his patients. They adored him. Bill told me, "Chuck Piper is one hell of a guy and one of the finest cardiologists in the state"—a particularly ironic comment since Dr. Piper was a general practitioner, not a heart specialist.

Blood tests later confirmed our diagnosis. Bill suffered another heart attack a few days later while still in the hospital, but we were there to treat him and he recovered. After a couple of weeks he went home—back to his farming community and, unfortunately, back to Dr. Piper.

SEVEN FACTORS AFFECTING THE QUALITY OF A DOCTOR'S CARE

Quality Factor 1. The Doctor's Level of Competence

The experience with Bill got me thinking. I wondered if physicians like Dr. Piper were common—doctors so incompetent that they couldn't even recognize a heart attack. My supervisor, Dr. Layton, was less than two years out of medical school, yet the diagnosis was *obvious* to him. I wondered how intelligent people like Bill could be so badly fooled. Finally, I wondered why Dr. Layton and the other medical residents laughed in private but never said anything to patients or to anyone who could do something about incompetents like Dr. Piper.

By competence I mean that constellation of skills, knowledge, and judgment necessary to practice medicine well. To practice competently, doctors must be able to recognize the symptoms of various diseases. They need to know which tests are necessary to diagnose and keep track of illnesses. They have to understand which drugs to prescribe and when. They need the skills to perform physical exams to detect accurately when something is wrong. Doctors need good communications skills to interview you about your symptoms and to help you understand tests, medications, and the nature of your medical problems. Surgeons and other doctors need the manual dexterity and technical skills to carry out procedures safely and effectively. The foundation of competence is formed in medical school and residency training, but good doctors constantly strive to improve their skills and keep their base of knowledge up-to-date.

Good judgment, like common sense, is more intangible. Some have it and others don't. It takes judgment to know when a drug or test is *not* needed, when the risk of intervening outweighs the likely benefit. A good doctor needs to be able to sense when things aren't adding up and when to reach out to others with more expertise in a particular area for help. **It is essential to medical competence that doctors know what they know and what they do not know.**

Many factors affect a doctor's competence. A doctor may never have received adequate training and simply lack the requisite knowledge. Some doctors who start out knowledgeable fail to keep up-to-date; as time passes, they become less and less competent. Other doctors become debilitated by illness or senility which they may not recognize or admit. One of my surgery professors had first-rate credentials and extraordinary book knowledge, but either because his Coke-bottle glasses couldn't fully correct his failing vision or because his coordination was poor, he simply could not carry out complex operations. I recall several surgery residents laughing among themselves in the hospital corridor about how dangerous he was in the operating room.

The stress of medical practice can also affect competence.

Doctor Heal Thyself: The Problem of Impaired Doctors

The practice of medicine has become more stressful in recent years. Doctors have fallen from their pedestals in the public eye. The "hassle factor" of medicine has greatly increased. With insurance companies and HMOs looking to reduce costs, doctors are increasingly having their judgments second-guessed. The paperwork gets worse every year. Many doctors have become too burned out and angry to deliver first-rate care. This burnout can lead to other problems.

Alcohol and Other Drug Abuse by Doctors

Researchers from the University of South Florida anonymously surveyed thousands of U.S. physicians regarding their use of alcohol and other drugs. The researchers found that doctors were less likely than other Americans to use cigarettes, marijuana, cocaine, and heroin but more likely to use alcohol, minor narcotics like Demerol, and tranquilizers like Valium. Almost 8 percent of doctors said they'd abused alcohol or other drugs or been addicted at some point in their lives, 2 percent in the previous year. Half of this 8 percent had problems with alcohol, one quarter with other drugs, and one quarter with a combination of alcohol and other drugs. The authors concede that because their survey relied on self-reporting and denial plays a major role in substance abuse, their numbers may underestimate the problem. Other studies, they note, estimate the alcoholism rate among doctors at between 13 and 14 percent.[1]

Not all types of physicians are at equal risk of becoming impaired. A Georgia study found that family or general practitioners in rural private practice were the most likely to abuse alcohol. Anesthesiologists, doctors who keep patients sedated during surgery, were the most likely to abuse other drugs, partly because of their easy access to them. Although the reason isn't clear, male physicians were more likely to have problems than female physicians.[2]

Physicians have traditionally been reluctant to report colleagues who abuse alcohol or other drugs. A few states, including Massachusetts, Oregon, and Minnesota, where laws mandate that physicians report impaired colleagues may be starting to make some inroads on the problem. The commonly applied name "snitch laws," a sort of childhood admonition against being a tattletale, reflects the profession's ambivalence about reporting potentially dangerous colleagues.

Bad Doctors

Perhaps it should come as no surprise that many doctors aren't good—there are plenty of lousy auto mechanics, bumbling government officials, and inefficient secretaries—but as a medical student I was surprised. I'd heard the malpractice horror stories: the botched surgeries, the neglected symptoms that turned out to be cancer, the operations where surgical instruments were left inside patients. I'd always believed these were isolated cases—the few bad apples. But when I worked in the university hospital in my third year of medical school, it seemed as if half the patients we saw owed their major problems to the inadequate care they'd received somewhere else before being transferred to us.

Since then I've learned that many doctors are less than competent. Dr. Piper was just the first of many dangerous physicians I've seen in my medical career. Almost all doctors have good intentions, but good intentions aren't always enough: **some of the most dangerous doctors I know are nice people.**

How Common Is Low-Quality Medical Care?

Researchers from UCLA and the Rand Corporation, an independent, nonprofit research institution, convened a panel of expert physicians to determine how often patients died due to poor medical care in the hospital. The panel found that 27 percent of the deaths overall were due to poor medical care. The numbers, however, depended on the condition: 18 percent of the deaths due to strokes, 24 percent due to pneumonia, and 37 percent due to heart attacks were blamed on poor medical care.[3]

When newspapers and TV cover bad medicine, they almost always focus on sensational malpractice cases, which is natural. But **most bad medicine is not malpractice.** Dr. Piper failed to diagnose Bill's heart attack, but from a *legal* standpoint he hadn't committed malpractice, because Bill wasn't harmed by the mistake (although he might easily have died).

Bad medical care takes many forms, often subtle. Bad doctors fail to examine patients thoroughly and miss diagnoses. They order too many tests, inflating medical costs and subjecting patients to needless risk. Bad doctors prescribe needlessly dangerous drugs. They perform unnecessary surgery. And they fail to prevent preventable disease. Considering all the varieties of bad medical care, its overall incidence is much higher than most people imagine.

Bad Doctors Can Be Hard to Spot

Polls show that most Americans are dissatisfied with our health care system but are happy with their own physicians. (I'm reminded of similar polls showing that most Americans blame Congress for many of the country's problems but like their own member of Congress. Recent elections suggest that trend is changing. Doctors may be next.) The sad truth is that many doctors—dearly beloved as they may be—are simply not very good. Whatever their intentions, they don't act in their patients' best interest.

Like Bill Carlson, most people have no idea when they've been victims of bad care. Other doctors certainly aren't going to tell them. The main reason for this silence is the near paranoia among physicians about malpractice suits. No doctor wants to say anything that might lead to a malpractice case against a colleague—no matter how justified such a suit might be. Collective silence seems to work.

How Often Does Medical Negligence Lead to Malpractice Suits?

Harvard researchers studying hospital records from the state of New York estimated that in a one-year period over thirteen thousand New Yorkers were killed and another twenty-five hundred permanently disabled due to medical care. More than 51 percent of the deaths were blamed on negligence.[4] If these numbers are extrapolated to the entire United States, twice as many Americans are dying from medical negligence as from car accidents. The researchers found, however, that the problem was largely invisible: more than 98 percent of people who were injured by negligent medical care did not sue their doctors. The authors concluded that only rarely does the legal system compensate injured patients or hold doctors accountable for substandard medical care.[5]

Many people assume that if a physician is licensed, he or she must be competent. State licensing boards, however, have proved ineffective in rooting out bad doctors. Consumers can't count on insurance companies either, because **doctors guilty of repeated malpractice usually have no difficulty obtaining malpractice insurance.** Large malpractice settlements are almost always shrouded by secrecy agreements that prevent any details from becoming public. Doctors with multiple malpractice settlements often go on practicing with none of their current and prospective patients aware of their records.[6]

Why do smart people have such a hard time telling a good doctor from a bad one? Perhaps, like Bill, many are fooled by good bedside manner. They figure a doctor who listens to them and who seems compassionate must be competent. As important as these qualities are, they don't make an otherwise incompetent physician good. In fact, some of the most charming characters you could ever meet are potentially dangerous. Remember Dr. Piper, and James Bond.

Quality Factor 2. The Doctor's Philosophy of Practice

Doctors vary enormously in their philosophy of medical practice—the collection of ideas, biases, and value judgments that inform the way they practice. You could see three different doctors for the same condition and end up with three widely differing recommendations. Study after study has shown huge variations in how often doctors prescribe drugs, how often they hospitalize patients, how often they operate. Your chance of having a particular operation might be three times or even ten times greater with one doctor than with his or her colleague down the block.

You might assume that your doctor's recommendation is based primarily on a scientific understanding of your condition, but the doctor's philosophy of practice can be as or more important. Here are a few areas in which doctors' philosophies of practice vary:

- *Patient involvement.* Some doctors believe that patients should do whatever the doctor says and not try to "interfere" in medical decisions. Others believe that their patients can make real contributions to their medical care and should take an active role.
- *Intervention.* Some doctors believe in aggressively employing drugs and surgery and other interventions, even in cases where the benefits are unproven. Other doctors are more selective in their use of high-tech fixes.
- *Preventive medicine.* Some doctors believe prevention is of vital importance. Others essentially ignore it and focus on treating people who are already ill.
- *"The latest thing."* Some doctors embrace trendy new therapies almost as soon as they're introduced. Others burned by experiences with past "breakthroughs" that ultimately proved more dangerous than helpful take a more cautious approach.

If your doctor makes a recommendation based on his or her beliefs or biases and not strictly on medical science, that fact usually isn't stated. You're simply presented with a recommendation. Most people never even consider what lies behind it. **Anytime a medical decision is based more on values than on**

science, you want to be sure that the decision reflects your values and not just your doctor's.

The Socialization of Doctors: The Hidden Curriculum of Medical School

The cornerstone of a doctor's philosophy of practice is formed in medical school. At the start of medical school most students are in their early twenties and impressionable, their beliefs and worldviews not yet fully formed. Most are idealistic. They want to help people and serve their communities. Contrary to popular belief, few students choose a career in medicine because they want to make big money. If that were their primary goal, it would be far more efficient to go to law school or get an M.B.A., so that after two or three years they could land a high-paying job. To become a physician requires four years of medical school after college, and, depending on the specialty, three to seven years of additional training. While their contemporaries in law and business have long since begun to reap the rewards of their professions, young doctors are often putting in eighty-hour weeks and living modestly. Meanwhile, their debts from medical school—these days often topping $100,000— accrue interest.

Whatever idealistic goals medical students start out with, most are profoundly changed by the time they finish their training. Much of this change is due to the strong socialization pressure they experience. Besides the official curriculum of medical school—the study of anatomy and various diseases— there is an unofficial curriculum of biases and attitudes inculcated into students every bit as methodically:

- *Professionalism.* Medical students are expected to work hard, be responsible, and put their patients' welfare above all else. This aspect of socialization is largely positive, although the work ethic can be carried to extremes. The doctors held in highest esteem by their professors and fellow students are usually workaholics whose lives are so unbalanced that they practically live at the hospital. To get the kind of grades that will further their careers, students are encouraged to emulate these workaholic role models and give up their outside lives as well. Doctors who follow this path may excel at the science side of medicine but sometimes don't do so well with the human side. Students are also taught to defend doctors' "rightful place" in society. Between lectures on the sounds of heart murmurs, professors warn about the dangers of socialized medicine and make snide comments about how lawyers are destroying the practice of medicine.

- *Malpractice.* A virtual paranoia about getting sued by patients is instilled in young doctors. Horror stories, such as the case of a woman supposedly awarded a million dollars after she claimed an X-ray of her head caused her to lose her psychic powers, are repeated ad nauseam. Students learn that "greedy lawyers" are responsible for the "malpractice crisis." Never is any mention given to the possibility that doctors practicing low-quality medicine might contribute to the problem. Young doctors are taught never to criticize another doctor in front of a patient, no matter how flagrant the mistake, for to do so would only invite a malpractice suit against the other doctor.

- *Specialization.* One reason we have a surplus of specialists in this country is that almost all professors in medical school are specialists and convey the message that the best doctors are specialists and the more specialized the better. General practitioners in the community are held up to ridicule. Good students are taught not to lower themselves by choosing a career in primary care. Several professors and one of the deans of my medical school went out of their way to dissuade a classmate of mine from going into family practice. She ended up choosing a surgical specialty.

- *Technology.* When it comes to diagnosis and treatment, students learn that newer and higher-tech is better. Death is the enemy and must be defeated at all costs: it is almost never better to let a patient die in peace if it is possible to extend life, regardless of the quality of that life. Students learn to disdain the "soft sciences" like psychology. The role of emotions and social conditions in medical problems, if not openly disdained, is largely ignored.

- *Alternative Medicine.* Students are taught contempt for everything alternative, dismissing it as unscientific, based only on anecdotal evidence. Professors routinely make disparaging remarks during hospital rounds and in lectures about alternative practitioners, such as chiropractors and acupuncturists. There's a double standard applied to alternative medicine. If a chiropractor misses a diagnosis or injures a patient, it's held up as proof that chiropractic is quackery. If an M.D. misses a diagnosis or injures a patient, that doctor may be criticized (in private) or the situation may be considered bad luck, but it's never held up as an indictment of the field.

- *Prevention.* By watching their professors in action, students come to believe that treatment is more important than prevention. It's not that anyone says, explicitly, that prevention is a waste of time. It's just that very little attention is paid to it. Students learn almost nothing about such vital subjects as nutrition. Professors in public health or preventive medicine are held in lower esteem than their colleagues in cardiology or neurosurgery.

- *Respect for patients.* Emulating their professors, students learn to value "good cases": patients with unusual diseases are considered interesting, while patients with the common chronic diseases that afflict our society are boring. Patients are objectified, thought of as the diseases that afflict them rather than as individuals. A patient might be referred to as "the gallbladder in room 502." Students learn to distinguish patients who are "innocent victims" from those who "bring their problems on themselves." They learn to differentiate desirable patients from the malingering *crocks*, the unkempt or sociopathic *dirt balls*, and the pain-in-the-neck, chronically ill *gomers* (an acronym for *Get Out of My Emergency Room*). Perhaps due to the stress of dealing with death and disease, doctors-in-training develop a black humor. You might be distressed to learn that because your critically ill father's condition is steadily deteriorating, his doctors joke that he's "circling the drain."

Not all students swallow the hidden curriculum without critical analysis, but most do. Think of the average doctor's attitude toward alternative healers. Students who at the beginning of their training are open-minded have no opportunity to investigate fields like acupuncture, because their time is monopolized. Saddled with heavy debt, most young doctors go directly into full-time or more than full-time practice. Few ever take the time later on to explore alternative medicine, but their general suspicion of it lingers.

Quality Factor 3. The Doctor's Agenda

Helping patients get better is only one of many, often competing, goals motivating physicians. The following are common items on doctors' agendas:

- *Help patients.* All doctors want to help their patients. Help can mean making a diagnosis, giving treatments, giving appropriate reassurance, being empathic, preventing disease, and educating patients about their medical conditions. Doctors vary in the importance they place on these different elements and in how much they're willing to compromise these goals in favor of other items on their agenda. In general, doctors want to satisfy their patients because it's both personally rewarding and good for business.

- *Provide high-quality care.* Almost all doctors try to provide high-quality care to all their patients. In order to do so, doctors need to spend time with patients. The more time they spend, the fewer patients they see and the lower their income. To practice high-quality medicine also requires a constant effort to keep up with the developments in medical science. **Because time invested in keeping up-to-date comes out of either free time or income-generating time, some doctors just don't do it.**

- *Make money.* Let's face it. Doctors want to make money. For some, money becomes the dominant consideration. They may order high-profit tests or recommend surgery to people who don't really need it. In managed care settings where their income is tied to reducing expenses, doctors may respond by inappropriately withholding tests and services.

- *Avoid getting sued.* Because doctors are constantly worried that someone is going to sue them, they shape the way they practice in an attempt to lower the risk. Within the profession, this mentality is referred to as CYA, for *Cover Your Ass.* What doctors fear in particular is being sued for missing a diagnosis or for failing to treat a treatable condition. **The primary ways that doctors try to lower their risk for malpractice suits is by ordering unnecessary tests and by prescribing unnecessary drugs.** Studies suggest, however, that this so-called "defensive medicine" does little to lower the risk of getting sued and serves only to inflate medical costs and to subject patients to the risks, expense, and hassle of tests and drugs they don't need.

- *Advance careers.* Doctors in university medical centers primarily advance their careers through research. They are often most interested in those patients on whom they can carry out research, if they're interested in patient care at all. Doctors working in HMOs will want to keep the administrators happy by keeping costs down and profits up. Doctors in group practices may want to keep their partners happy by doing a lot of procedures and thereby generating revenue.

- *Avoid hassles.* Doctors hate dealing with insurance company hassles, and they hate dealing with patients who hassle them. Doctors are trying to get through their schedules, and the less that slows them down the better. For some doctors this unfortunately means spending as little time as possible with patients. A patient who asks too many questions is considered a nuisance.

Some of the items on a doctor's agenda may be mutually exclusive. A doctor concerned with profits may rush patients, so that more can be seen in a day, compromising quality. Greedy doctors may order unnecessary tests or perform unnecessary surgery. A doctor who wants to satisfy a patient may agree to prescribe unneeded drugs that have no chance of helping while risking harm. **The simple truth is that low-quality medicine is often good for the bottom line.**

A doctor's agenda may also conflict with a patient's agenda. Patients want to know the doctor is concerned. They want emotional support. They want to be able to ask questions. They don't want to feel rushed. These things may take more time than the doctor wants to spend. Patients want to keep medical costs down, as long as their health isn't compromised. They don't want to wait too long to see the doctor.

Because their agendas differ from their patients', doctors may not wish to reveal theirs. What they say may not always be precisely what they mean.

What the Doctor Says and What It Sometimes Means

What the Doctor Says	*What It Sometimes Means*
We should get this test "just in case."	We should get this test just in case you decide to sue me.
We usually get an X-ray in these situations.	I can't think of a better reason to get one.
You need a cardiogram.	I just bought the machine and need to pay it off.
There is no medical reason for your problems.	It's all in your head (and I don't deal with that part of the body).
This drug has no side effects.	This drug is brand-new, so we don't know about its side effects yet.
This test is generally very safe.	If I told you about all the possible side effects, you might decide not to have it.
Here's a prescription.	Your appointment is over.
Here's something for your nerves.	You're getting on mine.

Quality Factor 4. The Doctor's Specialty

Primary Care Doctors

Primary care doctors are the ones you should generally see first for a medical problem. They are trained in general medicine and should be able to manage most medical problems without consulting a specialist. When the problem is more complicated or when it requires special expertise, a primary care doctor can recommend referrals to specialists and coordinate the recommendations of different specialists.

The three main types of doctors practicing primary care medicine are internists for adults, pediatricians for kids, and family practitioners for people of all ages. Doctors in all three fields are themselves specialists, having undergone three or four years of training after medical school, although they aren't usually referred to as specialists. General practitioners, who may have no training after a one-year internship—or in Louisiana, no training after medical school—are also considered primary care doctors. Some specialists like cardiologists spend some of their time seeing referral patients and some of their time doing primary care.

Primary care doctors have traditionally been the lowest-paid and the lowest-status doctors. This is changing as the country moves more in the direction of managed care. In HMOs, primary care doctors have taken on greater responsibility acting as so-called gatekeepers, granting or blocking access to specialists.

Specialists

Specialists focus on one particular organ system and are trained to manage the complex and rare disorders beyond the ken of most primary care doctors. But what specialists know about their field may come at the expense of their knowledge of general medicine. As Will Rogers put it, "Everybody is ignorant, only on different subjects."

The following table briefly describes what specialists do. The major fields are listed in bold type. Subspecialties of major fields are listed below them. To be a cardiologist, for example, a doctor must first train for three years in internal medicine, then do a three-year fellowship in cardiology.

What Different Specialists Do

Specialty	What They Handle
Family Practice	general medicine
Pediatrics	general medicine for children
Internal Medicine	general medicine for adults
Allergy	allergies, asthma
Cardiology	the heart
Endocrinology	hormone problems, diabetes
Gastroenterology	the stomach, liver, and intestines
Hematology	blood problems
Infectious Diseases	infections
Oncology	cancer
Nephrology	the kidneys
Pulmonary Medicine	the lungs
Rheumatology	arthritis and other joint problems
Surgery	general surgery
Cardiovascular Surgery	heart surgery
Colorectal Surgery	colon and rectal surgery
Neurosurgery	brain surgery
Ophthalmology	the eyes and eye surgery
Orthopedics	bone and joint surgery
Otolaryngology	ear, nose, and throat surgery
Plastic Surgery	cosmetic surgery
Thoracic Surgery	chest and lung surgery
Urology	urinary tract surgery, prostate problems
Vascular Surgery	surgery on veins and arteries
Anesthesiology	anesthetics for surgery
Dermatology	the skin

Emergency Medicine	emergencies
Neurology	the brain and nervous system
Obstetrics/Gynecology	pregnancy and delivery, female organs
Occupational Medicine	job-related and environmental illness
Psychiatry	psychological problems
Radiology	X-rays
Rehabilitation	rehabilitation after illness or injury

The incomes of doctors in different specialties vary widely. Most primary care doctors earn about $100,000 per year, general practitioners a little less, internists a little more. The higher-paying specialties tend to be the ones in which the doctors perform lots of procedures or operations, because it is by doing procedures that doctors make the most money. Endocrinologists do relatively few procedures and don't earn much more than internists. Cardiologists, on the other hand, perform stress tests and angioplasties; a few hours of procedures generate more profit than the rest of the week in their office. They average around $200,000 per year. Surgeons similarly earn most of their money in the operating room. Such surgical specialists as orthopedists and neurosurgeons make more than $300,000 per year.

Because of the enormous debts that most medical students now graduate with, more and more of the best students are seeking training in procedure-oriented fields, contributing to the relative glut of specialists. Fewer than a third of doctors in this country are in primary care, compared to 50 to 70 percent in every other developed country. The situation is bad and may get worse. Fewer than 15 percent of recent graduates plan on a career in primary care.[7]

Superspecialists

Superspecialists are doctors who not only have a specialty but focus their interest on a small area within that specialty. A superspecialist cardiologist, for example, might focus on heart rhythm disturbances. Superspecialists usually work in university medical centers.

Many books and articles advise consumers interested in high-quality medical care to seek out the nearest university hospital superspecialist whose area of expertise corresponds to their medical problem. I disagree. Rather than routinely consulting superspecialists for every problem that comes along, try to use them only when the specialists your primary care doctor refers you to are baffled or when they diagnose a "superspecialized" problem. **Superspecialists are absolutely the best doctors to see for particularly bizarre or complicated problems but not for more common conditions.**

Because superspecialists are authorities in their particular area of interest, people falsely assume they know a lot in general. They are often primarily researchers who may not be as skilled in the day-to-day practice of medicine as doctors who practice full-time. Many renowned superspecialists I've come across have been laughably deficient in their knowledge of general medicine. They are what the Germans would call *Fachidioten,* literally, "specialist-idiots." With increasing specialization the expert knows more and more about less and less, until finally he or she knows everything about nothing.

If you've consulted a primary care doctor and one or more specialists and they can't figure your problem out, or if you're diagnosed with a rare condition your doctor doesn't have much experience with, consider seeing a superspecialist. If you can find a superspecialist with a particular interest in your case, that doctor may be able to offer invaluable assistance.

Are Specialists Better?

In the United States specialists and particularly superspecialists are held in especially high regard by both their colleagues and the public. Many American consumers have become accustomed to self-diagnosing their problems, bypassing their primary care doctor, if they have one, and directly consulting the specialist who seems most appropriate. Many HMO members resent having their access to specialists impeded by primary care gatekeepers.

But are specialists better than primary care doctors? Is a hammer better than a screwdriver? It depends on the job. In general, primary care doctors are better at day-to-day medicine. It's what they've trained in and what they're presumably interested in. Primary care doctors tend to be better at the human side of medicine and at preventive medicine. They are in the best position to coordinate medical care and decide when referral to a specialist, and to which specialist, is advisable. Many patients who decide for themselves which specialist they need to see end up guessing wrong, wasting time and money.

Some specialists who spend part of their time doing primary care do a good job at it, but others lack enthusiasm for general medicine. More interested in patients who have problems in their specialty, they may not make the effort to keep up-to-date with advancements in general medical practice.

Compared with primary care doctors, specialists and especially superspecialists tend to intervene more.[8] They order more tests, particularly high-tech tests, prescribe more drugs, and hospitalize patients more often. Whether more is better depends on the specific condition, but the general tendency of American physicians has been to intervene too much.

Certain problems are clearly best handled by specialists. Cancer chemotherapy is almost always coordinated by an oncologist. Hard-to-control cases of diabetes should probably be managed by an endocrinologist. But even in these instances it's usually still a good idea to have a primary care physician overseeing things. The specialist or specialists can forward their recommendations to the primary care doctor, who can be sure that nothing slips through the cracks.

People who get all their care from various specialists with no one coordinating can suffer. Tests may be unnecessarily repeated. One specialist may order a drug that counteracts the effects of a drug another specialist has prescribed. Some things may be forgotten entirely. If a woman's cardiologist is taking care of her blood pressure, an orthopedist her arthritic knees, and a dermatologist her psoriasis, but nobody's doing a Pap smear or encouraging her to get a mammogram, she isn't getting optimal care, no matter how state-of-the-art each specialist is in his or her own right.

Nurse Practitioners

When you visit many HMOs and other clinics for a checkup, the chances are the person in the long white coat examining you, ordering tests, and handing you a prescription is not a doctor but a nurse practitioner. Nurse practitioners are registered nurses having completed four years of undergraduate nursing school who receive extra training in primary care. There are currently about fifty thousand of them in the United States. HMOs use nurse practitioners to save money, since their average pay is around $40,000 per year.

Because they have much less training than primary care physicians—typically nine to twenty-four months after college, compared with seven or eight years for doctors—nurse practitioners cannot be expected to manage some complex medical problems. They may handle such common problems as sore throats and bladder infections and manage some chronic diseases as well or better than some physicians. Due to their training as nurses, many of them practice a more personal brand of care and place more emphasis on prevention than most doctors. On average they spend 50 percent more time with patients. In studies nurse practitioners consistently score better in patient satisfaction than doctors.[9]

As with doctors, the quality of nurse practitioners varies. Since the field is relatively new, most of them will be up-to-date. The key thing nurse practitioners must know is when they have sufficient knowledge and skills to handle a situation and when they need help. Ideally, nurse practitioners should work in close collaboration with primary care doctors.

Physician Assistants

Many HMOs and private doctors' offices also employ physician assistants (P.A.'s) to function in roles essentially indistinguishable from those of nurse practitioners. The typical P.A. program requires students to have completed the equivalent of two years of college for admission, although many students enter with undergraduate degrees. P.A. programs average around two years, the first half devoted to book studies, the second to physician-supervised clinical training.

Whereas nurse practitioners study in nursing schools, which emphasize a holistic approach to patients, the training of P.A.'s more closely resembles a *Reader's Digest* version of medical school. P.A. programs are usually affiliated with medical schools, and physicians do most of the teaching. The values and biases of P.A.'s therefore end up being more like those of physicians than those of nurse practitioners. P.A.'s, for example, typically spend about the same amount of time with patients as do physicians.

There are currently around twenty-five thousand P.A.'s practicing in the United States. Every state except Mississippi recognizes them. Their average annual salary is over $50,000. Since their training is often less than one-fourth as long as physicians', P.A.'s have many of the same limitations in their knowledge and skills as nurse practitioners. Unlike nurse practitioners, who sometimes work independently of physicians, P.A.'s must work at all times under the close supervision of doctors.[10]

Quality Factor 5. The Doctor's Credentials

Credentials are one way to assess a doctor's competence. Many people, in fact, equate stellar credentials with state-of-the-art medical care. Doctors on the faculty of a medical school, for example, are likely to be up-to-date, at least in their specialty, and well-versed on the latest developments in high technology.

While credentials are important, great credentials don't guarantee a great doctor. A doctor educated at a prestigious medical school may know a lot but lack judgment. Credentials also say little about a doctor's agenda or philosophy of practice. Ultimately, it's how well a doctor practices that matters. Many fine doctors may have less-than-stellar credentials. **Good credentials increase the odds a doctor is good, but they aren't as important as is commonly assumed.**

How Do People Choose a Doctor?

A friend of mine joined an HMO a few years ago and was sent a booklet with photographs of the doctors and a brief description of where they went to school and what their specialties were. Finding it difficult to decide, my friend and his wife finally chose the only doctor on the page who was smiling.

There's no foolproof way to choose a doctor. Some of the common methods are:

- *Recommendations of friends and family.* The problem with this method is that friends and family members may not know how to evaluate a doctor's abilities. Studies suggest that most people rate doctors by their interpersonal qualities: how nice they are, how concerned they seem, and the like. These qualities are important but they do not guarantee competence.

- *Referrals from other physicians.* Referrals from one doctor to another may reflect institutional affiliations, friendship, or reciprocal (you refer to me and I'll refer to you) arrangements more than assessments of quality. **Doctors commonly refer patients to doctors they wouldn't choose for themselves or for their families.**

- *Physician referral services.* Perhaps you've seen ads for physician referral services on TV or in newspapers. Free of charge, you can call a local or an 800 number and be given the name of one or more doctors in your area. These services are generally for profit. They charge doctors to be listed and usually do little or no screening of the doctors. **Most physician referral services are nothing more than glorified advertising.** Hospitals similarly offer referral services for the doctors on their staff. When you call, you'll simply be given the name of the doctor currently at the top of the list. The next person who calls will get the next name on the list. None of the services give critical evaluations of the skills of the different doctors.

- *Potluck.* Some people take whatever doctor their health plan assigns them or simply open the Yellow Pages and take their chances. In fact, "Physicians and Surgeons" is the most-consulted heading in the Yellow Pages, used more than a billion times per year. Its closest competitor is "Auto Parts, New and Used."[11]

- *Recommendations from insiders.* The most objective source of information on the quality of doctors comes from the people they work with. Residents and hospital nurses are often the best sources. Most would be reluctant to comment on-the-record about the quality of different doctors but might be willing to tell you whom they see or to whom they'd send a sick relative. A man who recently moved to Boston walked into the emergency room of a prestigious hospital, cornered a resident, and walked out with the names of three highly respected internists.

Where the Doctor Went to Medical School

The value placed on where a doctor went to medical school within the United States reflects hype more than reality. All U.S. medical schools are accredited and offer a good education. Someone who went to Harvard or Johns Hopkins may have had better college grades or higher exam scores than the average medical student, but whether he or she will make a better doctor is far from clear. All U.S. medical schools turn out some excellent doctors and some not-so-hot doctors. Whoever graduated last in Harvard's class is still billed as a Harvard M.D.

In addition to schools granting M.D.'s, schools of osteopathy grant D.O. degrees. Doctors of osteopathy receive similar training to M.D.'s, but they are taught spinal manipulation similar to that practiced by chiropractors and a somewhat more holistic approach to medical care. Osteopaths have all the same legal rights to prescribe drugs and perform surgery as M.D.'s. Some D.O.'s train in the identical residency programs as M.D.'s but in general these doctors are frowned on by the medical establishment and are discriminated against in training opportunities. I have seen both excellent and poor osteopaths. The majority of osteopaths are general practitioners working in small towns.[12]

Medical schools outside the United States are more variable in quality. Some are excellent, others not so great. Doctors trained in medical schools in other countries include some of the best and some of the worst doctors I've seen. Though its hard to generalize, doctors trained in less developed countries may not have much exposure to the high-tech medical practice favored in this country.

Many Americans who don't have the grades or test scores to get into stateside medical schools enter programs in the Caribbean specifically designed to educate Americans. Some of the schools are decent, although they generally lack facilities, while others are little more than diploma mills. Similarly, many Americans enter medical schools in Mexico and occasionally in other countries. Unless you inquire, it might never occur to you that these doctors were educated outside the United States.

Although a doctor trained at Johns Hopkins certainly receives a better education than one trained at a medical school in Granada, the predictive value of knowing where a doctor was educated is often overstated. Even a doctor who trains in a second-rate medical school may overcome its shortcomings through hard work. Conversely, physicians trained in excellent schools may not have the temperament or common sense to practice medicine well. It's worth finding out what school your doctor attended, but ultimately, each doctor should be evaluated individually.

Where the Doctor Trained After Medical School

The first thing most physicians want to know when evaluating other doctors' credentials is where those doctors trained. In other words, in what hospital or hospitals did the doctors do their internships and residencies and, in the case of specialists, fellowships? In the United States the quality of different residency and fellowship programs varies more than the quality of different medical schools. University-affiliated hospitals are considered more prestigious than community hospitals without medical school affiliations. Prestigious university hospitals are more oriented toward superspecialization, however, and tend to turn out doctors with a similar bent.

Training programs generally consider graduates of American medical schools as more desirable, and the more prestigious programs usually have more luck attracting them. You can therefore roughly gauge how prestigious a program is by the percentage of American grads among their trainees. This method is not completely reliable, however, because some prestigious programs attract star students from all over the world—students more talented than the average American.

Where a doctor trained is important, but once again, it's what the doctor does with that training that matters most.

Board Certification

About four-hundred thousand of the six-hundred thousand physicians in the United States are board certified.[13] In order to receive board certification in a specialty, a doctor must complete a training program and pass a rigorous examination. Board certification means that a doctor has sufficient knowledge to pass the exam, or at least had it at the time the exam was taken. Since medical knowledge is constantly growing, a doctor who was last certified in 1970 may be twenty-five years out-of-date. Some specialty boards require that doctors be regularly recertified, but mandatory recertification is not yet universal.

Some older doctors may have trained before board certification was common, but these days board certification is becoming a minimal standard for physicians. Almost all doctors desire board certification, but many don't attain it because they haven't had the required training or haven't passed the exam. If your doctor isn't board-certified, ask why not.

Are Board-Certified Doctors Better?

Researchers from UCLA and the Rand Corporation examined medical records to determine how well different doctors in New Mexico treated people with sore throats. The researchers established minimal criteria for acceptable care, then measured how often different doctors met these minimal criteria. The following table summarizes their results:[14]

Type of Doctor	Percentage That Met Minimal Standards
Board-Certified M.D.	60
Board-Certified D.O.	24
Uncertified M.D.	42
Uncertified D.O.	27

Many doctors who list themselves as specialists in the yellow pages aren't really specialists, they've just decided to call themselves one. Many have neither completed the required training nor passed the rigorous certifying examination. The phone company makes no effort to verify the credentials of the doctors they list.[15]

Deceptive Specialist Listings in the Yellow Pages

Doctors from Harvard Medical School and the University of Connecticut investigated the credentials of all doctors who listed themselves as specialists in the Hartford, Connecticut, Yellow Pages. Here's what they found.

Claimed Specialty	*Percentage of Doctors Not Board-Certified in Specialty*
Allergy	67
Plastic Surgery	43
Family Practice	30
Colorectal Surgery	25
Hematology	19
Internal Medicine	18
Nephrology	17
Pediatrics	17
Cardiology	15
Endocrinology	14
Dermatology	13
Psychiatry	13
Gastroenterology	7
Pulmonary Medicine	7
Rheumatology	7
Ophthalmology	4
Orthopedic Surgery	2
Radiology	2
Surgery	2
Obstetrics/Gynecology	1
Infectious Diseases	0
Neurology	0

Neurosurgery	0
Otolaryngology	0
Thoracic Surgery	0
Urology	0

With the exceptions of plastic surgery and colorectal surgery, surgeons listing themselves as specialists were more likely to be certified than medical doctors, perhaps because many hospitals require that surgeons be board-certified in order to obtain hospital privileges.[16]

Some doctors list themselves as being "board-eligible," implying that they've completed the required training for specialty certification but have not yet taken or not yet passed the certifying examination. This is legitimate for a doctor who has just completed training, but the term is abused indefinitely by some doctors who never are able to pass the exam.

You can check on an M.D.'s board certification by consulting the *Directory of Medical Specialists* in your public library. **The easiest way to find out if an M.D. is certified is to call the toll-free number of the American Board of Medical Specialties, (800) 776-CERT.** They'll ask a few questions, then tell you what specialties a doctor is certified in and the year of certification.

Hospital Affiliation

In order to admit patients to a hospital, a doctor must have admitting privileges. Before granting these privileges, the hospital must consult a national data bank on physicians—unfortunately currently inaccessible to patients—which summarizes any disciplinary action against the doctor as well as the doctor's history of malpractice problems.

What hospital administrators do with the information is up to them. More prestigious hospitals may refuse admitting privileges to doctors with bad records. Doctors, though, are cash cows for hospitals. Hospitals need to fill their beds to be profitable, and it is doctors who direct patients into these beds.

Hospitals have a strong incentive to grant admitting privileges to a doctor with a large practice whose patronage could mean hundreds of thousands of dollars in business every year.

Membership in the Local Medical Society

At one time membership in the local medical society was considered an important indication of a doctor's standing in the community. In today's world it means next to nothing. It is sometimes possible to call local medical societies to check on a doctor's credentials, but they are not good sources of information on quality. Some medical societies will simply read the information the doctors provided, without making any effort to verify its accuracy.

The National Practitioner Data Bank

Since 1990 the National Practitioner Data Bank has collected information on all physicians in the United States. Any malpractice payments, any disciplinary actions by state licensing boards or medical societies, or any revocation or limitation of a doctor's privileges by a hospital or clinic must be reported. One of the goals of the Data Bank is to prevent physicians who are disciplined in one state from relocating to another state to avoid penalties. In the past doctors who had their licenses revoked in one state would simply move across the state line and open a practice, their past problems hidden from their patients and from the authorities in the new state.

In part because of the strong objections of the American Medical Association, the information in the National Practitioner Data Bank is not accessible to consumers. In fact, the AMA favors eliminating the data bank entirely, rather than see the information it contains get into the public's hands.[17] In lieu of the information in the data bank, **the best source of information on disciplinary actions by state medical boards or the federal government against physicians is published by the Public Citizen Health Research Group.** Their address is 2000 P Street NW, Washington, D.C. 20036.

Quality Factor 6. How the Doctor Is Paid

In exchange for their services, doctors in the United States usually receive:

- a fee for each service they provide
- a flat monthly fee for each patient cared for, or
- a salary or hourly wage

Each method of reimbursement contains incentives that can profoundly influence how a doctor practices. In addition, insurance companies and health plans frequently pay doctors bonuses and impose penalties in an attempt to shape the medical care they provide.

Fee-for-Service

The fee-for-service system is the traditional form of reimbursement in American medicine. The doctor bills for all services provided, including checkups, lab tests performed in the office, or surgical procedures. The more a doctor does, the bigger the bill. In the traditional fee-for-service system, some things are reimbursed more than others. Insurance companies pay doctors relatively little to sit with a patient and explain things or to conduct an in-depth interview. But **every time the doctor sticks in a needle or a tube, the cash register rings.**

As a result, fee-for-service doctors tend to order too many tests, especially ones where the profit margin is high, and to perform too many surgeries. Because unnecessary interventions can lead to complications, the potential harm is often greater than the potential benefit. Some people consider it a conflict of interest that the person who is advising you about whether to have a test or an operation stands to profit from it.

Testing in Fee-for-Service Versus HMOs

When Harvard University researchers compared the test-ordering patterns of doctors in private group practices, reimbursed under the fee-for-service system, with doctors in HMOs, whose pay was not affected by the number of tests they ordered, they found that private practice doctors ordered 50 percent more EKGs and 40 percent more chest X-rays, the two tests that they perceived as being highly profitable. There was virtually no difference in test ordering for blood counts and urinalyses, the low-profit tests.[18]

Because of the poor reimbursement for services other than procedures, fee-for-service doctors are in essence penalized for spending time getting to know you, carefully interviewing you about your symptoms, or performing a meticulous physical examination. These are precisely the areas where many American physicians are most deficient.

Another disadvantage of the fee-for-service system is that doctors may not want to care for patients who have no insurance or insurance from the government, like Medicaid, that pays only a part of their fees. Many fee-for-service doctors flat out refuse to see Medicaid patients, partly for financial reasons and partly out of a dislike for caring for poor people.

There are some advantages to the fee-for-service system too. Doctors who run their practices like small businesses have more incentive to work hard and keep their customers satisfied. Fee-for-service doctors know that you have the option of changing doctors anytime you wish and may therefore provide better service than you might find in a hospital clinic or an HMO.

Fee Per Patient

Doctors are sometimes paid a flat fee for each person they care for. So-called capitation payments—literally, "by the head"—are common in HMOs. When a doctor receives the same amount of money whether or not a patient comes in for visits or has tests done, there are no financial incentives either for or against providing services. Doctors may be tempted to take on more patients than they can handle—leading to less time with each patient and longer waits to see the doctor—because the more patients a doctor sees, the more money the doctor makes. Such doctors may also favor younger and healthier patients, who require less time.

Salary

With the growth of both group practices and HMOs, more and more doctors are working these days for a salary. Doctors who are paid a straight salary by a hospital or clinic have no direct financial incentive to order too many or too few tests. Some would argue that they may not feel they have the same personal stake in the care of their patients as private practitioners. Others would say that doctors who work for a salary may be less mercenary than doctors whose decisions are swayed by the bottom line: they may be motivated to provide only those services the patient needs—no less and no more.

Penalties and Bonuses

Most doctors I've talked with deny money plays *any* role in their decisions. They do not believe that getting paid more for doing more in the fee-for-service system leads them to order more tests or perform more surgeries. Managers of hospitals, clinics, and HMOs know better, however, and actively manipulate financial incentives to affect physicians' behavior.

Doctors Respond to Financial Incentives in Walk-in Clinics

A study in the *New England Journal of Medicine* compared test ordering by physicians at Health Stop, at the time the nation's largest chain of walk-in medical clinics, before and after a bonus plan was instituted. Health Stop administrators had been concerned that their salaried doctors lacked the financial incentives of traditional fee-for-service doctors to increase per-patient revenue. Under the plan, the more tests a doctor ordered, the bigger the bonus. After the bonus plan was instituted, the doctors ordered 23 percent more lab tests and 16 percent more X-rays. Those doctors earning bonuses increased their income by almost 20 percent.[19]

The entire fee-for-service system can be thought of as a bonus plan: every service provided yields a small—sometimes not so small—supplement to the doctor's income. Financial incentives, however, can work the other way too.

Financial Incentives in HMOs

In order to encourage doctors to keep costs down and profits up, HMOs offer them a strategic package of bonuses and penalties. Most HMOs withhold a certain percentage of a doctor's pay, often 15 to 30 percent, until the end of the year. If the plan turns a profit—primarily because all the doctors have kept costs down by limiting the services they provide to patients—the withheld amount is returned. Some HMOs pay bonuses when doctors keep down referrals to specialists and hospital admissions, two particularly costly items.

HMOs vary in how they structure the incentives. Some tie the return of the withheld money and bonuses to the performance of the HMO overall. In this system, the financial benefit to the doctor for withholding services is indirect, since the overall record of all the doctors determines the bonus, not the physician's individual record.

A more pernicious system, unfortunately too common in HMOs, ties a doctor's pay *directly* to how little he or she spends on patient care. Many HMOs set a yearly budget for each doctor, then pay yearly bonuses to those who come in under budget. In some HMOs if a doctor exceeds his or her yearly budget, plan administrators can place a lien on the doctor's future earnings or even drum the doctor out of the plan. **About 40 percent of primary care doctors in HMOs must pay for any lab tests they order out of their yearly pay. This system pits doctors against their patients: every time the doctor orders a $50 dollar test, that doctor's paycheck is $50 smaller.**[20] The doctor-patient relationship is soured, because even when a doctor legitimately feels a test or a referral to a specialist is unnecessary, the patient may suspect the doctor is doing nothing more than protecting his or her income.

Most physicians are well-intentioned. When the proper course of action is obvious—say someone needs to have their appendix removed—any good doctor, regardless of the reimbursement system, will take the same action. Much of medicine, though, is not clear-cut. Often there are many possible ways of treating a problem and not enough scientific evidence to distinguish reliably their relative effectiveness. Doctors are more likely to be influenced by financial incentives when the best approach is unclear. Financial incentives—both to do too much and to do too little—may unconsciously color a doctor's judgment.

Quality Factor 7. The Setting in Which You See the Doctor

Private Doctors' Offices

Doctors in private practice generally work on a fee-for-service basis, although in recent years many have begun to accept HMO patients as well. A private practice is a small business and, as such, depends for its survival on satisfying its customers. Since so many people equate the quality of their medical care with the quality of their interpersonal relationship with the doctor, a good bedside manner is vital to a financially successful practice.

Patient Satisfaction With Private Doctors

Researchers reporting in the *Journal of the American Medical Association* interviewed patients who visited doctors in different settings to determine which were most satisfied with the care they received. Doctors working in their own private offices, so-called solo practitioners, fared the best, with 65 percent of patients rating the visit as excellent. Doctors in HMOs and in large multispecialty group practices, on the other hand, were rated as excellent about half the time. Solo practitioners were rated as better in both personal and technical skills. They were also judged to be more accessible on the telephone, to explain things better, and to spend more time with patients.[21]

There are disadvantages to solo private practice. Doctors working alone have less contact with their colleagues and are more likely to fall behind in their medical knowledge. Since most patients tend to judge doctors based on their bedside manner and how nice their office is, being out-of-date doesn't necessarily hurt business much.

Group Practices

There are several advantages to dealing with a group practice as opposed to a solo practitioner. By having day-to-day contact with other doctors, group practitioners get feedback on their practice, their colleagues functioning as a form of quality control. Doctors in group practice are more likely to be up-to-date. In groups containing different types of specialists, referrals are often easier than they might otherwise be. Each doctor in the practice uses the same medical chart, meaning that all the lab results and all the notes by the other doctors in the practice are accessible, reducing the risk of redundant or fragmented medical care.

A recent AMA study showed that **doctors in group practice usually charge slightly more for an appointment, even though they spend less time with patients.** Patients of group practice also average a twelve-day wait for an appointment, compared with seven days for patients of solo practitioners.[22]

In my experience, when it comes to group practice, like attracts like. Excellent doctors tend to associate with other excellent doctors, whereas doctors of more dubious quality seem to find associates of similarly dubious quality. If you can discern the quality of one doctor in a group practice, you've got a strong clue to the quality of all the others.

HMOs and Other Forms of Managed Care

HMOs are the most common type of managed care plans. You or your employer pays an annual fee in advance to cover all your medical care for the year. In exchange for some restrictions, such as limited access to specialists, HMOs usually offer more comprehensive coverage at a lower price than traditional health insurance. Since HMOs receive the same amount of money regardless of whether you use services or not, they at least have a theoretical incentive to keep you well by practicing preventive medicine.

There are different types of HMOs. Some hire staff doctors, nurses, pharmacists and locate their offices, labs, and pharmacies under one roof. Others HMOs, sometimes referred to as independent practice associations (IPAs), contract with private doctors or group practices in the community to provide services to their patients.

Doctors in HMOs are paid in different ways. Primary care doctors are paid by salary, by fee-for-service, by capitation, or by a combination of the three. Specialists are usually paid by fee-for-service. Bonuses and incentives for keeping costs down, like withholding a portion of pay, also vary from plan to plan. Some pay their doctors a straight salary and offer no incentives whatsoever.

If you belong to an HMO or are thinking of joining one, be sure to ask how the doctors are paid and what bonuses and penalties are operative. Otherwise you may not fully appreciate the financial incentives that could be influencing your doctor's decisions. Interestingly, in a recent survey by *Consumer Reports,* the highest-rated HMOs paid their primary care doctors by fee-for-service.[23] Perhaps the countering financial incentives of fee-for-service and the various tactics HMOs use to keep expenses down lead to the best balance of services. Or perhaps many HMO members mistakenly believe that more medical care means better medical care and that fee-for-service doctors, even in HMOs, provide more.

To keep their costs down, HMOs try to limit high-cost items like hospitalization, referrals to specialists, mental health services, and certain high-tech tests. Although doctors in HMOs do not want to do so little that they risk lawsuits for missing diagnoses, they are pressured to be frugal. HMOs are not completely arbitrary in denying services. They refuse some discretionary surgery or save money by performing minor operations outside the hospital.[24] In most instances where surgery is necessary, they approve it. In the gray region where an operation might be helpful but isn't definitely required, they are more likely to say no.

How Good Are HMOs?

Researchers reporting in the *Journal of the American Medical Association* summarized the results of more than fifty studies to compare the performance of HMOs with that of traditional medical insurance plans. HMOs were found to use an average of 22 percent fewer tests that were expensive or had less costly alternatives. HMOs hospitalized fewer patients and discharged them sooner. People in HMOs had a somewhat higher number of doctor visits per year, although they had fewer visits to mental health specialists like psychologists. Most studies have found that the quality of care in HMOs is roughly comparable to that of traditional insurance plans for such diseases as high blood pressure, diabetes, and colon cancer. People with mental health problems, however, seem to do worse in HMOs. The one area where HMOs consistently perform better is in providing such preventive services as cancer screening and counseling to quit smoking. Overall, HMO enrollees tended to be less satisfied with the quality of their care and less satisfied with their interactions with doctors but more satisfied with the cost.[25]

The disincentive HMO doctors have to use medical services may be compensated for by the lack of disincentives patients have to visit the doctor. People with traditional insurance have annual deductibles and often must pay a certain percentage of the cost of a visit. HMO patients have no deductibles and often only pay a few dollars every time they see the doctor. Many HMOs also provide low-cost prescriptions and more complete coverage for such preventive care as Pap smears and mammograms than do traditional fee-for-service insurance plans.

Because primary care and specialist services are tightly coordinated in HMOs, the fragmentation and redundancy so typical of private practice fee-for-service medicine can be avoided. Access to physicians can be more difficult, however, both for appointments and on the telephone. There also tends to be more physician turnover in HMOs.[26]

HMO patients have to choose from a limited number of doctors. If you have a particular doctor you want to see, that can be a problem. Good HMOs attempt to screen out doctors of low quality, so the limited choice could be to your advantage. HMOs also engage in ongoing quality control of their physicians, less frequent in private practice.

So-called Preferred Providers Organizations (PPOs) are another form of managed care that has achieved some popularity in the last few years. PPOs, offered by many insurance companies and large employers, are loose-knit groups of doctors who provide medical care at a discount to members. Members are not required to choose a primary care physician and can directly consult specialists if they choose to. Unlike the situation in HMOs, you can still use doctors outside the plan, but you'll have to pay substantially higher fees.

Walk-in Medical Clinics

In the last several years walk-in clinics, also known as "doc-in-the-box" clinics, have mushroomed in shopping centers and on main drags all over the United States. Walk-ins offer convenience—no appointment is necessary—and millions of people choose these clinics for routine care rather than traditional doctors' offices. These clinics are typically free-standing—that is, not affiliated with a hospital—although some hospitals have added such clinics to offer a cheaper alternative to their emergency rooms. Walk-in clinics usually provide on-site X-rays, EKGs, and simple lab tests, although available services vary from clinic to clinic.

Most of these clinics operate for profit. They run efficiently; patients are often checked in and seen by the nurse and then the doctor in less than an hour. Waiting time is largely a function of how many other people are seeking care at the same time. Since no one has an appointment, service is first-come, first-served. Busy periods vary, but the late afternoon and early evening, when most people get home from work or school, are often jammed. Before seeking care in a walk-in clinic, you may want to call ahead to find out if they are busy.

The quality of the doctors who work in these clinics varies enormously. Some work full-time, while others are moonlighting residents. Many of the doctors in walk-in clinics lack board certification and do not have admitting privileges at any hospitals.

Doctors in walk-in clinics are typically paid an hourly wage, but many clinics offer doctors a bonus, the size of which depends on how many tests they order. Walk-in clinics profit greatly from lab tests, and these physician kickbacks lead to unnecessary blood tests, X-rays, and cardiograms. One doctor wrote an article in the *New England Journal of Medicine* a few years ago describing how he'd been fired from a major chain of walk-in clinics, not for practicing badly, but simply because he hadn't run up the patients' bills enough.[27]

Walk-in clinics use other techniques as well to generate revenue, especially when the patient has insurance. Unnecessarily frequent followup visits may be suggested. In a clinic where I once worked, they used a ploy called "the suture check." Anyone who got stitches (sutures) was instructed to return two days later to make sure the wound wasn't becoming infected. The doctor typically examined the patient for only a few seconds, but the patient's insurance company was billed for another visit. For most patients simple instructions about the warning signs of infection given at the time of suturing would have sufficed.

These clinics are best-suited for minor problems like bladder infections, ear infections, or sprained ankles. Since it's sometimes difficult for patients to judge the severity of their medical condition, a walk-in clinic affiliated with a good hospital is often the best choice. If they need more intensive services, transfers can easily be arranged. Walk-in clinics are less appropriate for chronic problems like diabetes or high blood pressure, which are better managed by doctors with whom you can establish a long-term relationship. At a walk-in clinic you may see a different doctor each time you visit. Chronic problems are poorly managed with such fragmented care.

Walk-in centers can provide good care for routine problems, especially if you can't get an appointment in a doctor's office quickly enough and your problem is not severe enough to require a visit to an emergency room. But the rule of thumb should be caveat emptor, "let the buyer beware." And remember, you don't have to agree to any lab test you don't feel is necessary.

Other Types of Clinics

Community health centers are often located in areas where the population has been traditionally underserved, such as inner-city neighborhoods. They often target their programs to meet the needs of their clientele and tend to focus on primary care. The doctors who work in these clinics are usually paid either a straight salary or an hourly wage and thus have no financial incentives to do too much or too little. Some of the doctors working in community health centers are fulfilling an obligation to work in an underserved area in exchange for financial aid during medical school. Many of these clinics deliver excellent care to people who would have a tough time getting it otherwise.

Many hospitals have large outpatient departments, where patients are cared for by staff doctors. These doctors are usually paid a straight salary. In the case of teaching hospitals, the doctors who see the patients are usually interns and residents, although they are supervised in varying degrees by more senior doctors. The quality of the care depends both on the competence and experience of the doctors-in-training and on the thoroughness of the supervision. One problem with teaching hospital clinics is that the residents only stay one to three years before moving on. Once you've gotten comfortable, you may discover you've been reassigned to another, usually greener, doctor.

Emergency Rooms

Emergency rooms are attached to a hospital. If a patient needs to be admitted to the hospital for further care, transfer is simple. If there is a strong likelihood you will be admitted to the hospital for your problem, then it is a good idea to know something about the hospital before going to its emergency room. In a true emergency, however, the nearer the hospital, the better. Once your condition is stabilized, you can usually arrange to be transferred to another hospital if you want.

Emergency rooms, as the name suggests, handle emergencies best. An ER is the place to go for a heart attack, a severe asthma attack, or a broken bone. ERs are not the place to go for routine or chronic medical conditions, although many patients, especially those with no health insurance, do just this. One reason is that if you truly have an emergency, an ER can not legally turn you away, whether you can pay or not. Under the federal COBRA law, ERs are required to perform a "medical screening exam" on all patients to determine whether an emergency exists before refusing to treat them or transferring them somewhere else.

If you go to an emergency room because your knee has been bothering you for six months, you are likely to end up with a cursory examination, a big bill, and a referral to another doctor to evaluate your problem. ER doctors get annoyed with patients seeking care for nonemergency problems. Among other disadvantages, ERs are expensive: for most the minimum charge, without lab tests or X-rays, is about $100. The waiting time is often excessive. In a big city ER, it is not unusual to wait five or six hours to be seen. Patients are not seen in the order they arrive but according to the severity of their problem. If you have already waited four hours with your knee pain and a man suffering a heart attack is rolled in, he will be seen first—as he should be. Because ER doctors typically work in shifts, the doctor who begins a patient evaluation may not be the one who finishes it. Faulty transfer of patient information from one doctor to another can compromise patient care.

The competence of doctors working in ERs varies enormously. Some hospitals are staffed twenty-four-hours a day by board-certified specialists in emergency medicine, but you can't realistically expect this ideal situation in smaller or more rural hospitals. In the Harvard study on medical negligence mentioned earlier, a high percentage of medical injuries sustained in emergency rooms were due to negligence. The researchers speculated that the reason may have been that emergency rooms are often staffed with doctors who are not well trained in emergency care.[28]

Many hospitals rely on part-timers or on moonlighters, who may be residents from local training programs earning extra money while off-duty. Moonlighting residents, unfortunately, may not have the requisite knowledge and skills to manage all emergencies. A resident at my hospital told me a horrifying story about the night he'd just spent moonlighting in a small ER outside of town. An ambulance had come in with a pregnant woman who was near her delivery date when she was severely injured in a car accident—a situation that he as a resident in internal medicine was clearly unqualified to handle. Despite his best efforts both she and her baby died before his eyes.

Most doctors working in ERs are paid either hourly or by salary. These doctors have no financial incentive to order unnecessary tests but may do so out of fear of being sued. Unfortunately, in true emergencies there is little opportunity for patients to influence which tests are ordered.

Different Types of Hospitals

The quality of medical care varies from hospital to hospital. Some problems that may be well handled in some hospitals are poorly handled in others. As with different types of specialists, different types of hospitals have relative strengths and weaknesses. In general, the more a hospital handles a particular problem, the more proficient it becomes at dealing with that problem. Practice may not make perfect, but it helps. Large hospitals that perform many heart bypass operations tend to have much lower death rates than hospitals that do only a few. Similarly, people with AIDS are more than twice as likely to die if they are treated in a hospital inexperienced in treating AIDS patients.[29]

As with choosing a doctor, you want to decide on a hospital before you get sick. Often when you choose a doctor or a health plan, the hospital you will use is already decided. In that case you may want to weigh the quality of the hospital when making your choice. In true emergencies you usually should go to the nearest hospital, even if it's not your preferred hospital, since a delay could prove harmful. For less urgent situations, you may have the luxury of traveling to the hospital you prefer.

The Joint Commission on Accreditation of Healthcare Organizations (JCAHO) inspects hospitals periodically to make sure they are meeting minimal standards of excellence. The inspections are voluntary, and not all hospitals comply. **Any decent hospital should be accredited by JCAHO and should be willing to prove accreditation status if asked.** The telephone number for JCAHO is (708) 916–5600.

The major types of hospitals in this country are as follows, although there is some overlap in the categories:

• *Teaching hospitals.* University medical centers and other teaching hospitals have three main missions: to educate young doctors, to conduct research, and to take care of patients. The bulk of the day-to-day care is delivered by doctors-in-training—interns and residents—who are supervised by private or staff physicians.

Because doctors-in-training need to gain experience, you are more likely to undergo multiple interviews and exams. Multiple exams can be of benefit in that one doctor may pick something up that another doctor missed, but they are also a nuisance. You may not have the energy or desire to repeat your story and subject yourself to examination by several different doctors. Although it's not always a good idea to do so, you have the right to refuse to be examined repeatedly.

As interns and residents become more skilled, they take on progressively more responsibility for patients. Be advised, however, that they sometimes do things they're not adequately trained to do. It is reasonable to ask a resident or medical student who plans to do a procedure on you, "How many of these have you done before?" If surgery is planned, you could ask the head surgeon, "Will you be performing this operation yourself, or will the residents do it?"

Teaching hospitals keep up on the latest advances in medical thinking and technology. They typically have more sophisticated equipment for diagnosis and treatment on site. Doctors in teaching hospitals tend, however, to order more tests than necessary—some more for teaching or research purposes than out of any strict medical need—and to use high-technology fixes when they aren't necessary. For these and other reasons, teaching hospitals tend to be more expensive.

That said, **teaching hospitals, particularly university hospitals, are often the best place to go if you have a rare or complex medical problem—the type of problem best handled by superspecialists.** Almost all of the most prestigious hospitals in the country are teaching hospitals. When deciding on whether to use a teaching hospital, keep in mind that **every July 1 a new crop of inexperienced**

interns and residents replaces the last group. You are
therefore more likely to get good care at a teaching
hospital in the late spring than in the early summer.

- *For-profit hospitals.* Hospitals run on a for-profit basis, such
  as those owned by large companies like Humana or the
  Hospital Corporation of America (HCA) are becoming more
  common. In my experience, for-profit hospitals pay a lot of
  attention to the amenities: they feature well-appointed
  rooms and nice-looking lobbies replete with large ferns and
  modern art. These attractions have little to do with the
  quality of care these hospitals provide but may affect their
  patients' perceptions of quality. If you don't have insurance,
  you may have a tough time getting in a for-profit hospital.
  They often try to ship poor patients off to public hospitals.

- *Community hospitals.* Most of the small- to medium-sized
  hospitals in this country are referred to as community
  hospitals. Many nonprofit community hospitals are run by
  religious organizations. Some are teaching hospitals. Community hospitals probably handle routine medical problems
  better than complex ones. **For common conditions like
  pneumonias or hip fractures, a good community hospital
  is often the best choice.**

- *Public hospitals.* These include VA hospitals and large mu-
  nicipal hospitals like Boston City Hospital and Cook County
  Hospital. Due to funding problems, the infrastructure of
  many of these hospitals is crumbling and they are sometimes
  understaffed. Because they care for many poor people, some
  more well-off people avoid them. The quality of the doctors,
  however, can be quite good in those public hospitals affiliated with medical schools.

- *HMO hospitals.* Some HMOs use hospitals in the community, contracting with them to provide services. Other,
  particularly larger, HMOs run their own hospitals. These
  hospitals are generally as good or bad as the doctors and the
  HMO that run them.

The Quality of Care at Different Types of Hospitals

Researchers at UCLA and the Rand Corporation examined medical records from almost three hundred hospitals in

different areas of the country to see if there was a relationship between the type of hospital and the quality of care. They compared rural and urban hospitals, teaching and nonteaching hospitals, small and large hospitals (based on the number of beds), and for-profit and nonprofit hospitals. They also looked at large public city and county hospitals that typically serve the urban poor. For each type of hospital they predicted what the death rate should be, based on how sick the patients were, then compared that number with the actual death rate. The following table lists the differences between the actual and the predicted death rates. Hospitals with positive numbers had more deaths than expected, those with negative numbers had fewer deaths than expected.

Type of Hospital	Difference Between Actual and Predicted Death Rates, By Percent
rural	1.4
small city	0.6
large city	− 1.1
nonteaching	0.7
limited teaching	− 0.8
major teaching	− 2.5
public	1.2
for-profit	− 0.4
nonprofit	− 0.5
<100 beds	1.9
100–200 beds	− 0.5
201–400 beds	− 0.1
>400 beds	− 0.8
large city/county	− 1.3

In general, patients in larger, urban hospitals fared better. The greater the hospital's involvement in teaching, the better. Public hospitals did less well, except for large city and county hospitals, which tended to be major teaching hospitals.[30]

As important as the quality of a hospital is, the quality of the doctor may be even more important. The authors of the above study speculated that patients in rural hospitals do worse because these hospitals have difficulty attracting skilled doctors and that the doctors who work in rural hospitals may not have enough contact with other physicians to remain up-to-date. Another study showed that while the more bypass operations a hospital does, the lower the death rate, the number the individual surgeon does is even more important.[31] Even if the nursing and support staff in a hospital are great, an incompetent phyician can still do a lot of damage. Even otherwise excellent hospitals may have a few turkeys on their medical staffs.

Putting It Together

The best time to choose a doctor is when you are well. Sometimes it's impossible to anticipate when you might get sick or injured. You don't want to find yourself in that situation without a doctor you know and feel you can trust. Regardless of a doctor's reputation, it's only after you've met that you can assess whether the doctor is someone you can work with.

Some of the seven factors affecting the quality of a doctor's care are easy to determine. It's usually possible to ascertain a doctor's specialty and credentials before your first visit. How the care is paid for is usually a function of the type of medical

---

Seven Factors Affecting the Quality of a Doctor's Care

1. The doctor's level of competence.
2. The doctor's philosophy of practice.
3. The doctor's agenda.
4. The doctor's specialty.
5. The doctor's credentials.
6. How the doctor is paid.
7. The setting in which you see the doctor.

coverage you have. You have some choice in the setting where you get medical care, although a managed care system may restrict your choice. Determining a doctor's competence, agenda, and philosophy of practice takes more doing. You need to scrutinize how well the doctor interviews you, orders tests, prescribes drugs, practices preventive medicine, and does all the other things that make up a doctor's work. Helping you make these determinations is what the rest of this book is all about.

In the coming chapters I'll systematically explain how to evaluate the quality of your medical care and how to play a more active role in the medical decisions that affect you the most. More than anything else, I will try to explain how to think about medicine and its proper practice, so that you can better evaluate your doctor's recommendations and give yourself the best chance of getting the best medical care possible.

2

IS YOUR DOCTOR TAKING THE TIME TO DO THE JOB RIGHT?

SEVERAL TIME-CONSUMING ACTIVITIES, VITAL TO PROVIDING GOOD medical care, pay doctors nothing or next to nothing. These include:

- conducting careful medical interviews
- performing thorough physical exams
- educating patients
- staying up-to-date with medical advances

In effect, these activities cost doctors money, since the time they require could otherwise be spent seeing more patients and performing more procedures—that is, generating more revenue. The result is that many doctors skimp on these important activities.

The interview and exam are where doctors collect most of the data important to good medical care. The less carefully they collect this data, the less accurate their predictions will be about what you have, what tests you'll need, and what treatments should be tried. Doctors who cut corners during the interview and physical exam may order the wrong tests because they weren't looking in the right place. They may also order tests to rule out diagnoses that could have been eliminated—more safely and inexpensively—by the interview and exam.

Computer experts have dubbed this phenomenon Garbage In, Garbage Out, or GIGO for short: if data collection is sloppy, even the most sophisticated analysis of the information is likely to lead to the wrong answer.

Skimping on patient education also undermines the quality of care. Patients with a poor understanding of their medical conditions are less likely to follow a doctor's instructions, make suggested lifestyle changes, take prescribed medicines, and recognize side effects of therapy. They are also less likely to feel satisfied with their medical care.

Since doctors have little financial incentive to spend time with you and in many instances are actually penalized for it, **the amount of time a doctor spends interviewing you, examining you, and explaining things reflects how genuinely concerned that doctor is for your welfare.** Luckily, you can directly observe how much time your doctor devotes to these activities.

Judging whether your doctor is staying up-to-date is more difficult. Because of the ongoing expansion and revision in medical knowledge, doctors must constantly strive to stay current. Within a few years of completing medical school, doctors discover that dozens of new drugs have come on the market, new high-technology tests have been invented, and important new diseases have come to light. A doctor's patients can't benefit from these advances if the doctor fails to keep up-to-date. By paying attention to clues during your appointment, you can usually figure out whether the doctor is making the effort.

Case History: If You Don't Look, You Can't See

Annie O'Malley was the troubled child of an alcoholic father, a little girl who found her only refuge in food. Starting at the age of ten, she was placed by her mother on strict diets. Annie would exact her revenge by retreating to her room to gorge herself on an entire box of cookies.

Despite her difficult childhood, Annie has found happiness and success in adulthood. She's the owner of a busy travel agency, has a wide circle of friends, and gives of herself freely. When a friend developed AIDS, she nursed him in the months before his death. She and her husband, Lionel, take in foster children too emotionally disturbed to have made it with other families, kids one step away from being institutionalized. Several of them have blossomed while living with her. Annie has always been good at taking care of others, but it's taken her years to learn how to take care of herself.

Ever since I met Annie in college, she'd had pain in the back of her hip that at times shot down her leg. She walked strangely, with a kind of waddle, pivoting her hips from side to side with each step. Her mother says she's always walked that way. In the mid-1970s Annie was a construction worker but had to quit because her leg hurt too much. She'd seen a series of doctors for the problem, starting with her family physician. They'd performed cursory exams and ordered X-rays of her back, always telling her she had a lower back problem—nothing severe enough to warrant surgery. Annie tried their suggestions but nothing, including losing weight, helped. The pain only got worse.

In 1983, my last year of medical school, Annie asked me if I would take a look at her back. She told me how frustrated she'd been with her doctors. As a fourth-year student I wasn't all that knowledgeable, but I had done a rotation on the orthopedics ward a few months earlier and had learned how to do a basic examination of the back and joints. I examined her and agreed that she probably had some problems with her back, but I was struck by how much pain she had in her hip. To examine her hip, I had her lie on her back, and, with her knee bent, held her calf in my hands and gently rotated her hip in the socket, moving the leg up and down. Even the slightest movement hurt her. The situation wasn't much better on the other side. I recommended she have her hips checked out by a superb orthopedist I'd studied with at the medical school. I even reminded her once, but she never went.

Instead, about a year later, she saw another orthopedist, a Dr. Peters, who hospitalized her for a series of tests, including a CAT scan—a computer-assisted X-ray—and a myelogram, a test in which the back is X-rayed after a dye is injected into the fluid surrounding the spinal cord. These days myelograms have largely been replaced by a less invasive test, the MRI scan, which uses magnetic fields instead of X-rays to take pictures.

The morning after the myelogram, Dr. Peters arrived at Annie's hospital room. He said the test showed that while there was some stress on her lower back, it was not more severe than many people experience every day. He told her she wouldn't require treatment unless her condition drastically worsened.

"My friend, who's a medical student, thinks the problem may be in my hips," she said. "Could you examine them before you discharge me?" He looked at her, stonefaced. "And my brother-in-law is a physician, and he thinks it could be my hips too. He wants me to get them checked out."

Dr. Peters glanced down at Annie. "What kind of physician is your brother-in-law?"

"A psychiatrist," she said. That was the wrong answer. In my experience, of all specialists, psychiatrists are probably held in the lowest esteem by their medical colleagues.

"There is no problem with your hips. We have them on X-rays and they're fine." He left without examining her. (He was wrong, by the way. Her hips had never been X-rayed.)

Two months later Annie had an appointment with another orthopedist to get a second opinion. On the day of her appointment, the doctor had a heart attack and retired from practice.

Annie waited three years before seeing another doctor. Meanwhile, her pain steadily worsened. When she described the pain, Annie tipped her head as if to look straight at you but held her eyes closed as she spoke. She couldn't take a vacation because she was unable to walk more than one block. She couldn't swim laps, which she'd previously done every morning. She couldn't go to the movies, because it required sitting in one position for more than a few minutes. She'd given up sex, because it hurt too much.

In 1987 Annie became more assertive. She saw another orthopedist, Dr. Orlovsky, and told him she thought she'd been misdiagnosed by Dr. Peters. She asked him to examine her hips. Annie agreed to have an MRI scan, because she thought it was going to be of her hips, but when the results returned, Dr. Orlovsky informed her that the scan was of her back. The good news, he said, was that the problem didn't look that severe. The bad news was that she was going to have to lose weight—a near impossibility given her inability to exercise. This time she wasn't going to settle for that answer.

Through a friend Annie got a referral to a specialist in joint problems, a rheumatologist. She told this doctor that she did not want her back examined, thank you, she'd already had every test known to man on her back. She wanted him to examine her hips. After examining her for less than a minute, he said, "The problem is obviously in your hips."

The final diagnosis was congenital dislocation of the hips, meaning that her hip bones had never really been in the sockets since birth. Due to the hips' abnormal position, Annie walked strangely and the cartilage wore down. Arthritis set in, which is what caused her pain. Because the arthritis had advanced so far before it was caught, the only thing the doctors could offer was to replace her hips surgically.

Any doctor who bothered to do a basic one-minute hip exam should have spotted that Annie had a hip problem. In fact, Annie's problem should have been recognized at birth or shortly thereafter. A check for dislocated hips is a standard part of the examination of all newborns. Dislocated hips, while occasionally difficult to recognize at birth, become obvious in the first six to twelve months of life and should be picked up by the pediatrician during routine checkups. If a dislocated hip is caught in the first year of life and if a simple nonsurgical treatment is given, 96 percent of children end up with perfectly normal hips.[1] Failure to make the diagnosis is a common cause of malpractice suits against pediatricians. But Annie, like most people who receive poor medical care, isn't interested in suing her doctors.

In 1988 Annie had the operation, first on one hip, then a few months later on the other. Everything went fine. The following year I received a postcard from the Cook Islands in the southwest Pacific near Samoa. Annie and Lionel were touring the islands, swimming and hiking and having a great time.

SEVEN WARNING SIGNS OF AN INADEQUATE INTERVIEW

Several things can tip you off to an inadequate medical interview. While there is no one right way to conduct an interview, some practices are clearly preferable to others. For minor problems a doctor's failure to conduct a proper interview may not affect the quality of care much. At other times a careful interview can be life-saving.

Interview Warning Sign 1. The Doctor Spends Too Little Time to Interview You Thoroughly

For some medical problems the interview alone is enough to make a diagnosis or at least to rule out certain possibilities. Migraine headaches are so classic in their symptoms that a careful history may be the only thing needed to make the diagnosis. At other times, as with the heart pain of angina, the interview can help decide whether or not further testing is warranted.

The Importance of the Interview

How important is the interview in making the correct diagnosis? Researchers at West Virginia University studied the relative contribution of the interview, the physical exam, and laboratory tests in eighty patients who came to a medical clinic with previously undiagnosed conditions. They found that after just the interview, the doctors could make the diagnosis 76 percent of the time. The physical exam resulted in another 12 percent of the patients being diagnosed. Lab tests resulted in another 11 percent of the diagnoses. Although the interview was the most important tool in making the correct diagnosis, the physical exam and the lab tests helped rule out certain conditions and strengthened the doctors' confidence in their diagnoses.[2]

In order to conduct an adequate medical interview, the doctor must devote sufficient time to it. Doctors who spend a few rushed minutes with you, ask a series of rapid-fire questions, glance at their watch, and scurry out of the room are unlikely to provide first-rate care. Neglecting to obtain vital bits of information may lead them to miss diagnoses, order the wrong tests, or prescribe the wrong drugs. You probably won't end up feeling very good about the encounter either.

Some doctors fail to spend enough time with patients out of

financial considerations, while others may simply be victims of their own success. These in-demand doctors are so overcommitted and spread so thin that they can't do any of their patients justice.

Other doctors, like the harried interns of teaching hospitals, have long working hours imposed on them. In teaching hospitals apprentice doctors—the interns and residents—are often deprived of sleep and stressed out by their grueling schedules. Recently there have been improvements in their working hours, but medical residents still often work in excess of eighty hours per week. Surgery and obstetric residents often work more than one hundred hours per week in jobs that have become more hectic. Harried residents are known to cut corners when it comes to patient care. If a nurse calls a resident requesting that a patient be evaluated, the resident will often deflect the request, telling the nurse something like, "Give her a couple of Tylenol, and if she still looks bad in an hour, call me back." A telephone order takes thirty seconds; a trip to the ward to evaluate a patient and to write a note in the chart can take half an hour.[3]

Waiting for the Doctor

Surveys of patients show that the single biggest determinant of their satisfaction with medical care is the amount of time spent in the doctor's waiting room. A long wait can signal that a doctor is overcommitted or disorganized. Consistently long waits can also reflect a clinic's or doctor's lack of respect for your time. Appointments may be spaced so tightly, in an effort to maximize the doctor's efficiency, that delays are inevitable.

Remember, though, that a well-organized doctor can fall behind schedule because he or she has wedged someone with an emergency into an already full schedule or has spent longer than anticipated with a patient who had an emotional reaction to a diagnosis—consideration you yourself might want some day. My recommendation is to **judge quality more by what happens while you're with the doctor. A doctor who makes the effort to probe your concerns carefully may be worth the wait.**

But if you wait an hour for a five-minute appointment that feels like a pit stop at the Indianapolis 500, you've got a right to be angry.

Since delays in a doctor's schedule are routine, planning for them is often the best approach. You may want to consider some of the following strategies:

- *Call ahead.* Before leaving for your appointment, call the clinic to find out if the doctor is behind schedule and if so, when you might reasonably expect to be seen.

- *Speak with the receptionist.* As soon as you arrive for your appointment, ask again if the doctor is running late. Tell the receptionist how long you're able to stay. Courteous receptionists will routinely inform patients if the doctor is behind schedule.

- *Schedule the first appointment of the day.* The earlier in the day you see the doctor, the less chance there is for other things to have put the doctor behind schedule. This method is not foolproof, since doctors often visit hospitalized patients before their office hours and can be delayed. Scheduling the first appointment after lunch also decreases the odds of a long wait.

- *Bring something to read or do.* Despite your best efforts, you may have to wait. Perhaps it seems obvious, but it's a good idea to bring something to do or to read. Ideally, read something about your medical problems while you wait, so you can ask better questions when you're with the doctor.

Interview Warning Sign 2. The Doctor Uses Poor Interview Technique

Experts studying medical interviewing have discovered that doctors vary greatly in the methods they use to interview patients. Some examples of poor interview technique are:

- *The doctor interrupts you.* There is an old saying, God gave you two ears and one mouth. Listen twice as much as you talk. Doctors would do well to heed the advice. Most don't allow their patients to fully tell their stories.

Doctors Interrupt Patients

Researchers at Wayne State University in Detroit tape-recorded office visits to analyze how doctors interviewed patients. They found that doctors typically interrupted patients within the first few seconds of the interview. The average time until the first interruption was eighteen seconds. The doctors allowed their patients to finish their opening statement less than a quarter of the time. Typically the doctors interrupted to ask a series of yes or no questions and effectively took control of the conversation. Doctors interrupted patients to save time, but most patients who were allowed to complete their opening statement took less than a minute to do so. None took longer than two and a half minutes. Once interrupted, less than 2 percent of patients went on to finish their initial statements. The researchers concluded that when doctors interrupt, they cut off the spontaneous flow of information and, in effect, deny patients the opportunity to raise important concerns.[4]

- *The doctor asks mostly yes or no questions.* Studies show that a string of yes or no questions is a poor way to conduct an interview. Important information may be missed. Doctors may jump to premature conclusions about the cause of the symptoms. Skillful interviewers, on the other hand, begin with open-ended questions like "What's the matter?" or "How can I help you?" and allow patients to tell their stories in their own words. As these doctors hone in on a diagnosis, they may ask more pointed questions, like "Is there any relation between eating and the pain?" and then even more specific questions, like "Did antacids help?"

- *The doctor asks leading questions.* "Do you still beat your wife?" is the archetypal inappropriate leading question. Experts believe that less obviously inappropriate leading questions, like "The pain didn't wake you up at night, did it?" may lead to inaccurate answers.[5]

- *The doctor uses medical jargon.* The problem with the fancy Latin and Greek terms doctors throw around is that their patients may not understand them. For most people, "Have you noticed your heart pounding hard or fast or skipping beats?" is preferable to "Have you noticed any palpitations?"

- *The doctor seems rushed or distracted.* Although a busy doctor may have a lot on his or her mind, you should have the sense that while you're together, you've got the doctor's undivided attention. It's best if the doctor isn't flipping through your chart or taking extensive notes while you speak. If the doctor's mind is elsewhere, the doctor may not hear what you say.

When you're evaluating a doctor's interview technique, remember that given time constraints, it isn't always possible for a physician to address every concern you might have. If you have more concerns than can reasonably be addressed in a single appointment, try to make an agreement with the doctor to deal with your most pressing problems first and, if necessary, schedule a return appointment to get to the others.

Interview Warning Sign 3. The Doctor Ignores Psychological and Social Causes of Illness

Many doctors seemingly prefer to think of people as the sum of their organs rather than as complex, thinking, feeling beings. They make little effort to get to know you as a person, to find out what you care about, what your family situation is, whether you have financial problems or other stress points in your life.

It's only in recent years that most doctors have even admitted the connection between emotions and health, a connection their patients have made intuitively for years. Almost reluctantly, the medical profession admitted the link between stress and ulcers, but many doctors just don't get how your emotional well-being can affect virtually every phase of your life. These days studies linking stress to various medical problems abound: people under stress are more susceptible to the common cold,[6] more likely to develop high blood pressure,[7] have a heart attack,[8] or suffer a recurrence of breast cancer.[9] **Emotional well-being is not only important to health, it can mean the difference between life and death.**

The Role of Emotional Support in Surviving a Heart Attack

Researchers at Yale University School of Medicine have found that elderly patients who have friends and family who provide emotional support are more likely to survive a heart attack. Of patients studied, thirty-eight percent of those with no sources of emotional support died in the hospital, compared with 12 percent who had two or more sources of support. By the end of one year, 55 percent of those who lacked supportive friends and family were dead, compared with only 27 percent of those with two or more sources of support. Controlling for the severity of the heart attack, the researchers concluded that the risk of death for patients who reported no emotional support was almost tripled.[10]

A person's emotions may determine not only if he or she will die from a particular condition but when. Just about every doctor has seen patients who have, as they say, given up the ghost and decided to die. As if by sheer force of will, many of them are dead within days.

Deciding When to Die

At the University of California researchers looked at the death rates of elderly Chinese women before and after the Harvest Moon Festival, an important holiday in the Chinese calendar. Traditionally, Chinese families have been male-centered, but during the Harvest Moon Festival the central ceremonial role is played by the oldest woman in the household. The researchers found that the Chinese women had 35 percent fewer deaths than expected the week before the Harvest Moon Festival and about the same number of excess deaths the week after. A similar study showed that Jewish men could delay their deaths until after Passover.[11]

Physicians often have the attitude that it is their duty first to be sure their patients don't have a "medical" cause for their symptoms. Only if all the tests come up negative will the doctors consider psychological factors—if they consider them at all. If doctors would only incorporate an appreciation of the psychological contribution to physical disease from the beginning of their analysis, unnecessary tests could be avoided and more patients would feel satisfied with the process. It is not negating a patient's real physical suffering or genuine medical problems for a doctor to postulate that stress or depression may be contributing factors.

Doctors may feel uncomfortable discussing such "unscientific" matters as emotions. Some feel they wouldn't know what to do with the information a patient gave them. Others worry that their patients will feel insulted or think their complaints aren't being taken seriously. In my experience most patients are happy, even relieved, to discuss these matters and to understand their contribution to their medical problems.

Recognizing Depression

Doctors do a notoriously poor job of recognizing depression. According to studies, doctors fail to recognize anywhere from 45 to 90 percent of the psychological illness they see.[12] Most people who suffer from depression don't go to psychiatrists, they turn up in the offices of primary care doctors like family practitioners or internists. And often these patients don't complain of depression. Like many people who aren't depressed, they mention headaches, stomach problems, or fatigue. Since the symptoms of depression and many medical conditions overlap, it's often appropriate for the doctor to run a few tests to rule out various medical conditions, to avoid prematurely attributing all the symptoms to depression. But if the doctor fails to recognize the depression—and simply conducts a series of tests or gives some medicine to suppress symptoms—the consequences can be tragic.

Case History: A Writer's Depression

In 1985 the writer William Styron sank into a major depression that nearly cost him his life. Darkness Visible—A Memoir of Madness,* *his moving account of his descent into a suicidal depression and his subsequent recovery, should be required reading for all physicians.*

After years of abusing alcohol, Styron developed a sudden physical aversion to it. Without the elixir that had smoothed the

---

* New York: Random House, 1990.

*rough edges of his troubled life, life brought less and less pleasure.
He became somber and fidgety and began to fixate on various
"twitches and pains" that he was convinced heralded serious
disease.*

*For years he'd been using high doses of Valium-like tran-
quilizers to help him sleep at night. One doctor had prescribed one
at three times the usual dose and told him he could take it with no
more thought than if it were aspirin. Normally these drugs
shouldn't be used for more than a week or two. In someone who
abuses alcohol, they are especially problematic, given the additive
depressant actions of tranquilizers and alcohol.*

*After months of suffering Styron sought medical attention. He
visited an internist who conducted a three-week series of high-
tech tests and told him there was nothing wrong with him.
Initially pleased with the clean bill of health, Styron was within
days spiraling back down the vortex of an agitated depression. He
continued to take high doses of another Valium cousin, Halcion,
to get a few hours of dreamless sleep each night. Within a few
months he was on the verge of suicide. He'd gone as far as
attempting to pen a suicide note (but a writer to the end, he was
never satisfied with the results) and had carefully disposed of his
personal journal so that no one could read it after his death.
Luckily, just before carrying out his plan, he confessed his
intentions to his wife, who called the doctors. After months of
hospitalization, he recovered.*

*Styron's doctor apparently never considered depression as a
cause for his symptoms: he was fixated on finding a medical
explanation. The doctor should have also considered the possibility that Styron's symptoms were the side effects of the high
doses of tranquilizers or at least that the tranquilizers contributed
to the problem. His doctor might have known that long-term users
of tranquilizers frequently have other substance abuse problems
or undiagnosed depression.*[13]

Failure to diagnose depression leads to unnecessary laboratory tests. More importantly, it leads to unnecessary suffering
and, in too many cases, suicide. Depression is almost always
treatable. Every year thousands of people like William Styron

are brought back from the brink of suicide to live satisfying and productive lives.

Depression is often straightforward to diagnose if the doctor takes the time to ask a few simple questions: How's your appetite? How well have you been sleeping? Have you been sad? Crying a lot? Have you thought of suicide? Sometimes all the physician needs to do is to create an atmosphere where the patient feels permission to talk. If a woman says, "My marriage is on the rocks," the doctor might respond, "What's going on?" encouraging her to elaborate. If the doctor responds, "I see. Now where was the pain?" she'll probably keep quiet about her marital problems and the opportunity to detect her depression may be lost.

Since doctors can't be depended on to diagnose depression, you should try to help them. If you think you may be depressed, say so. If your doctor won't listen, find another doctor.

Interview Warning Sign 4. The Doctor Ignores the Possibility of Job-Related or Environmental Illness

Job-Related Illness

When some people say, "My job makes me sick," they mean it. Each year in the United States over 50,000 people die of job-related medical conditions. Another 350,000 people become ill because of their work.[14] Occupational diseases are often mis-diagnosed, and when the connection between your job and your symptoms is missed, so is the opportunity to treat you properly and to prevent further problems.

Job-related medical problems span a wide range—from lung cancer due to asbestos exposure, to fatigue from working the night shift at the factory or hospital, to carpal tunnel syndrome (a nerve problem causing numbness and pain in the hands) from typing at a keyboard too much. Unfortunately the average U.S. medical student gets about four hours of training in occupational medicine during four years of medical school.[15] The result is that most doctors, except for the few who've taken the time to learn on their own, know little about job-related illness.

Your primary care doctor should incorporate a few questions concerning your work into your initial interview, because—as with most medical problems—the interview is the best tool to diagnose job-related illness. Some of the things the doctor should ask are:

- *What do you do for work?* How long have you done it? How stressful is it?
- *What are your working conditions like?* Do you lift heavy boxes? Apply pesticides to the lawn? Sit at a desk all day and type? If you are working in hazardous conditions, they may be able to suggest possible remedies or refer you to another doctor who can.
- *Have you had any previous jobs that exposed you to hazardous conditions?* Since some hazardous exposures may not cause problems for years, doctors should also ask about any jobs you've had in the past where you might have been exposed to such things as chemicals or asbestos or loud noise.
- *Is there any relationship between your job and your symptoms?* If you are seeing a doctor for a new symptoms that aren't readily explained, the doctor should ask if there is any association between it and your work. Some people who suffer from so-called sick-building syndrome, for example, get headaches and fatigue that start a few hours after they arrive at work and begin to breathe the stale air. Symptoms fade a few hours after they go home. On weekends or if they work somewhere else for a day, they have no symptoms at all.

Environmental Illness

A doctor should also explore the potential link between your symptoms and your environment. Most of us live surrounded by plastics, solvents, detergents, and pesticides. In exploring unexplained symptoms, doctors should ask you what chemicals you come into contact with in your day-to-day life and what precautions you take against accidental exposure. They should ask too about your hobbies, as they can be a source of environmental illness—from the paint stripper you've been applying to that chest of drawers to the lead you use to fashion homemade fishing sinkers.

Interview Warning Sign 5. The Doctor Ignores Your Opinions and Concerns

There are several reasons why it's important that doctors solicit their patients' concerns, beyond simply satisfying the customer.

- *Your perspective may be essential in making the correct diagnosis.* Sir William Osler, the turn-of-the-century British physician whom many consider the "father" of modern American medicine, advised his colleagues, "If you listen to your patients, they will give you the diagnosis." Annie O'Malley asked two doctors point-blank to examine her hips. Neither complied. They were so busy pursuing what they thought was wrong, they gave no serious consideration to what she thought.

    Because many people won't volunteer information without being prompted, it's often helpful if the doctor asks an open-ended question, such as "What are you concerned this might be?" or "Is there anything else about this that you're worried about?"

    A good interaction with a doctor facilitates trust. If patients sense that a doctor is interested in their opinions and concerns, they are more likely to share vital pieces of information that they simply wouldn't mention to another doctor.

- *Emotional support is itself therapeutic.* One reason that people visit doctors is for emotional support, which is at times more therapeutic than drugs or surgery. Dialogue between doctors and patients can be, as the writer Anatole Broyard put it, "mouth-to-mouth resuscitation." Ironically, the modern doctor's failure to meet patients' emotional needs has led to an erosion of public satisfaction with medical care at a time when medical care is more effective than at any time in history. The desire for a better human connection leads many to seek care from such alternative practitioners as acupuncturists, homeopaths, and herbalists. Alternative practitioners listen to their patients and invite the patients' perspective. Their popularity in part reflects the fact that they provide what many conventional physicians do not, time and attention—whether or not their treatments are otherwise effective.

- *A doctor's failure to solicit your point of view undermines the effectiveness of therapy.* Studies have shown that people who have a good relationship with their doctor are more likely to follow suggestions, take prescribed medication, and agree to recommended tests. A doctor who doesn't ask may not find out that a patient has no intention of taking a prescribed medicine due to a fear of side effects. A doctor who understands the patient's concerns can often assuage them by providing more information or substituting a less objectionable therapy.

   Due to cultural differences, superstition, or alternative belief systems, the patient's understanding of the disease may be different from the doctor's. A woman who believes she has hypertension because she's "hypertense" may fail to understand the rationale for drug therapy. She may simply need to be told that stress is just one factor elevating blood pressure and that even if she eliminates it from her life, she'll probably still need treatment. A man who believes that vengeful ancestors are causing his arthritis may be skeptical of the doctor's proposed remedies. While not necessarily agreeing with the man's beliefs, if the doctor can acknowledge them respectfully, he or she may be able to find a mutually satisfactory treatment plan.

- *A doctor who doesn't understand your concerns will have a hard time addressing them.* Say a young woman visits her doctor complaining of a lump under her arm. After feeling it, the doctor is certain the lump is a benign fatty growth known as a lipoma. Unless the doctor specifically asks her, the doctor may not realize she's worried about cancer. Without that information the doctor may not be able to give her the reassurance she's seeking.

   Many people go to the doctor with a hidden agenda.

They're worried they've got a particular disease but don't say so. They don't want to appear foolish. They're just plain scared. Patients with a hidden agenda may neglect to volunteer information important to making the diagnosis. To get the information, doctors have to ask. Here's a case in which at first I didn't ask, because I accepted a patient's self-diagnosis of a cold, but the information fortunately came out.

Case History: Larry Turner's "Cold"

Larry Turner, a young actor who had just finished college, came into my office one afternoon several years ago complaining of a "cold." He'd had a cough for a couple of weeks, he said, and had noticed that he was having breathing problems just walking around. What he didn't say was that he was gay and worried that he might have AIDS. While examining him, I became suspicious that things weren't adding up. He was taking about twenty-five breaths per minute, about twice the normal breathing rate, just sitting on the edge of the examination table. It's unusual for a young man to be that short of breath without there being something seriously wrong. Among other possibilities, I wondered if he might have pneumocystis carini pneumonia (PCP), a common opportunistic infection associated with AIDS. When I listened to his lungs through the stethoscope, I heard crackling sounds. At that point I asked him about risk factors for infection with HIV, the virus that causes AIDS: Had he injected drugs? Was he gay? Had he had unprotected sex? He was forthcoming and admitted his concern about AIDS. I told him that I was concerned too. I referred him to the emergency room of a local hospital, where a chest X-ray unfortunately showed findings consistent with PCP. The diagnosis of AIDS was confirmed within the next few days. Although his fear about AIDS was confirmed, there is effective treatment for PCP. After a brief hospitalization Larry was discharged in much better shape.

Interview Warning Sign 6. The Doctor Avoids Embarrassing Questions

Given the findings on his physical exam, I probably would have referred Larry Turner to the emergency room even if I hadn't asked him about his sexual history. The information about his sexuality might not have been absolutely essential, but it certainly facilitated his quick diagnosis and treatment. There are times, however, when **the doctor's avoidance of potentially embarrassing topics leads to missed diagnoses, lost opportunities to treat, and even the death of patients.**

Some topics that doctors may be reluctant to broach are:

- *Sex.* Sexuality can be difficult to talk about, for both doctors and their patients. It's hard for many doctors to ask a patient, "Have you had anal intercourse?" or ask a sexually active teenager, "Do you use condoms?" It may be even more difficult to ask teenagers the follow-up questions to make sure they know how to use condoms correctly. But these questions are essential, because teenagers who don't use them correctly may end up the parent of an unwanted child or infected with HIV.

Doctors Often Fail to Take a Sexual History

Researchers at Boston University Medical School found that doctors asked less than one-third of new patients if they had any sexual problems or concerns. A sexual history was included in the interview for 43 percent of men but only 21 percent of women. Doctors were less likely to ask older people about sexual problems. Interestingly, the researchers found that the age and sex of the patient did not influence the likelihood of sexual problems. Ninety-eight percent of patients asked about sexual difficulties considered the questions appropriate. The sexual history often improved the doctor's understanding of the patient. Perhaps most importantly, it yielded important medical information 26 percent of the time and led to changes in treatment or follow-up 16 percent of the time.[16]

When asking about sexuality, doctors should be nonjudgmental and not jump to conclusions. Doctors frequently assume young lesbians are heterosexual and give them undesired advice about birth control. Similarly, doctors may assume that older patients are no longer sexually active. Faulty assumptions may undermine trust and lead to mistaken diagnoses. If patients feel they are being judged for their behavior, they may be unwilling to talk about it.

Doctors who neglect the sexual history are either reluctant to devote the required time, can't overcome their inhibitions, or assume that sexual functioning is not important to a particular patient. By not asking, the doctor may fail to learn of discord in the patient's marriage or other significant relationship, of sexual abuse or of other problems that could affect the patient's health. Sexual problems can provide clues to diabetes, hormone problems, or depression.

Doctors who fail to take a sexual history may not recognize when their patients are suffering a side effect of a prescribed medicine. Several medications for high blood pressure, for example, can cause impotence, difficulty with ejaculation, or loss of interest in sex.[17] Unless the doctor asks, the patient may continue to suffer these side effects when a simple change in medication could solve the problem. Some people, not realizing that their problem is a side effect of medication, falsely attribute their difficulties to old age or a loss of interest in their partner. Others make the connection but, rather than mention it to their doctors, simply stop taking their medication, leading to poorly controlled blood pressure and an increased risk of heart attack or stroke.

- *Incontinence.* Many older people, particularly women, suffer from incontinence but are too embarrassed to bring it up with their physicians. When a concerned doctor asks, though, most of them will speak freely. This vexing problem is often amenable to treatment ranging from simple exercises to drugs to, in some extreme cases, surgery.

- *Drug and alcohol use.* Doctors should routinely incorporate questions about drug and alcohol use into the interview, even with people who show no signs of having a problem. If the physician suspects a problem, he or she may need to ask a few direct questions, such as "Have you ever felt you should cut down on your drinking?" or "Has anyone ever annoyed you by criticizing your pot smoking?" Perhaps

William Styron's doctor missed the contribution drugs and alcohol played in his depression because he never asked.

- *Childhood sexual abuse.* In recent years some of the consequences of childhood sexual abuse have come to light. The problem appears to be much more common than previously believed and may have major repercussions on the subsequent behavior and health problems of the victims. These people have been shown to have higher-than-expected rates of depression, anxiety, and various medical conditions including pelvic pain and intestinal problems.

Medical Consequences of Sexual Abuse

Doctors at the Mayo Clinic surveyed over five hundred women who came for routine care at a rural family practice clinic. Over 20 percent of the women admitted a history of childhood sexual abuse. Besides having more current medical problems, these women were more likely to have begun smoking at an early age, smoke more, abuse alcohol, have multiple sexual partners at a young age, and forgo Pap smears, all factors that put them at higher risk for later health problems. Strikingly, fewer than 2 percent of the women had ever told their physicians about the abuse.[18]

If a doctor can sensitively broach the subject of sexual abuse, important clues to current behavior and health problems can be obtained. If the patient does reveal a history of abuse, then interventions that go to the source of the problem, like therapy, may in the long run be much more effective than isolated efforts to suppress each symptom or modify each unhealthy behavior.

- *Domestic violence.* It's estimated that one in seven women visiting a primary care doctor and one in three visiting an emergency room are victims of domestic violence. Besides the obvious connections with bruises and broken bones, domestic violence may underlie such diverse symptoms as fatigue, headaches, eating disorders, intestinal problems, and difficulty sleeping. Because partner abuse is so common, experts now recommend that primary care doctors *routinely* incorporate relevant questions into the interview.

The doctor might ask, "Since the last time I've seen you, has anyone hit or threatened you?" If the partner accompanies the patient into the office, the doctor may need to be creative to find a way to talk with the patient in private.

- *Issues surrounding resuscitation and interventions near the end of life.* Death is another topic that's difficult for both doctors and patients to discuss. To someone who is healthy or at least in no imminent danger of death, questions like the following can seem morbid: "What would you want done if you were in an irreversible coma?" "If you were terminally ill and your heart stopped beating, would you want an electric shock that might resuscitate you?" Only by posing these tough questions can a doctor learn about your values and, if the time comes when you're unable to communicate your preferences, hope to give you the care you would have wanted.

Keep in mind that **if your doctor doesn't ask you about CPR while you're healthy, he or she may never get the chance.** People can be struck by heart attacks or strokes or accidents without warning. Faced with the decision to perform CPR or to hook you to a mechanical ventilator, in the abscence of instructions the doctor may decide for you. And doctors often aren't very good at predicting patients' wishes.

Consulting Patients About CPR

Doctors at the Beth Israel Hospital in Boston looked at how often physicians talked with their patients about cardiopulmonary resuscitation (CPR). In the hospital, CPR involves placing paddles on the chest to deliver a strong jolt of electricity to try to restart the heart, sticking a breathing tube down the throat to deliver oxygen, and rhythmically compressing the chest with great force to circulate blood. The doctors discovered that less than 20 percent of patients who had been resuscitated with CPR had discussed it with their doctors beforehand.

Of twenty-four patients who survived CPR, fifteen had wanted it, one was ambivalent, and eight had not wanted it done. The patients who didn't want CPR were worried about further suffering or a life hampered by chronic disease. Significantly, only one of the sixteen doctors who cared for the patients who hadn't wanted CPR correctly anticipated the patient's desire. Some doctors apparently can't imagine that a rational person could refuse throttle-to-the-floor medical technology. One of the doctors even said, "Who wouldn't want to be resuscitated?"[19]

Interview Warning Sign 7. The Doctor Fails to Treat You With Respect

Don't forget that the doctor works for you. Whether you pay for your health care directly out of your pocket, have insurance, or receive government assistance, by walking into the doctor's office you have in effect hired the doctor. **You are not a burden to the doctor; you are the doctor's source of livelihood and deserve to be treated accordingly.**

A doctor who barely knows you should not call you Bob or Mary or Darnell without your permission, unless you have conveyed an informality that makes it natural. Many elderly people in particular find it insulting and patronizing for someone they may never have met before to address them by their first name. In the hospital this form of inappropriate familiarity is more the rule than the exception, particularly with elderly or demented patients. The rule of thumb should be: If you wouldn't feel comfortable addressing the doctor by his or her first name (or if they wouldn't feel comfortable with it), then the doctor shouldn't be doing it to you, unless you request it.

Similarly, I believe the medical interview should at least begin with you fully clothed and sitting with the doctor. For many people it's intimidating to be interviewed dressed in a skimpy medical gown or even worse in one of those disposable gowns that look like giant paper napkins. Of course, if during the physical exam more information comes out, it's fine to continue the interview in the exam room. I realize that the reality is that in many clinics the nurse routinely asks you to change before you meet with the doctor. If you feel uncomfortable with this practice, I suggest you politely complain to the nurse, doctor, or clinic administrators.

Disrespect harms the patient's trust and confidence in the doctor. As we've seen, trust facilitates open communication and can be vital to the success of both diagnosis and therapy. People who have bad interactions with a doctor are also less likely to return for needed follow-up.

Seven Warning Signs of an Inadequate Physical Exam

After the interview, the physical exam is the doctor's most important tool to diagnose medical problems. During the exam the doctor begins to test hypotheses formed during the interview. Annie O'Malley's doctors made the mistake of not testing their initial hypothesis that she had a back problem with a careful physical exam. This error caused them to miss the true diagnosis and to pursue a costly and fruitless series of tests. Remember the dictum garbage in, garbage out. Not even the incredible resolution of an MRI could diagnose Annie's hip condition because the doctor ordered the scan on the wrong part of her body.

In the discussion that follows I'll focus on the physical exam as it's used to diagnose people who have symptoms. Another use of the physical exam, discussed elsewhere, is to screen for various medical conditions, such as breast cancer or high blood pressure, in people who have no symptoms.

There is no one right way to conduct a physical exam, but some methods are preferable to others. The following warning signs could tip you off that your doctor is performing a less-than-adequate physical exam.

Examination Warning Sign 1.
The Exam Isn't Thorough

As with the medical interview, to perform an adequate physical exam, a doctor must devote enough time to it. It's difficult to generalize about how detailed an exam should be, since requirements vary with your symptoms, past medical problems, age, and other factors. As you deal with different doctors, however, you'll probably notice that some are more thorough than others: they examine more of you and spend more time on each area. Since a physical exam is cheap and safe, there is much to be gained and little to be lost from being meticulous.

This is not to say that you should expect a complete physical exam every time you visit the doctor. Instead, based on information from the interview, the doctor decides which parts of the physical exam to focus on. One basic rule of thumb is to look where the symptoms are. If your arm hurts, it should be examined. If you have a cough, the doctor ought to look at your throat and listen to your lungs. After hypothesizing that Annie O'Malley had a low back problem, her doctors should have performed an examination of her back. Even if they hadn't thought to examine her hips, if they'd performed a thorough back exam, her hip problem would have come to light.

Let me illustrate. To examine an aching back, the doctor usually starts by simply looking at it. In serious back problems, the normal inward curve of the lower back can be lost due to muscle spasms. The doctor may ask the patient to bend forward and backward and side to side to check how well the spine moves. Next, the doctor feels the back to see if the spine or muscles are tender when they're pressed on. A crucial part of the back exam is the straight-leg raise. The patient lies on his or her back and allows the doctor to lift one leg as high as it will go while the other rests on the table. A herniated disc in the lower back can push on the roots of the sciatic nerve, causing the back, buttock, or leg discomfort known as sciatica. A straight-leg raise stretches the sciatic nerve and can reproduce the pain. Had Annie's doctors performed the straight-leg raise, they would have noticed that even the slightest movement of either leg at the hip joint caused her excruciating pain. At that point they would have been alerted that a more detailed hip exam was in order.

The last part of the back exam is a quick neurologic examination. The doctor tests the muscle strength and skin sensation in the legs and the reflexes at the knee and ankle, all of which can be affected by sciatic nerve problems. Finally the doctor watches the patient walk. People with back problems often walk stiffly, avoiding any unnecessary movement, as if the entire lower back were encased in cement. Here again, an observant doctor might have been alerted to Annie's hip problems, because of they way she waddled.

This back exam is usually sufficient to diagnose common back problems like sciatica and muscle spasms. There are less common causes of back pain that need to be looked for in older patients and in those with suggestive symptoms. Cancer of the spine, perforated intestinal ulcers, and ruptured aneurysms of large arteries such as the aorta, for example, all can cause back pain. When the interview and the patient's medical history raise these as possibilities, the physical exam needs to be even more extensive.

Teaching the Physical Exam to Medical Students

One reason that American doctors fail to perform thorough physical exams is that the value of the exam is no longer stressed in medical schools. Students instead are taught to depend on high technology. The result is that most young doctors never develop the bedside diagnostic skills physicians once routinely possessed. Medical school faculty tend to be researchers who spend little time in the examining room exercising and honing their diagnostic skills. Whatever skills they have tend to atrophy. More importantly, the message they pass on to young students—whether directly or implicitly—is that the physical exam isn't reliable enough to base decisions on, so why bother learning it well.

Teaching the Physical Exam to Young Doctors

Researchers at Duke University, one of the country's most prestigious medical schools, studied their doctors-in-training—medical interns and residents—to see how well they could diagnose various abnormal heart conditions based on the physical exam. The doctors examined "Harvey," a high-tech mannequin bearing a vague resemblance to the "Annie" mannequins used in CPR classes and engineered to simulate the physical findings of various heart conditions. For example, when the doctors put their stethoscopes on Harvey's chest, they would hear the classic loud rumbling sound of a certain type of heart murmur. When they felt the pulse, it too would be altered in the classic manner described in cardiology textbooks. The doctors were allowed examine the mannequin at their leisure in a quiet room. In real life doctors are rushed, most patients don't have all the classic findings and the wards and clinics where examinations take place resonate with the sounds of beepers and telephones. Even given ideal circumstances, for the three heart conditions simulated, the doctors were wrong in their diagnoses between 46 and 63 percent of the time. Perhaps the saddest finding of all was the lack of improvement with time: doctors in their final year of training did no better than the interns.[20]

In my last year of medical school I spent two months as a visiting student at the University of London. Britain spends considerably less per capita on health care than the United States. One reason is that doctors there rely more heavily on the physical exam to make diagnoses and to follow a patient's progress. Before graduating, English medical students must pass a rigorous examination in which they interview and examine a series of patients they know nothing about. They must evaluate patients with complex heart murmurs, for example, and within a few minutes emerge from the room with the diagnosis—without the benefit of any laboratory or other high-tech tests. I was amazed at how much more skilled the professors over there were at bedside diagnosis than my own professors back in the States and how much more competence in performing physical exams they expected from their students.

Examination Warning Sign 2.
Vital Signs Aren't Taken

The first part of the physical exam is the taking of the vital signs: the temperature, the pulse, the blood pressure, and the breathing rate. The name *vital signs* is appropriate: they are vital. **People are rarely acutely ill if their vital signs are normal, and a change in the vital signs can be the first signal that something is not right.** I have seen a jump in the pulse or in the breathing rate be the only sign heralding a pneumonia or a blood clot in the lungs. A seemingly minor alteration in a vital sign can alert your doctor that further questions, examination, or tests may be necessary.

Failure of a doctor (or a nurse) to measure your vital signs may signal an inadequate physical exam. Some doctors don't pay much attention to them; this is part of the general devaluation of the physical exam in favor of blood tests and X-rays and other high-tech interventions. There are times, of course, when it isn't necessary to take all four vital signs. If you twist your ankle playing basketball, the doctor probably won't take your temperature (although it certainly doesn't hurt, and the result may be surprising and lead to something else being discovered).

In clinics and doctors' offices nurses are generally good about taking the temperature and blood pressure but only check the pulse rate sometimes and rarely bother to measure the number of breaths per minute. It was Larry Turner's elevated breathing rate that provided the first clue that something was seriously wrong with him.

In the hospital nurses are supposed to measure the breathing rate along with the other vital signs, but in everyday practice they often just guess. I remember the day a distraught nursing student rushed up to me in the hall. She'd been assigned to take the vital signs of a patient and was worried because his breathing rate was only twelve per minute. Looking back through his bedside chart, she'd discovered it had been consistently recorded as twenty for a week. I reassured her that a breathing rate of twelve per minute was normal. Perhaps I should have told her that I suspected she was the first nurse actually to measure the patient's breathing rate since his admission to the hospital.

Examination Warning Sign 3.
The Doctor Fails to Wash His or Her Hands

Since half a dozen people in Florida were said to be infected with HIV by their dentist, hundreds of news stories have focused on the possibility of catching AIDS from your doctor. At the time of this writing, there are no other known examples of a patient's getting HIV from a doctor or a nurse (although dozens of health care workers have been infected by patients), despite the billions of interactions each year. This is not to say that doctors shouldn't take precautions to protect themselves and their patients—they should—only that the risk has been greatly exaggerated for its headline value.

A far bigger problem is the risk of catching other kinds of infections from your doctor. According to the Centers for Disease Control, more than 2 million Americans annually acquire infections—from pneumonias to surgical wound infections—in the hospital. Each year these infections cause nineteen thousand deaths directly and contribute to another fifty-eight thousand. Yet how many stories have you seen about this risk, compared to the multitude on "AIDS-infected doctors"?

Many hospital-acquired infections are transmitted to patients from the hands of health care workers. This is not new information. In the 1840s the Hungarian Ignaz Semmelweis, while a medical student in Vienna, investigated why so many women who delivered their babies in the hospital died of childbed fever. Childbed fever was rare in women who delivered at home. Semmelweis concluded that germs carried on the hands of medical students, who went straight from dissections in the autopsy room to the maternity ward, infected the expectant mothers.

When Semmelweis instituted the practice of thorough hand washing with soap and water prior to examining the women in labor, the death rate from childbed fever plummeted. The physician-in-charge, however, was not impressed with Semmelweis's dramatic success—perhaps out of jealousy or ignorance—and prevented Semmelweis's promotion and eventually drove him from Vienna. Distraught over the failure of the medical profession to accept hand washing, a failure which led to countless unnecessary deaths, Semmelweis died at forty-seven, in an insane asylum. The medical profession still hasn't fully adopted the practice 150 years later.

How Often Do Doctors Wash Their Hands?

To follow standard infection-control practices, medical perrsonnel should wash their hands after every contact with a patient and every time they manipulate potentially contaminated equipment, such as IVs. Researchers at the University of Washington discovered that on average workers in intensive car units washed their hands only 38 percent as often as recommended. Many even failed to wash their hands after such activities as changing soiled dressings or manipulating urine bags. Respiratory therapists washed their hands about 70 percent as often as they should have, nurses and X-ray technicians each about 40 percent of the time. Physicians were the worst offenders, washing their hands less than 26 percent as often as recommended.[21]

The seemingly trivial action of hand washing is, according to experts, the single most important way to prevent hospital-acquired infections. It is recommended after every single contact with a patient, even contacts as simple as taking the blood pressure or touching a patient's hand. Failure to wash hands is a problem not just in the hospital but also in clinics and doctors' offices. I once spent an entire afternoon working with a specialist who examined dozens of patients and didn't wash his hands once.

Case History: Sick of Visiting the Doctor

Miriam Crosby is a ninety-one-year-old retired teacher and abstract painter who has lived alone for years since her husband's death. Last February she was feeling well, but at her doctor's suggestion, went to the doctor's office for a routine visit. Everything checked out well, but within forty-eight hours Miriam was laid up in bed with a terrible cold that lasted more than a week. She hadn't had contact with anyone else in the few days before her appointment, so she's certain she caught the bug in the doctor's office. In fact, the likelihood of catching an infection is probably the highest in the hospital and the doctor's office; they are, after all, where other people go when they're sick. In the hospital, especially, you can catch bugs that you can't find anywhere else in town.

Miriam speculates that she was infected in the waiting room, but it's possible the doctor was carrying a virus from a previous patient on her hands and passed it on to Miriam. Experts believe that most colds are spread by hand-to-hand contact, not by coughing or sneezing. A common scenario is that a person with a cold blows his or her nose, then a few minutes later shakes your hand or hands you a pen. If you then rub your nose or touch your finger to your mouth, you may become infected.

Although it's not always possible, the best way to protect yourself from a doctor-acquired infection is to make sure that the doctor washes his or her hands either before or after seeing you (after is okay, as long as the doctor did it after the last patient too). Doctors should lather their hands for a good thirty seconds. A quick rinse is not enough. If you don't have the opportunity to observe the physician directly, glance in the office sink. Is it wet? Has the soap dispenser been filled? This method isn't always reliable, since clinics may have multiple sinks. Another technique is simply to ask the doctor before you're examined, "Have you washed your hands?"

Examination Warning Sign 4. The Doctor Doesn't Follow Universal Precautions

Because of the possibility of spreading infection—either from the doctor to the patient or vice versa—doctors should wear latex gloves during certain parts of the physical exam, for example, if they'll be putting their fingers inside your mouth, examining a skin infection, or performing a genital exam. You should also expect doctors to wear gloves when drawing blood or performing invasive procedures, such as sticking tubes in various parts of your body. If there's a possibility that blood will spatter, they should wear eye protection. Any equipment used should be either disposable or properly disinfected after each use.

Since the AIDS epidemic began, the concept of universal precautions has taken hold. Because you can't look at someone and tell if they're infected with HIV, the safest course is to assume that anyone could be infected and to protect yourself accordingly. Don't feel insulted if practitioners—doctors or dentists—wear gloves while examining you it's for your protection and theirs. Be more concerned if they don't, because if they're not wearing gloves with you, they may not be wearing them with other patients whose infections you could catch.

Although AIDS is the infection people seem to fear most, hepatitis, a viral infection of the liver, is a far bigger risk. Although less often deadly than AIDS, hepatitis appears to be far easier to catch. A recent report in the *American Journal of Public Health* detailed an outbreak of hepatitis among the patients of a dermatologist in Fort Meyers, Florida, who failed to follow universal precautions. According to the report, the dermatologist's hands were often contaminated with blood; he did office procedures without gloves and failed to wash his hands after every patient. His hands and equipment were frequently contaminated with both HIV and the hepatitis virus. Even so, while thirty of his patients caught hepatitis, none developed evidence of HIV infection.[22]

A doctor should not only wear gloves during some examinations and procedures but change them between patients. Not to do so gives only the illusion of hygiene, since contaminated gloves can lead to the spread of infections just as surely as contaminated hands. Doctors should also wash their hands after they remove their gloves, since gloves can leak and contaminate their hands.[23]

Remember, though, that AIDS and the more serious forms of hepatitis are not spread casually. You can't catch them by shaking someone's hand or by sitting in the same waiting room. It is generally only through sex or by contact with infected blood that you can contract these viruses. So be sure your doctor is taking the proper precautions, but don't be paranoid.

Examination Warning Sign 5. You Aren't Asked to Change for the Exam

For anything beyond a minor complaint, a doctor usually can't do an adequate exam unless you change out of your street clothes. I have nonetheless often seen doctors examining the heart by sliding their stethoscope down the front of a patient's shirt or listening to the lungs through several layers of clothing.

Recently I was supervising a fourth-year medical student in a hospital clinic when a young construction worker came in complaining of low back pain shooting down to the buttocks. The student, a bright and energetic young man, interviewed and examined the patient, then came into my office to discuss the case. In a confident manner he pronounced that he doubted the man had sciatica. He thought it was just "muscle stiffness."

"Okay," I said, "let's go see him." We walked into the exam room, where the patient was sitting on the edge of the examination table, fully clothed in a thick flannel shirt, jeans, and steel-toed work boots, fully laced. I interviewed him briefly, then asked him to strip down to his underpants and to put on a hospital gown so that we could do a more complete exam. The student and I left the room to let the man change in private.

Back in my office I asked the student how he'd been able to examine the man with all his clothes on. He told me that he'd had the man lift up his shirt so he could examine his back. He'd tapped his knees through his jeans but hadn't done a straight-leg raise. Because the man still had his boots on, I knew the student hadn't checked his ankle reflexes, the strength in the muscles of his feet, or the sensation in his skin, essential elements of a back exam.

We returned to the patient's room and for the student's benefit I reviewed the proper technique for performing a back exam. I stressed that it can't be done properly unless the patient changes. The patient, by the way, did turn out to have sciatica.

Case History: Mary McDonald's Skin Cancer Checkup

Mary McDonald, a seventy-six-year-old Florida sun worshiper, visited her dermatologist for a six-month follow-up exam after having a skin cancer removed from her temple. Because of her fair complexion and constant sun exposure—Mary practically lives in a bathing suit—she is at about as high a risk for skin cancer as you can be. After she'd waited more than an hour, the doctor hurried into the room and within five minutes had burned eight different precancerous spots off her face. Perhaps because he was running behind schedule, he never asked her to change and didn't bother to inspect her arms or back or legs, common locations for skin cancer. Luckily, this time she didn't have cancer.

Examination Warning Sign 6.
Embarrassing Exams Are Skipped

Mary McDonald's dermatologist may have been in too big a hurry to wait for her to change and to do a more complete exam. Another possibility is that he was too embarrassed to ask this elderly woman to change or to examine her skin, as he should have, from head to toe. A dermatologist who is unwilling to look at the skin, all of it, should seriously consider finding a new field.

Doctors are most likely to defer rectal exams, gynecologic exams, and other tests that they and their patients find embarrassing. Doctors who skip a needed test to save their patients from embarrassment are doing those patients no favor. At times, they may be doing a grave disservice. I remember an elderly man with a drinking problem who complained for years of stomach pains. His doctor examined the man's belly on several occasions but never bothered to do a rectal exam, despite the man's ongoing symptoms. If the doctor had done the exam, a simple chemical test probably would have shown hidden blood in the man's stool, a warning sign for cancer. Instead, two years went by until the man turned up at a local hospital, where stomach cancer was diagnosed. By that time the cancer had spread extensively and was inoperable.

Doctors are more likely to forgo embarrassing exams on members of the opposite sex. A recent study in the *New England Journal of Medicine* showed that female physicians were twice as likely as males to obtain Pap smears on women patients. Young males doctors were found to be least likely to do the test.[24] I have seen several cases where male doctors failed to perform a gynecologic exam on young women with unexplained abdominal pain, an exam needed to rule out a pelvic infection or life-threatening tubal pregnancy. Consider the following case.

Case History: "It's Embarrassing"

A twenty-four-year-old woman went to an emergency room complaining that she was urinating more frequently than usual and experiencing a slight burning when she did so. The doctor examined her abdomen but skipped the gynecologic exam. Despite her normal urinalysis, he diagnosed a bladder infection and sent her home on antibiotics.

Two days later she was back in the ER with fever, headaches, muscle pains, and severe burning when she urinated. This time a pelvic exam was done and she was discovered to have genital herpes. It was so bad at that point that she needed intravenous treatment and had to be admitted to the hospital, where she spent an excruciating week. Had the doctor made the diagnosis when she first turned up in the ER, she could have been treated with oral medication and might have been spared the pain and expense of a week in the hospital.

Interestingly, it wasn't just the pelvic exam that was skipped. The doctor never took a sexual history, despite its potential relevance to her symptoms. It turned out she had a new sexual partner with whom she'd had unprotected intercourse five days before her symptoms began.[25]

Examination Warning Sign 7.
The Doctor Doesn't Respect Your Modesty

The flip side of a doctor's willingness to risk embarrassment in the interest of thoroughness is the doctor's respect for your modesty. During potentially embarrassing exams, a doctor should take care to drape the areas of the body being examined and to expose only as much as is necessary at a time. Doctors examining you in a hospital bed or in an emergency room should close the curtain separating you from other patients and, when possible, shut the door. A doctor who leaves the room while you change into a gown should knock before reentering to avoid barging in before you're ready.

When a male physician performs a gynecologic exam, it's reasonable to request that a female nurse or other female employee be present, to act as a chaperone of sorts. Many clinics do this automatically. If you feel more comfortable, you may request that a nurse be present for the entire physical exam.

If you don't wish to have an exam you find embarrassing or uncomfortable, it's your choice. Doctors should only recommend which exams to have. Doctors who think you're making a mistake by refusing an exam should explain why. If in spite of this information you refuse, they should respect your decision.

The doctor should respect your modesty to build trust and rapport, both of which can positively affect the outcome of medical care. Respecting your modesty as much as possible—while still being thorough—is also common decency.

Is Your Doctor a Good Teacher?

Doctors who skimp on the interview and the physical exam may also skimp on educating their patients. In Latin the word *doctor* means "teacher," and of all the hats the doctor wears, that of teacher is among the most important. After completing the interview and the physical exam, the doctor and the patient typically return to the interview room to talk. There the physician tells you what he or she has deduced, recommends further tests and treatment, and instructs you on what to do to get better. This is often the best time to ask questions.

It's important that the doctor speak in a language appropriate to your intelligence and level of education. Jargon should be avoided, but patronizing baby talk isn't much better. (I'm reminded of an Edgar Argo cartoon in which an elderly woman says to her doctor, "I appreciate you explaining it to me in terms I can understand—especially that part about Mr. Stomach and the food choo-choo.")

If you leave the doctor's office feeling that you didn't understand what the doctor told you or that your questions weren't answered, your doctor isn't doing a good job as a teacher. A good doctor will often ask his or her patients at the end of the visit if they have any other questions or concerns that weren't addressed. Again, if there isn't sufficient time to deal with them all, a return appointment can be scheduled.

In the following sections I'll list some rules of thumb to help you determine how well your doctor teaches. The degree of detail the doctor goes into will, of course, depend on the severity of your condition and on your level of interest.

The Diagnosis

Whenever possible, for each diagnosis made, the doctor should discuss:

- what it is
- how you got it
- how the diagnosis was reached
- how certain the diagnosis is
- what makes it better
- what makes it worse
- what to expect will happen
- what follow-up you'll need
- what would indicate your condition is worsening
- what to do if that happens

When doctors can't make a diagnosis, they ought to speculate on the possible causes of your symptoms and tell you how concerned they are. If they doubt your problem is significant, they should tell you why. Even when doctors are satisfied that there's nothing wrong with you, if they can't convey their reasoning effectively, you're unlikely to feel satisfied.

Planned Tests

For each recommended test the doctor should explain:

- how it's done
- what's being looked for
- what side effects it may have
- how the test's results will affect therapy
- alternative ways of diagnosing your condition
- the pros and cons of the alternatives

Drug Therapy

For any drug prescribed the doctor should outline:

- how and when it should be taken
- how long it should be taken
- why it's necessary
- what side effects are likely
- possible serious side effects even if they are less likely
- what to do if you feel you may be experiencing a side effect
- what to do if you miss a dose

Prevention

During the education phase of the office visit a lot of preventive medicine happens or ought to happen. The doctor should tell you how your habits of exercise, diet, and smoking, for example, influence your medical problems and how modifying your habits could benefit you. For people whose problems are related to environmental or occupational factors, the doctor should recommend how to prevent future hazardous exposures.

Written Instructions

Studies show that people forget about half of what a doctor tells them within a few minutes. It's therefore a good idea for the doctor to write out instructions, possible side effects, or other important points. It's also not a bad idea for you to take notes on what the doctor says. Preprinted handouts describing various drugs, tests, or medical conditions can be helpful, as long as they're written at a level appropriate to your education and avoid medical jargon.

Is Your Doctor Out-of-Date?

With the explosion in medical research and technology, there is more medical information out there than any doctor can master, and what is out there is constantly changing. Nonetheless, every doctor must make the effort to keep abreast of important new developments, particularly those likely to affect his or her patients. To stay current, physicians must read medical journals, attend conferences, and review new medical textbooks. This effort is more than many physicians are willing or able to make.

Do Doctors Keep Up-to-Date?

Over seven hundred internists, family practitioners, and obstetricians were surveyed regarding their knowledge of a test that has been around for more than ten years. The test, called a hemoglobin A1C, has proved invaluable in assessing how well controlled someone's diabetes is. Dozens of articles on how to use it have appeared in medical journals and in textbooks. Nonetheless, 65 percent of doctors in general practice and 36 percent of internists didn't understand how to use it correctly. Doctors were also ignorant of other widely disseminated advances. Over half didn't know that experts believed the drug digoxin should be discontinued or not used at all in many elderly patients with heart failure (more on this later). Almost 40 percent of obstetricians failed to offer their patients an attempt at a normal vaginal delivery before automatically repeating a cesarean section, even though experts have for years recommended they do so.[26]

When evaluating how up-to-date a physician is, keep the following in mind:

- *When doctors complete their training, they are generally well versed in current medical practice.* Although they may lack experience and the judgment and perspective that comes with it, newly trained doctors will be familiar with the latest drugs, have used the latest medical technology, and have treated patients with newly discovered medical conditions like AIDS or Lyme disease. Their knowledge may not remain current for long.

How Quickly Do Doctors Get Out-of-Date?

In a study in the *Journal of the American Medical Association,* almost three hundred doctors practicing in New York,

New Jersey, and Pennsylvania who had passed the board certification exam in internal medicine volunteered to be retested. The results showed that the doctors' knowledge dropped precipitously after training. Only 66 percent of the doctors who'd passed the test five or six years earlier scored a passing grade. Of doctors who'd been certified fourteen to fifteen years earlier, only 32 percent passed. Consider too that the doctors in this study were volunteers, who presumably thought their chances of passing were good. The failure rate among other doctors may have been even higher.[27]

• *Older physicians are more likely to be out-of-date, but those who make the effort to stay current combine their broad knowledge with a wealth of experience.* The world's most respected medical teachers and authorities tend to be gray-haired. On the other hand, the absolutely worst physicians I've ever seen were also older. There is no mandatory retirement age for physicians, which is as it should be, since some remarkable individuals retain their skills into their eighties and beyond. These doctors, though, are probably more the exception than the rule. According to the *Boston Globe*, 40 percent of the suspensions, censures, and other punishments for prescription violations in Massachusetts in one recent year were taken against doctors over sixty-five. Yet these doctors made up only 8 percent of licensed physicians, and many of them practiced only part-time.[28]

Older Doctors More Likely to Hospitalize Patients Inappropriately

Researchers at the Rand Corporation examined medical records to determine how often doctors of different ages hospitalized patients for inappropriate reasons. They discovered that doctors who'd been in practice more than fifteen years admitted patients inappropriately 27 percent of the time. Age wasn't the only problem, though. Younger doctors had an inappropriate admission rate of 20 percent.[29]

• *A doctor who is up-to-date in one area may be badly behind-the-times in others.* A cardiologist may be well-versed on the latest treatments for angina or high blood pressure but know little about developments in diabetes or in asthma. Since many specialists also deliver primary care, there is a greater risk of their being out-of-date when they step out of their area of expertise. This is particularly true of doctors whose specialties involve performing a lot of procedures, like cardiologists and intestinal specialists (gastroenterologists).[30]

- *The best way to discover if your doctor is up-to-date, is to know something about your medical condition.* The more you know, the better you'll be able to assess your doctor's knowledge. If you have asthma, for example, and you've been doing your reading, you'd know that expert opinion on treatment has changed radically in the last several years. The drug theophylline, which was once the mainstay of asthma treatment, has largely been supplanted by inhaled medicines, particularly inhaled cortisone-like medicines. Your physician should be aware of this change in thinking.

- *Asking questions can help you to assess how up-to-date your doctor is.* You could ask about a medical condition that's been in the news. Ask, for example, "If someone has an HIV test and it's negative, does it definitely mean they're not infected?" Any doctor who is even reasonably current will know that because of the so-called window period, the test can take up to six months to become positive. The correct answer is that the more time has passed since possible infection, the lower the chance of a false negative.

- *A doctor who prescribes the latest drugs or orders fancy high-tech tests is not necessarily up-to-date.* Doctors who are behind-the-times are often inordinately swayed by promotional efforts by drug companies and are more likely to prescribe the latest highly advertised drugs. When new drugs or tests are ordered by doctors who don't understand them well, the risk of improper use or unrecognized side effects increases. On the other hand, the use of outmoded drugs or tests can be a clear indication a doctor has not kept up.

- *As important as up-to-date medical knowledge is, it's probably overrated.* The diagnosis and treatment of many problems hasn't changed much in recent years. Given the resiliency of the human body, the self-limited nature of many medical problems, and the lack of effectiveness even today of many treatments, state-of-the-art care isn't always crucial.

The practice of medicine, like the width of ties, is subject to fashion. Decades ago doctors felt that blood clots played a major role in heart attacks, but this view subsequently fell from favor. Now the pendulum has swung back, and doctors are enthusiastically promoting aspirin and other blood-thinning drugs to prevent heart attacks. Early in this century and again in the 1940s researchers thought that a bacteria might be the cause of stomach and duodenal ulcers. By the 1950s this theory was dismissed, only to be resurrected in the last few years and now widely accepted.

Another example is the rise and fall and rise of the drug digoxin. Perhaps no drug has gone in and out of fashion as much as digoxin, first prepared from the leaves of the purple foxglove plant more than two hundred years ago by folk healers. In the study mentioned above, doctors were asked if they followed expert recommendations to discontinue digoxin in elderly people with heart failure. Those who had failed to stop using the drug were judged out-of-date. At the time the study was published, in 1989, most authorities believed that digoxin provided little benefit, despite its potentially serious side effects. Its side effects haven't changed, but digoxin's stock value has rebounded. A recent *New England Journal of Medicine* study showed that patients with heart failure who stopped taking it had worse symptoms, lower quality of life, and more hospitalizations than those who continued the drug.[31]

Up-to-date knowledge is sometimes equated with quality medical care. Yet it is just one element of quality care and in many cases not the most important. If you have a physician who is a little behind-the-times but who is otherwise thorough, compassionate, and communicative, you may be able to get excellent care. All things being equal, you'd like a physician who embodied these qualities *and* was up-to-date. Sometimes, however, you've got to compromise.

Staying Up-to-Date

States require that doctors update their medical knowledge on a regular basis. In my home state of Massachusetts doctors must earn one hundred hours of continuing medical education (CME) credits every two years in order to renew their license.

Much of the effort doctors make to keep current doesn't greatly affect how they practice. If they read medical journals— the most common way to keep up—they tend to read about areas in which they have an interest rather than areas in which they have deficiencies. Similarly, **doctors select which continuing education courses they take. The problem is that doctors often don't know what they don't know.**

Many doctors get their medical information from such low-quality sources as throwaway medical journals. My medical junk mail contains dozens of them, thick with glossy ads for new drugs, some containing articles that are either blatantly biased or thinly veiled promotions for a particular drug. Articles in these journals don't undergo the rigorous scrutiny that is standard in such high-quality medical journals as the *New England Journal of Medicine* and the *Journal of the American Medical Association* (whatever you think of the AMA, their journal is highly respected). Doctors, by the way, usually have to pay for high-quality journals out of their own pockets. Because a doctor's time to read is limited, any time spent reading the throwaways keeps them from reading the good stuff. Surveys indicate that older doctors, general practitioners, doctors who work in rural locations, those who work in smaller hospitals, and those with no contact with medical students are more likely to read throwaway journals. They are also less likely to rely on such high-quality sources of information as medical libraries or on-line medical databases.

If you get an opportunity, look around the doctor's office to see what medical journals are there. If throwaways like *Medical Economics, Hospital Medicine,* and *Private Practice* dominate, be concerned. Look also at the textbooks on the shelves. Are they current editions or are they old and dusty?

Putting It Together

Doctors who always seems to rush you, are difficult to contact, and are slow to return your phone calls may be overcommitted—too busy to provide the compassionate and thorough care you deserve. **No matter how much they know or how impressive their credentials are, doctors who don't take the time can't deliver first-rate care.** Less time spent with you usually means more tests, since ordering a test takes less of a doctor's time than a careful exam. The same principle applies to drugs. Less time means more drugs, since explaining why you don't need them can take twice as long as simply writing the prescriptions. Less time definitely means less prevention, and for many problems prevention is the most important thing a doctor can do.

If you sense your doctor is cutting corners during the interview, you can bring up information, assuming your doctor is willing to listen. This situation is far from ideal but can sometimes be workable. If your doctor fails to provide the opportunity for you to express your concerns, it may be time to find yourself a doctor who will.

The Seven Warning Signs of an Inadequate Interview

1. The doctor spends too little time to interview you thoroughly.
2. The doctor uses poor interview technique.
3. The doctor ignores psychological and social causes of disease.
4. The doctor ignores the possibility of job-related or environmental illness.
5. The doctor ignores your opinions and concerns.
6. The doctor avoids embarrassing questions.
7. The doctor fails to treat you with respect.

The Seven Warning Signs of an Inadequate Physical Exam

1. The exam isn't thorough.
2. Vital signs aren't taken.
3. The doctor fails to wash his or her hands.
4. The doctor doesn't follow universal precautions.
5. You aren't asked to change for the exam.
6. Embarrassing exams are skipped.
7. The doctor doesn't respect your modesty.

Unfortunately, some doctors feel threatened by assertive patients and may respond in a hostile or defensive manner. Do your best to be polite and nonthreatening. Another problem is that doctors who neglect the physical exam may not be very good at it. Physical diagnosis is not like riding a bike. A doctor must continually practice examination skills or they tend to atrophy.

If your doctor doesn't tell you what you need to know about your diagnosis, tests, or therapy, try asking questions. Sometimes it's helpful to write a few questions out before your office visit. If the appointment is almost over and you're not satisfied, you can simply say, "Before I go, could I ask you a couple of questions?" You can also try to make up for gaps in what your doctor teaches you by reading about your medical conditions, planned tests, or recommended treatments. Again, this is a less-than-ideal situation, but it's sometimes tenable.

If you sense that your doctor is behind-the-times but you're otherwise satisfied, you may want to consult with other physicians every now and then to make sure your case is being handled well. If you feel your physician is missing something, get a second opinion.

Whatever their reasons, doctors who fail to devote enough time to their patients compromise the quality of care they provide. These same doctors may be lacking in other ways too. A doctor who is motivated by financial considerations to rush patients, for example, may also tend to order unnecessary but profitable tests. More on this in the next chapter.

3

IS YOUR DOCTOR ORDERING THE RIGHT TESTS?

DOCTORS OFTEN ORDER TESTS ILLOGICALLY. SOMETIMES THEY FAIL to order necessary tests, but more commonly they order unnecessary ones. By ordering tests poorly, doctors run up medical bills, expose their patients to unnecessary risks, and fail to diagnose treatable conditions. Part of the problem is that many patients expect tests, believing more competent physicians order more tests. Some people feel that if a doctor doesn't order a test, their problem isn't being taken seriously. Ordering a test is one way for a physician to answer the question, What are you going to do for me, doc?

Once upon a time in America, money for health care seemed limitless. The prevailing sentiment was Do everything you can, whatever the cost. But our economy has slumped, health care's bite out of the gross national product has tripled, and realities are changing. No one likes to think of money when their health is on the line. But the fact is, with increased pressure to contain costs, doctors must consider the economic ramifications of their decisions. If there's a one-in-a-million chance you've got cancer and a million-dollar test can give the answer, no doctor could order it. When it comes to our own health, though, we all want to know and we want to know now. As understandable as that attitude is, it no longer reflects economic realities.

Case History: A $300 Cold

When Martha Samuels woke up, her neck and shoulders and her lower back ached. Her throat felt raw. Her nose was running.

97

She had a dry cough. She told herself she probably had the same thing her husband, Bill, had had the week before. Aspirin helped, but Martha didn't feel up to her hectic job as a legal secretary, so she called in sick.

Her husband hadn't seen a doctor at all and was already better, but Martha had noticed a new walk-in clinic in the shopping center up the road and decided to try it. Martha was generally healthy: she was thirty-two-years old, didn't smoke, and jogged a couple of times a week. She worried a lot, though. She read articles on health in various magazines, and every time she read about a new disease, she became convinced she had it. As she checked in to the clinic, she told the nurse it was probably just a bad cold but she just wanted to be sure.

The nurse led her to a room separated from the others by a curtain and had her sit on the edge of the exam table. The nurse slid a thermometer under Martha's tongue, pumped up a blood pressure cuff, then took a throat culture with a cotton swab. She told Martha the doctor would be with her soon and pulled the curtain closed.

Twenty minutes later the doctor arrived, asked her a few questions, and performed a brief exam. He recommended a complete blood count, a Monospot test to rule out mononucleosis, and a chest X-ray. Martha had the tests, then waited for the results.

The news was good. Her blood count was normal and the mono test was negative. There was no evidence of pneumonia on the chest X-ray. Throat culture results would be back in two days. Martha gratefully accepted a prescription for the antibiotic Ceclor and another for the cold remedy Bromfed and went home to bed. Two days later she felt well enough to return to the law firm.

I saw Martha a week later for an unrelated problem. She had developed a small patch of red skin on her arm and just wanted to be sure it wasn't anything serious. It wasn't. During our talk, she expressed her satisfaction with the care she'd received the week before. As I read through her chart, though, I realized she'd had several unnecessary tests.

In the clinic the week before, Martha's temperature and blood pressure were normal. Her pulse rate of eighty beats per minute was only slightly higher than usual, suggesting she was mildly dehydrated and needed to drink more fluids. In his note the doctor described her throat as red, but he didn't see any white spots on her tonsils that might have suggested strep throat. Her ears showed no signs of infection, and she didn't have any swollen glands in her neck. Her lungs sounded normal.

Considering her symptoms, the fact that her husband had a similar illness the week before and was now well, and the findings on the doctor's exam, there should have been little doubt about the diagnosis—a common cold. Just what Martha had predicted to the nurse as she checked in.

To understand why none of the tests was necessary, let's go through them one at a time:

- *The complete blood count (CBC)* consists of two main components, a white cell count and a hemoglobin, a measure of red blood cells. The white cell count goes up in certain infections, but there was little to suggest Martha had a serious infection, so the test was unlikely to provide useful information. The hemoglobin is used to detect anemia. Nothing in the interview or the doctor's exam suggested that Martha was anemic.
- *The Monospot* is a blood test used to diagnose mononucleosis. Given Martha's age and relatively mild symptoms, the chance she had mono was remote. Even when someone has mono, the Monospot usually remains negative until the second week of illness. Thus, the negative result on the first day of her illness was no guarantee she didn't have mono. There was no justification for performing the test.
- *The throat culture* detects the presence of a type of bacteria called streptococcus—strep for short—a frequent cause of sore throats in children. Untreated strep throat can lead to rheumatic fever, a serious illness which can destroy heart valves. In adults, less than 10 percent of sore throats are caused by strep. Martha had no known exposure to anyone with strep throat, and she lacked all three of its cardinal features: high fever, swollen lymph glands in the neck, and

an inflamed throat with white spots on the tonsils. In someone with none of these signs, strep throat is rare. Martha also had a cough and a runny nose, symptoms not usually associated with strep, lowering the likelihood of a positive throat culture even further. As expected, Martha's culture turned out negative. Even before he had the results of the throat culture, however, the doctor prescribed Ceclor. While the choice of this particular antibiotic was not a good one, for reasons we'll discuss in the following chapter, Ceclor is effective against strep throats. Thus, the test was doubly unnecessary: even a positive culture would not have changed therapy.

- *The chest X-ray* was done to look for pneumonia. Patients with pneumonia typically appear acutely ill, have problems breathing, or have high fever. Martha had no such worrisome symptoms and her lung examination was normal, making pneumonia improbable. While blood tests and throat cultures carry minimal risk, X-rays expose patients to radiation, a real, albeit small, risk. Unless clearly needed, X-rays are a particularly poor idea for women of child-bearing age who could be pregnant, since a developing fetus is inordinately susceptible to radiation injury.

Seven Principles of Appropriate Medical Testing

Martha Samuels's doctor ordered $158 worth of tests, none of which was essential (and that was in addition to the $59 fee for the visit and almost $90 for the prescriptions). Had Martha asked a few questions and understood the basic principles of medical testing, she might have been able to avoid some or all of the unnecessary tests.

Although there can be no cookbook approaches to deciding which tests are appropriate, the proper use of diagnostic tests is based on simple principles. Good doctors rely on such principles, either consciously or subconsciously, when deciding which tests to order. In the following section, I lay out the principles of appropriate medical testing as I see them. With this information—and even without any medical training—you can begin to judge how well your doctor orders tests. The idea is not to take over for your doctor but to equip yourself to participate in medical decisions—to be sure you get the tests you need and avoid the ones you don't.

Test Principle 1. Use Tests Selectively

Sensible test ordering involves obtaining a few specific tests to confirm or to rule out what the doctor hypothesizes. A shotgun approach to testing—ordering a wide array of tests and seeing what you come up with—is almost always a bad idea. In order to be sure you're not getting unnecessary tests or the wrong tests, keep the following in mind:

- *Begin with a thorough interview and exam to narrow the possibilities.* An inadequate interview and exam increase the likelihood of inappropriate testing. Only after the interview and exam can a doctor make an informed guess about what's wrong with you and recommend the appropriate tests. Martha Samuels had one test, the throat culture, before she even saw the doctor. To save time, nurses often obtain blood tests, EKGs, or X-rays before the doctor evaluates the patient. Sometimes the nurse anticipates what the doctor wants, sometimes not. I've seen a nurse send a patient for a knee X-ray when what the patient needed was an X-ray of the ankle. Other times, patients have had several tests when none was needed. The nurses' intentions are good. They're trying to save the patient and the doctor time, but the result of this "Shoot first and ask questions later" approach is a load of unnecessary tests. Except in emergency situations, my advice is to politely refuse tests until you've been examined by the doctor.
- *Use as few tests as possible to establish the diagnosis with reasonable certainty.* Sometimes your doctor may feel fairly certain of his diagnosis but want to order more tests "just to be sure." This approach may be appropriate when there is a lot at stake, for instance if he or she thinks you have cancer

and is recommending chemotherapy. For most medical problems, however, the belt and suspenders approach to diagnosis (to make doubly sure your trousers stay up) isn't a good idea. Many doctors, however, seem to believe the more, the better. When more data can be collected without major risk or expense, as with a careful interview and exam, this philosophy may be reasonable, but excess testing comes at a cost, both financial and otherwise.

• *The best test may be no test.* Part of a doctor's job is to decide when a patient's symptom is serious and when it's nothing to worry about. If a patient complains, "My right elbow itches every time I eat pastrami," the doctor shouldn't be ordering a lot of tests. Many people mention unusual symptoms that don't sound serious and that no amount of testing is likely to explain. A healthy shrug of the shoulders is probably the best response the doctor can give. If, on the other hand, the patient complains, "I get a sharp pain in my belly every time I eat pastrami," a few tests out may be in order.

Occasionally a symptom that doesn't sound serious at first turns out to be significant. It simply isn't prudent, however, to chase after every symptom with a battery of tests. In the early stages of many diseases, the symptoms may be vague and of short duration. Early tests may not pick up the disease. As time goes on, the picture becomes clearer and the diagnosis can be made.

Some patients have a million symptoms. It is impractical and inappropriate to do a test for every one. Instead, after careful follow-up questioning and a thorough exam, the doctor should order those few tests that may help to pin things down. If there's reason for concern, it's always possible to schedule a return visit. **Sometimes the best course of action is watchful waiting or, as it's sometimes called, tincture of time.**

Doctors are trained to think scientifically. Many of them expect there to be a physical reason for every symptom, definable by a number or by an abnormal test result. Given the litigious atmosphere in health care these days, doctors often feel they at least need to look for a physical reason for each symptom. In their scientific zeal many doctors ignore the role of psychological and social factors in disease. If a young patient who is unemployed and having marital problems feels dizzy, a bunch of expensive tests may not be the best way to proceed.

• *At times, it's preferable to forgo tests and, based on the results of the interview and the exam, simply begin treatment.* Doctors refer to this practice as *empiric therapy.* Empiric therapy is often appropriate when a diagnosis seems likely, when the test to diagnose it is expensive or has potentially serious side effects, and when the treatment is relatively safe and effective. For example, a forty-year-old man, working in a high-stress job, complains that a gnawing upper-abdominal pain has awakened him each morning for a week. He tells his doctor he sometimes gets a similar pain during the day and finds that eating relieves it. These are classic ulcer symptoms. After determining that the man's condition is stable, many doctors would order an endoscopy, a test in which a fiberoptic tube is passed down the throat to view the stomach and upper intestines.

Since endoscopy entails a small risk of infection or bleeding and rarely even precipitates a fatal heart rhythm, a safer and cheaper approach would be to forgo the test and to simply start treating the man with antiulcer medication. He could also be instructed to try to reduce those things that make ulcers worse, like stress, smoking, coffee, and alcohol. If after a few weeks on medicine he's no better, an endoscopy could still be done. If he improves, he might never need the endoscopy at all.

The Rate of Inappropriate Endoscopy

Researchers at the Rand Corporation and UCLA studied over fifteen hundred patients who had undergone the procedure. They judged an endoscopy appropriate if the expected benefit—increased life expectancy, reduced anxiety, or relief of pain—outweighed such negative consequences as potential side effects, time lost from work, misleading or false diagnoses, and the anxiety and pain of having the procedure. By these criteria, only 72 percent of the tests were found to be appropriate. Of endoscopies done in a doctor's office, only 63 percent were appropriate. In fact, the actual percentage of appropriate endoscopy might be lower, because when in doubt the authors labeled a test as appropriate. Apparently millions of these high-cost, high-profit tests are being done inappropriately every year.[1]

With the recent discovery that a bacterium may be responsible for many cases of ulcers, the standards about when endoscopy is appropriate are beginning to change. The above study was done before the role of bacteria in ulcers was widely appreciated. Whatever happens with developments in the diagnosis and treatment of ulcers, the principle of empiric therapy endures: for some conditions, it can make sense to forgo testing and simply treat.

- *The law of diminishing returns says that the more certain a diagnosis, the less useful information will come from a diagnostic test.* Say that after the interview and exam your doctor is 80 percent sure you have a pneumonia; after a blood test, 90 percent sure; after an X-ray, 99.5 percent sure. Is it worthwhile to have a CAT scan to raise the probability to 99.9 percent? The law of diminishing returns also applies when it's fairly certain you *don't* have the condition in question. As we'll explore later in this chapter, when the likelihood that you've got the condition in question is low, the odds that you'll get a spuriously abnormal result from a lab test—a false positive—dwarf the chances of actually finding the condition.

- *Labs tests give the most useful information when the odds of your having the condition in question are exactly fifty-fifty.* As more data come in, raising or lowering the odds of the diagnosis, each successive test tends to yield less helpful information.

- *Doctors order unnecessary tests because they're worried about getting sued.* When doctors say they want to get a test "just in case," it often means the likelihood of your having the problem is minuscule. Before agreeing to go along, particularly if the test is invasive, find out how likely the problem is. Ask, "Would it be risky if I didn't have the test right away? Could I come back if my symptoms persist?"

"Just in case" can be a tip-off that the test is defensive, as in, "I'd like to get this test just in case you decide to sue me later." Any action by a physician designed to reduce the risk of being sued for malpractice is called *defensive medicine.* Doctors these days are, not completely without justification, paranoid about malpractice suits. In a climate of multi-million-dollar awards to plaintiffs and skyrocketing malpractice insurance premiums, many physicians have changed the way they practice. Some of these changes may be to your benefit, as when the doctor is more thorough or better explains the side effects of treatments. But not all the changes are desirable.

Defensive Doctors

Researchers from Harvard University surveying physicians in New York determined that doctors greatly overestimate their odds of being sued for malpractice. On average, doctors perceived they had about a one-in-five likelihood of being sued in a given year, about three times the actual rate. The doctors estimated that if they were negligent and the patient was harmed as a result, they'd get sued 60 percent of the time. In fact, the researchers discovered that fewer than 2 percent of such negligent events lead to a malpractice suit. The doctors' estimates were thirty times too high. In response to their fear of malpractice suits, four out of five doctors admitted ordering extra tests and procedures.[2]

When doctors order tests they know aren't necessary to lower their risk of lawsuits, their patients may be subjected to potentially dangerous tests and may worry needlessly that they have the medical condition being looked for. Medical costs go up too. According to the AMA, the cost of defensive medicine in the United States is $20 billion annually and rising. The funny thing is that these efforts by doctors to protect themselves from lawsuits probably don't work. For the most part, patients sue doctors they don't like. If a patient finds a doctor arrogant, withdrawn, or unconcerned and *then* something goes wrong, the result may be a lawsuit. But if the relationship is good, patients seldom sue.

• *"Routine" tests are often unnecessary.* A doctor may order a routine test simply out of habit. Given the high rate of false positives, tests should be done only when the doctor has good reason to suspect you have a specific condition and when diagnosing it will benefit you. Batteries of routine tests are often little more than fishing expeditions.

Studies suggest that routine chemistry panels, which include such tests as blood sugar, sodium, potassium, and calcium, are of little use, although when the doctor suspects a particular condition, some of the individual components are worth checking.[3] Routine blood counts have proven to be almost worthless.[4] Routine EKGs are probably only worthwhile for elderly patients or for those with known heart disease,[5] although obtaining a single baseline EKG sometime in mid-life may be worthwhile.

Another commonly unnecessary routine test is the chest X-ray.

"Routine" Chest X-rays

An article in the *Annals of Internal Medicine* reviewed fifteen published studies on the value of routine chest X-rays taken before operations and on admission to the hospital. The authors concluded that the X-rays almost never helped. In fact, misleading results were much more likely than helpful ones. The authors recommended the practice of obtaining routine chest X-rays be stopped, unless the patient has symptoms of chest disease or is going to have surgery of the chest. In the absence of symptoms, even decades of cigarette smoking were insufficient reason for an X-ray. The authors write, "Patients in whom chest radiographs are likely to improve outcome are best identified by a careful history and physical exam."[6] Sound familiar?

The potential impact of eliminating unnecessary routine chest X-rays is enormous: an estimated 30 million routine chest X-rays are taken in U.S. hospitals per year, at a cost to consumers of $1.5 billion. Thirty million X-rays also mean a great deal of unnecessary radiation exposure.

I recall that on Christmas eve of my internship year, while on duty in the emergency room, I became acutely ill with an intestinal infection. I lost so much fluid so quickly that the nurse hooked me up to an IV and poured in three liters of saline solution. Even then, I felt so lightheaded that I nearly passed out just trying to sit up. I knew I'd have to be admitted to the hospital at least overnight. On the way to the ward, they rolled my gurney into the X-ray suite for a routine chest X-ray. Even in my compromised condition, I knew the X-ray was inappropriate. I was a healthy non-smoker with an intestinal infection and not so much as a cough. I politely refused the test and a day and a half later was well enough to go home.

Many unnecessary routine tests are ordered on hospitalized patients, both on admission and during their stay. Emergency room nurses often obtain unnecessary tests. In teaching hospitals the decisions about which tests to order are often made by interns and residents. These apprentice doctors work an incredibly hectic schedule, and to save time they routinely order a battery of tests without much thought. By and large, they would rather order unnecessary tests than have to explain later why they didn't order some test a supervisor deems important.

"Routine" Tests in the Hospital

Sevral studies have shown that two routine blood tests, the PT and the PTT, which measure the ability of blood to clot, have little value in asymptomatic patients and have recommended their routine use be abandoned. Investigators at the University of Pennsylvania wanted to see how well doctors at their university hospital followed this recommendation. They found that the tests were ordered on 81 percent of all patients admitted to the medical ward and that 70 percent of these tests were unnecessary. Many doctors apparently ordered the tests out of habit, even though the best way to determine clotting abnormalities is to interview and examine the patient.[7]

- *Even one unnecessary test can initiate a cascade of events that could ultimately harm you.* You might ask, What's the harm in an inexpensive lab test, even if it's unnecessary? Maybe it'll pick up something the doctor didn't suspect. First of all, these inexpensive tests, done millions of times, contribute to the surge in medical costs. There is a human cost as well. Remember, for a test you don't really need, the odds of finding an unsuspected problem are dwarfed by the odds of a false positive result. **Besides worrying you, a false positive result may lead to further unnecessary testing or to unnecessary treatment, each with its attendant cost and risk.**

  In the study cited above, for example, one of the patients had an abnormally high PTT caused by a condition that doesn't lead to abnormal bleeding. His doctors, however, worried he might bleed during a test and gave him a transfusion of several units of blood plasma—an inappropriate and potentially dangerous decision. The patient could not have benefited from the transfusion yet was subjected to the risk, albeit small, of contracting hepatitis or even AIDS.

Test Principle 2. Results Should Affect Prognosis or Therapy

If the results of a test won't affect your prognosis or treatment, there's usually no reason to do it. Martha Samuels's chest X-ray is a case in point. Here is an imagined dialogue illustrating how Martha might have handled this situation.

Martha: What's the X-ray for?

Doctor: To make sure you haven't got pneumonia.

Martha: What are the odds that I've got pneumonia?

Doctor: Only slight, but I just want to be sure.

Martha: What do you estimate? A one-in-ten chance? One-in-a-hundred?

Doctor: Considering that you don't have fever and that your lungs sound clear, I'd guess one in a hundred.

Martha: I see. What would you do if I had pneumonia?

Doctor: Probably send you home on antibiotics. You're not sick enough to be hospitalized.

Martha: Would you prescribe an antibiotic if I didn't have pneumonia?

Doctor: Yes, I probably would.

Martha: Then the X-ray isn't really affecting the decision?

Doctor: Well, no, not really.

Martha: I think I'll pass on the X-ray then, but I'll come back if I'm feeling worse.

Some frequently ordered tests have absolutely no benefit in making diagnoses or in assessing prognosis. They may appeal to physicians who want to do something or to give the appearance they're doing something but who don't have much else to offer. Consider the following example.

Chronic fatigue syndrome (CFS), a disabling illness that has struck in near-epidemic proportions in the last several years, offers an example of useless testing. Its victims, often in the prime of their lives, experience chronic headaches, sore throats, swollen glands, low-grade fevers, muscle aches, difficulty concentrating, and fatigue so overwhelming that it may be difficult to get out of bed. A number of viruses, including Epstein-Barr and herpes, have been postulated to cause the syndrome, but scientists disagree as to what role they play, and so far the cause remains unclear. No tests have proved of value in people with CFS. None can clinch the diagnosis, guide treatment, or affect prognosis. The diagnosis of CFS, as with many other illnesses, is based almost entirely on the interview and physical exam.

Sensing an opportunity to cash in, however, one national lab mailed a promotional flier to physicians advertising an expensive battery of tests for CFS. The battery included tests for antibody levels to several viruses and a few measures of the immune system's functioning. Because doctors feel so helpless with CFS patients, many of them ordered these worthless tests. As the doctor who reported this promotional campaign in the *Journal of the American Medical Association* wrote, "The (potentially lucrative) commercial marketing of irrelevant laboratory tests...is useless to both physicians and patients, expensive and distracting."[8]

Tests to Determine Prognosis

Even when treatment decisions are not influenced, tests can be appropriate if they help predict what will happen in the future. For many, information on prognosis or reassurance that everything's all right is a legitimate reason to have a test.

For example, Huntington's disease is an inherited disorder that usually starts in middle age. As it advances, the person develops flicking movements of the arms and legs, bizarre grimacing, and a progressive loss of brain function. People with an affected parent have a fifty-fifty chance of getting it. So far there is no effective treatment. When a test was developed that could predict who would develop the disease, many people faced a dilemma. Would they rather know or not know? Some chose to have the test; some decided against it.

The Benefits of Knowing Your Prognosis

Researchers at the University of British Columbia studied the reactions of people who had a test that predicted whether they would develop Huntington's disease. Before the test was offered, there was concern that those given bad news would break down or even commit suicide. As expected, the researchers found that the group which received favorable results showed a marked improvement in psychological health. Perhaps surprisingly, the group receiving the bad news showed no major deterioration in well-being and actually had a slight decrease in distress and depression one year later. The people who did the worst psychologically were those in whom the test results were inconclusive. It seems that certainty, even if it's bad, can yield psychological benefits. The test is not for everyone, however: a small percentage of those in *both* groups—good news and bad—had trouble coping with the results.[9]

Diagnosis for the Sake of Diagnosis

The practice of medicine is based on diagnosis. The idea is to find out what's wrong with the patient and to plan treatment accordingly. It isn't always possible to make a diagnosis, but that's the goal. A precise diagnosis, however, doesn't always benefit the patient. Before agreeing to a test or a series of tests designed to make a diagnosis, ask yourself, How will I benefit from knowing the diagnosis? Peace of mind? A change in therapy? If the condition being looked for is not treatable, sometimes it doesn't make sense to look for it.

Case History: Do We Really Need to Know?

Helen Shea was an elderly woman who was hospitalized late one winter night. She was fiercely independent, the kind of person who'd chosen to avoid doctors most of her life. She'd only come to the hospital when she couldn't go on—short of breath and racked with pain.

She was emaciated and clearly near death. We could feel a rock-hard tumor, the size of a cantaloupe, taking up much of her abdomen. We knew it was cancer, but no one was sure what kind. Regardless of the type, though, nothing could be done to save her: things had gone too far. Nonetheless, several of the doctors were pushing for a biopsy, just to make the diagnosis. Her family, however, decided against the procedure, and within a few days, she died in her sleep.

Diagnosis for Research Purposes

Doctors at major medical centers and university hospitals are often primarily researchers. If your problem is in their area of interest, they may recommend tests not because the results will help manage your condition but because the results interest them or further their research. If the primary rationale for a test is research, you should be told. If you decide to endure the discomfort and risk the side effects of a test for research purposes, that's your choice, and in fact, the advancement of science depends on the generosity of volunteers. You shouldn't, however, feel obligated to undergo tests you don't want in exchange for the doctor's care. The doctor or hospital should also pay for any such tests and for treatment of any side effects you experience.

Test Principle 3. Weigh the Risks and Benefits

Whether a test is appropriate is often a matter of judgment. Having a test entails both risk and expense. Forgoing a test often means accepting some uncertainty, since a diagnosis could be missed or delayed. In Martha Samuels's case, the risk of a chest X-ray, even if small, was not justified given the minor nature of her illness. Had she been sicker, the risk-benefit equation might have shifted, making the X-ray a good idea.

When evaluating the risk and benefits of a proposed test, keep the following in mind:

- *The test shouldn't be worse than the disease.* Any invasive test can cause a side effect. Liver biopsies occasionally lead to fatal hemorrhages. X-ray studies of the kidney can precipitate kidney failure. I once treated an elderly man who nearly died when he went into anaphylactic shock (the most serious type of allergic reaction) after being injected with contrast dye for a CAT scan of his head. His doctor had ordered the test because the man was depressed, which experts consider an insufficient reason to order a CAT scan—particularly one with contrast dye. Luckily, shots of adrenaline and other medicines raised his dangerously low blood pressure and saved his life.

- *It's not always better "to do the tests and to know."* It may be preferable to tolerate a remote chance that something will go undiagnosed than to risk a serious side effect of a test. If there's a one-in-a-thousand chance you've got cancer and the test to diagnose it kills one in five hundred, the odds favor not doing the test.

- *Even tests with potentially serious side effects are advisable if the risks are outweighed by the benefits.* If there's a one-in-ten chance you've got a curable cancer and the test to diagnose it kills one in five-hundred, the risk is well worth taking. Although a CAT scan of the head is considered inappropriate for someone whose only symptom is depression, if other symptoms pointed to the possibility of a brain tumor, the test would be advisable.

- *Think ahead.* Good chess players anticipate the next several moves before making a decision. When evaluating the risks and the benefits of a test, consider what you would do if the test came back abnormal. Ask the doctor what he or she would likely recommend. Then try to anticipate how you'd feel. If the test were abnormal, would you proceed to have a more invasive test or an operation, if recommended? If you're certain you'd refuse to take the next step, it sometimes makes sense to avoid the first one.

- *Your values matter the most.* Different people will look at the same information on the risks and benefits of a test and will come to opposite conclusions. Individuals differ in the value they place on resolving uncertainty and in how they tolerate risk.

Consider the case of a healthy thirty-five-year-old man who notices a little blood on the toilet paper while wiping himself after a bowel movement. Recognizing a warning sign of colon cancer, he visits his doctor. The doctor discovers a hemorrhoid and is reasonably certain it's the cause of the bleeding. The doctor tells him colon cancer is rare—though not unheard of— in a healthy man his age without a family history of colon problems. To rule out colon cancer completely, the man would have to undergo a test or a series of tests that are uncomfortable, expensive, and while generally safe, not without risk. Without the tests he will have to accept the remote chance, say one in ten thousand, that he has an undiagnosed cancer. In this circumstance some people would say, "If there's a one-in-ten-thousand risk of cancer, I want the tests." Others would say, "You're not doing those tests to me. I'll take my chances." The decision is a value judgment. There is no right answer.

For a sixty-five-year-old man in the same situation, almost all doctors would recommend the tests, since colon cancer is common at that age. If the man were twenty-five, few doctors would recommend them. The proper course of action is clear at the extremes of age, but there is a substantial gray area. Different doctors will draw the line at different points. Remember, though, a doctor's recommendation that you have a test may be colored by many factors, including concern over a potential malpractice suit. **The question should not be "How much uncertainty is your doctor willing to accept?" but rather "How much uncertainty are you willing to accept?"**

Test Principle 4. Go Where the Money Is

When asked why he robbed banks, Willie Sutton reportedly answered, "That's where the money is." The same principle applies to medical diagnosis: Look where you're likely to find the payoff.

- *Look for common conditions before rare ones.* Common problems are common. Rare ones aren't. The money says look for common problems first. Only if the search comes up empty should rarer causes be sought. There are, of course, exceptions. In an emergency, as with an unconscious patient, a doctor may have to cast a wide net and look for many possible causes simultaneously. In general, however, things can be done in an ordered fashion.

  Imagine if the doctor examining Martha Samuels had wanted to be sure her sore throat and cough weren't due to throat cancer. He might have recommended a CAT scan or that someone look down her throat with an endoscope. These tests would, of course, be absurd in a young non-smoker who had just developed her symptoms. The risk would clearly outweigh the benefit.

- *Avoid hunting for zebras.* Some specialists have seen so many unusual cases in their careers that they tend to overestimate how common these problems are in the general public. When something comes along that looks like a horse and walks like a horse and smells like a horse, they think, *This could be a zebra!* Watch out when your doctor wants to order a lot of fancy tests to rule out a condition that almost nobody ever has.

  In medical school, we were taught that when patients developed high blood pressure, you needed to do a series of sophisticated tests to be sure they didn't have a rare tumor called a pheochromocytoma, or a pheo for short. This tumor secretes hormones that raise blood pressure. I remember as a student and later as a medical resident ordering dozens of these tests. Considering that 60 million Americans have high blood pressure, I presume I wasn't the only one.

Finally, in my last year of residency training, I took care of a patient in whom we discovered a pheo. He had classic symptoms: sky-high blood pressure that hadn't responded to standard blood pressure medicines and repeated episodes in which his heart beat hard and fast and his face flushed beet red. After interviewing him, we put a pheo at the top of our list of possibile diagnoses. We ordered the tests, and sure enough he had it.

I remember discussing the case with the specialist involved, a middle-aged endocrinologist who had trained at one of the country's top hospitals. He told me that in all his years of training and practice, this was the first pheo he'd ever seen. His comment made me wonder about the wisdom of all those tests we'd done looking for pheos. This was an exceedingly rare disorder. The case was the buzz all around the hospital, and no one else I spoke with had ever seen one before either. In the one patient who did have the tumor, we had a pretty good idea of it before we'd even ordered the tests.

• *Rule out emergencies.* The price for missing a diagnosis when someone is in immediate danger of death or permanent harm can be immense. If a sixty-year-old man complains to his doctor of a heavy pain in his chest, his doctor may consider dozens of possible causes—a pulled muscle, a bronchitis, a stomach ulcer, or, as the man probably fears, a heart attack. The highest priority is to make sure it isn't a heart attack, since any delay in treatment could prove fatal. By simply asking the man a few questions, the doctor may be able to determine that the pain isn't coming from the heart. Sometimes the doctor will need to do an EKG. And, if suspicious enough, the doctor may admit the man to the hospital until it's determined whether he's suffered a heart attack. Once a heart attack has been ruled out, the search for other causes can begin.

Not all life-threatening conditions, however, are emergencies. Only those conditions that if not treated promptly could lead to permanent disability or death need be ruled out before considering more likely diagnoses. Cancer is potentially life-threatening in the long term, but a delay of a few days in diagnosis is generally not critical. The same cannot be said of a heart attack. Even when cancer is a possibility, it is sometimes appropriate to wait a week or more to see if your symptoms subside before proceeding to invasive tests.

Test Principle 5. Start With Less Invasive Tests

The more invasive a test is, the more likely it will cause a serious side effect. In making the decision between tests that differ in safety, consider the following:

• *In general, you should obtain the least invasive test that can provide the necessary information.* If a diagnosis can be made with a simple blood test, why get an X-ray and be exposed to radiation? If a CAT scan can provide much the same information as exploratory surgery, why risk an operation?

  Say you have a heart murmur, a whooshing sound heard through a stethoscope caused by turbulent flow across the heart's valves. Some murmurs are benign, some are serious. It's the doctor's job to differentiate one from the other. The place to begin is with the least invasive test of all, the physical exam.

  Before the advent of high-tech tests, doctors relied almost exclusively on their bedside skills to diagnose heart murmurs. They would inspect a patient's fingernails and lips, place their hands on the chest and feel the lift of each heartbeat. With their stethoscopes they would listen to the *lub-dub, lub-dub* of the pumping heart and make the correct diagnosis. The increased sophistication of medical tests has unfortunately led to dependence on them. While some physicians remain adept at the physical exam, it is more and more becoming a lost art. The reality is that you can no longer count on a physician's ability to differentiate one type of murmur from another.

So, assuming you need a test to evaluate your murmur, which should you have? An echocardiogram, in which sonar waves are bounced off the heart to create a picture? Or a cardiac catheterization, in which a catheter is threaded through blood vessels in the arm or leg and into the heart, allowing dye to be injected while X-rays are taken? A cardiac cath yields more accurate results, but this accuracy comes at some risk. Serious complications—such as heart rhythm disturbances, even cardiac arrest—result up to 4 percent of the time. About one person in five hundred undergoing the procedure dies, though healthier patients tend to have a lower rate of complications. The echocardiogram, on the other hand, while providing less accurate pictures, appears to be safe. Because of its safety, the less invasive echocardiogram is considered the preferred initial procedure to assess a heart murmur.

- *If a more invasive test is going to be necessary no matter what, you can often skip the less invasive test.* If your heart condition were so serious that you're going to need surgery, a cardiac cath may be necessary to precisely define the problem. The less invasive but less accurate echocardiogram may therefore be a waste of time and money.

Sometimes the less invasive test, while not inappropriate per se, gives a falsely reassuring result that may lead to disaster. Say a forty-four-year-old woman discovers a lump in her breast that wasn't there previously. To evaluate the lump, the doctor could order a mammogram. Even though the majority of such lumps turn out to be benign, the decision could be a mistake. The problem is that mammograms, best used to screen for breast cancer in women without symptoms, miss some cancers, so in this case even a negative result is not reassuring enough. If a woman has a lump and a negative mammogram leads to the decision *not* to biopsy, the diagnosis of cancer could be delayed for months, even years. Such a delay can be deadly. I have seen cases where physicians were falsely reassured by a negative mammogram, only to have the poor woman return some months later with breast cancer that had spread to other areas of the body and was no longer curable. Failure to diagnose breast cancer is in fact the second most common reason that doctors are sued and leads to the largest malpractice settlements.

The Accuracy of Mammograms in Evaluating Breast Lumps

In a study reported in the *Journal of the American Medical Association,* researchers looked at over one hundred women under the age of forty-five who developed breast lumps that turned out to be cancer. Prior to having a biopsy, fifty-two of the women had a mammogram. The mammogram failed to show the cancer 63 percent of the time. In fifteen instances the normal mammogram led to the decision to defer surgery; all fifteen of these women had more advanced tumors when eventually operated on.[10]

If a new breast lump is found, experts recommend that the doctor try to remove fluid from the lump with a needle. If the lump is a benign cyst, when the fluid is removed, the lump disappears. If the doctor is unable to remove any fluid at all, the lump could be a tumor—in which case a biopsy should be done. According to an editorial in the *New England Journal of Medicine,* the only good reason to order a mammogram in this instance is to look for other suspicious areas.[11] Whether to have the biopsy, of course, remains the woman's choice. The doctor should estimate the odds of cancer and the woman can decide what degree of uncertainty she's willing to accept.

Test Principle 6. Think Twice About Surprising Results

When evaluating surprising test results, consider the following:

- *An abnormal test result is sometimes a false positive—that is, abnormal even though you don't have the condition in question.* False positive results might more appropriately be called false alarms, because unexpectedly abnormal results can alarm both doctors and patients. False positives can also lead to unnecessary tests or treatment.

Let me illustrate. My sister Debbie called me one Friday a few years ago, crying so hard she was coughing. She was expecting her second child and had just been informed by her obstetrician that her baby might have Down's syndrome (the birth defect formerly referred to as mongolism). He recommended she come in the following Monday for an amniocentesis, in which a long needle would be passed into her belly to remove fluid for genetic testing of the baby. Debbie had already agreed to the test.

Her doctor had informed her that one of the blood tests, the alpha fetoprotein (AFP) was low, which suggested Down's syndrome. Debbie was devastated, worried about her baby, and facing an invasive procedure which itself causes a miscarriage as often as one out of two hundred times—even in healthy pregnancies. I advised her to cancel the amniocentesis until she had the AFP level repeated.

Debbie went in the following Monday and had the blood test redone. The result was normal, and she never needed an amniocentesis. The baby, my niece Jacqueline, was fine.

- *If a test gives an unexpected abnormal result, repeat it before proceeding to a more invasive procedure.* If you have any questions about the accuracy of the lab where the test was done, consider repeating it elsewhere. Of course, something can go wrong with the second test as well. If two results differ greatly and a lot is at stake, repeat the test again.

There was, by the way, another problem with the doctor's recommendation of an amniocentesis for my sister: a safer, less invasive test should have been done first. AFP levels generally rise during pregnancy. If Debbie's doctor had overestimated how many weeks pregnant she was—a common error—he might have expected a higher AFP level. A recent editorial in the *New England Journal of Medicine* recommended that women with low AFP levels undergo an ultrasound examination to be sure the doctor hasn't inaccurately estimated the date of conception.[12] According to the authors, with the much safer ultrasound exam, half of all women with low AFP levels can be spared an amniocentesis.

- *Many things lead to inaccurate results.* You might ask, "What happened with the first AFP test?" It's hard to know for sure, but there are several possibilities. The calibration of the machine could have been off at the time the first specimen was run, leading to the error. Perhaps another patient's blood tube got switched with my sister's. Maybe a technician copied a number incorrectly. All of these mistakes occur, more often than most people are aware.

  Other factors can affect the results of various tests: how the technician drew the blood, how long the tube sat on the counter before the test was run, when you last ate, if you just exercised, what medicines you've taken in the last few days. For most tests no adjustment is made for your age, sex, or size, even though they can affect results. A common error is to assume that the elderly will conform to the "normal" range determined for younger people.

- *A false positive result is not necessarily due to lab error.* For many diseases, there is an overlap between the test results of the sick and the healthy. A line between abnormal and normal must be drawn somewhere, and the decision where to place it is based on statistics. A cutoff is often chosen at a level where a normal person will get a normal result 95 percent of the time. In other words, 5 percent of normal people will get an abnormal result. For some the result will be abnormal every time they take the test. This does not necessarily mean that they need more tests to figure out the reason. If the likelihood of a problem is remote, sometimes nothing further need be done.

- *The more tests done, the greater the likelihood of at least one false positive result.* Consider routine chemistry tests often run in panels consisting of up to twenty individual tests. The cutoff point between normal and abnormal for each individual test allows a 5 percent false positive rate. If six tests are done, more than one quarter of normal people will have at least one abnormal result. In a battery of twenty tests, two-thirds of normal people will have at least one abnormality.

- *The less likely a problem is, the more likely an abnormal test result is a false positive.* This is a basic principle of test interpretation, yet many physicians don't seem to understand it. Let me explain. Say that only one person in a thousand has disease X and that the test for it yields a false positive result 5 percent of the time. If we tested one thousand randomly chosen people, we would expect to find one person with the disease. But fifty people (5 percent of one thousand) would get false positive test results. In other words, only one person in fifty-one with an abnormal result would actually have the disease. This is not the impression many patients get when they're told their test results are abnormal. Doctors may not be much better at interpreting abnormal results.

How Well Do Doctors Interpret Abnormal Test Results?

Researchers stood in the hallways of four Harvard Medical School hospitals and quizzed resident physicians, fourth-year medical students and faculty members about the hypothetical disease and test described above. The doctors were asked to assess the likelihood that someone with a positive result had the disease. Only 20 percent of the faculty members gave the correct answer of one in fifty-one. Almost half the participants answered that 95 percent of the people with a positive result had the disease—an estimate almost fifty times too high. If the answers at Harvard Medical School were this bad, we can only guess how well the average doctor would do.[13]

- *Some tests have extremely high rates of false positives.* The newly developed screening test for prostate cancer, the PSA, is notorious for its high rate of false positives. In other words, many people who don't have prostate cancer come up with abnormal results.

Another example is the blood test for Lyme disease. The antibody test for the tick-borne infection is inherently inaccurate. Because there are so many false positives, experts recommend that the tests should only be done on people who've been in areas known to harbor infected ticks or who have suggestive symptoms. These symptoms include a characteristic skin rash early on and, if the person isn't treated with antibiotics, arthritis and certain heart and neurological problems months later. Doctors don't always follow the experts' advice. The diagnosis of Lyme disease has in fact become trendy, with many people misdiagnosed based on false positive tests. Some of them end up being treated with expensive and potentially dangerous drugs that have no chance of benefiting them.

The Overdiagnosis of Lyme Disease

Researchers at the Lyme disease clinic at the New England Medical Center studied almost eight-hundred patients referred to them for Lyme disease. They found that in only 23 percent was Lyme disease causing their symptoms. Another 20 percent had had Lyme disease in the past and still had antibodies to it, but their symptoms were caused by other medical conditions. The remaining 57 percent had never had Lyme disease. Many of these people who were incorrectly diagnosed had had false positive test results at other labs and had already been treated without benefit before being referred to the clinic.[14]

- *The more abnormal the result, the greater the likelihood of a problem.* Say the normal range for a test extends from 10 to 30. A result of 31 or 32 is much more likely to be a false positive than a result of 132. When you're in doubt and there's no emergency, repeat the test a few weeks or a few months later. If you are healthy and a test result is slightly abnormal, it will tend to stay about the same or improve slightly. If you are developing a problem, the results will usually worsen over time.

- *The more likely a problem is, the more likely a normal test result is a false negative.* False negatives are also a big problem. In the example mentioned earlier, false negative mammograms led doctors to miss the diagnosis of cancer in women who had developed lumps in their breast. Doctors and patients alike tend to accept uncritically the results of sophisticated tests. If the odds of a serious problem, like cancer, are great enough, you may need additional tests to be sure the diagnosis is not missed.

Test Principle 7. Examine
the Financial Incentives

The traditional reimbursement system in the United States rewards intervention by paying doctors a fee for each service rendered. The doctor in the walk-in clinic that Martha Samuels visited ran up over $150 worth of tests for a simple cold. In my experience walk-in clinics regularly "churn" patients by ordering unnecessary tests and scheduling excessive return visits to generate extra profit. Doctors in private solo and group practice often have similar incentives to run up the bill.

The incentives are the opposite in health maintenance organizations (HMOs), which bill patients a fixed amount each year, regardless of how much is done. Although doctors in HMOs do not want to do so little that they risk lawsuits for missing diagnoses, they are pressured to be frugal. As we've seen, many HMOs pay yearly bonuses to doctors who spend less on their patients.

Although the comparison is perhaps a little harsh, you can think of your doctor in the same way you'd think of a car dealer. **Having tests done in a private practice is analogous to purchasing options on a new car: you may want some, but the more you get, the higher the profit to the dealer. Having tests in an HMO is like trying to get the dealer to fix your car on warranty: the more the dealer does, the lower the profit.** This is not to say that most doctors (or car dealers) are unscrupulous, only that it pays to know where the incentives lie.

It's logical, perhaps, to assume that fee-for-service doctors order too many tests and HMO doctors too few. I believe that in many instances they both order too many. The norms of American medicine concerning test ordering evolved under the fee-for-service system that rewarded intervention. These norms still influence the practice of many doctors who have since moved on to HMOs. Doctors in HMOs, like those in private practice, may also order unnecessary tests because of their concern about malpractice suits.

Testing in the U.S. Versus England

In a study involving patients with uncomplicated high blood pressure, Harvard researchers compared test ordering by American physicians with that of their counterparts in England. The English doctors, all part of the National Health Service, received a flat yearly payment per patient, regardless of how much or little was done. At the time the study was conducted, malpractice suits were uncommon in England, so test ordering there was unlikely to be affected by the fear of a lawsuit. The researchers found that American physicians performed five times as many blood counts, seven times as many chest X-rays, and forty-one times as many EKGs.[15]

Tests in the Doctor's Office

A doctor generally makes no profit for referring you to a hospital to have an X-ray or lab test done. The same test performed in the doctor's office can yield a handsome payoff. When evaluating the recommendation to have a test performed in a doctor's office, consider the following:

- *Once a doctor makes an investment in medical equipment, there is a natural tendency to use it.* Doctors in private practice commonly purchase such testing equipment for their offices as blood analyzers, X-ray machines, EKG machines, or more fancy heart monitoring equipment. Roughly one quarter of all lab tests are performed in doctors' offices. Approximately 75 percent of all X-rays taken outside the hospital are performed in the offices of doctors who are not radiologists.

   My office junk mail (about five times the volume I get at home) regularly contains advertisements for various office testing equipment. Prominently featured on many of the brochures are words like "income potential." Here's a typical blurb: "It takes only a few tests a month to recoup the cost of an IMEXLAB 9000. Most physicians perform many more, and because tests are reimbursed by Medicare and by third parties, each one builds profits!"

The Frequency and Cost of X-rays in Doctors' Offices

Investigators reporting in the *New England Journal of Medicine* found that doctors who performed X-rays in their own offices ordered them more than four times as often as doctors who have to refer their patients elsewhere, and they consistently charged higher fees. At the time the study was done, an ultrasound on a pregnant woman performed in a doctor's office, for example, averaged more than $300. The same test done by an X-ray specialist, a radiologist, averaged $185.[16]

- *The quality of tests done in doctors' offices is often not good.* X-rays done in doctors' offices on average are not as safe or as accurate as those done by radiologists. Office doctors often train their receptionists or secretaries to take the X-rays. Unfortunately, neither the doctors or their staffs may fully appreciate the dangers of radiation or apply adequate safeguards against excessive exposure. Because they don't understand the equipment as well, they tend to deliver more radiation than necessary per film, to take more films than necessary, and to repeat more X-rays due to poor technique.[17]

Until recently office labs weren't regulated by the federal government or by most states. As with X-rays, the lab tests are often done by nurses or billing clerks who have no formal training in laboratory technology. The accuracy of the results is questionable.[18]

The Accuracy of Tests in the Doctor's Lab

The College of American Pathologists studied the proficiency of five-thousand labs across the country by sending them a blood sample with a known level of cholesterol. A lab was judged acceptable if its results were less than 5 percent off. Almost 90 percent of commercial and hospital labs met the standard of quality. Fewer than 30 percent of the labs in doctor's offices did so. Almost one-third of doctors' labs were more than 15 percent off, more than three times the acceptable level. The key factor that predicted accuracy was the skill of the operators; in doctors' offices they weren't as reliable.[19]

- In general, the more tests a doctor's lab does, the better the accuracy. Doctors' labs vary in how busy they are. A lab in a large group practice probably performs many more tests per week than a similar lab in the office of a solo practitioner. Hospital and commercial labs that run hundreds of tests per day tend to be the most proficient.

A Dangerous Test in Some Doctors' Labs

A test called a prothrombin time (PT) is commonly used to evaluate the effectiveness of blood-thinning drugs given to prevent a recurrence of a heart attack or stroke. Researchers at the University of Alabama postulated that an inaccurate result could lead a physician to prescribe an inappropriately high or inappropriately low dose of blood thinners, which could *cause* strokes or heart attacks rather than prevent them. Studying the records of almost fifteen thousand patients, they found that those patients who had PTs in doctors' labs that performed the fewest tests per month had twice as many strokes and three times as many heart attacks in the week following the test as those whose PTs were done by commercial labs. The more PTs a doctor's lab did per month, the more closely results approximated those of commercial labs.[20]

- *Tests in the doctor's office are, of course, not necessarily inappropriate.* You simply need to be aware of how the profit motive can affect a doctor's test recommendations. Because of accuracy problems in doctor's labs, you may be more inclined to repeat surprising test results, possibly at a commercial or hospital lab. As the government increases its scrutiny on doctors' labs, the quality should improve, although these labs probably won't, anytime soon, reach the level of accuracy of labs with certified laboratory technicians. Nevertheless, at times the convenience and timely availability of test results in the doctor's office may be worth the added expense and the risk of inaccurate results.

Tests in Outside Labs

Financial incentives can also influence doctors who order tests at outside labs. Many doctors own or have partial interest in diagnostic laboratories where blood and urine analyses, X-rays, and other tests are performed. Although they don't receive a direct payment for each test they order, the more tests they order, the better the yield on their investment. Some particularly questionable limited partnership arrangements are not offered to the general public—only to doctors who can refer patients to the labs—and pay doctors more than a 100 percent annual return on their investment.[21] Critics have blasted these schemes as nothing more than indirect kickbacks.

Physician Ownership of Health Care Facilities

A comprehensive survey, mandated by the Florida state legislature and reported in 1992 in the *Journal of the American Medical Association,* revealed that at least 40 percent of practicing Florida physicians had an investment in a health care business to which they refered patients. The researchers who conducted the survey felt the number might have been even higher, because those physicians who refused to answer the survey were probably more likely to have been investors. Over 90 percent of diagnostic imaging centers (such as MRI facilities) and over 75 percent of ambulatory surgery centers in Florida were owned wholly or partially by referring doctors. Referring physicians were investors in half the clinical laboratories and radiation therapy centers and in almost 40 percent of the physical therapy centers. In most of these facilities the majority of patients were referred by their physician investors.[22]

Concerned about the potential conflict of interest, in 1992 the AMA took a position against physician ownership of medical facilities. The AMA concluded that "in general, physicians should not refer patients to a health care facility outside their office practice at which they do not directly provide care or services when they have an investment interest in the facility."[23] The AMA later reversed itself, saying that such referrals would be okay if the patient is informed of the doctor's financial interest in the facility and of available alternatives.

In 1992 the federal government began prohibiting doctors from referring Medicare patients to clinical laboratories they own or hold an interest in, a practice sometimes called self-referral. As of the beginning of 1995 the ban was extended to include Medicaid patients and to prohibit self-referral to X-ray and radiation therapy facilities, home health care services, and physical therapy and rehabilitation centers. (Medicare, by the way, is the government's insurance program for the elderly, while Medicaid is for the poor.) So far there are few restrictions on self-referrals to kidney dialysis centers, weight loss clinics, or drug treatment programs or for patients with private insurance. Proposed legislation may fill some of these gaps.

Putting It Together

Beyond helping you to decide whether to have a particular test, I hope awareness of the seven principles of appropriate medical testing will increase your understanding of how your physician practices medicine. When you analyze your physician's use of tests, you begin to gain an appreciation of his or her beliefs and biases. All doctors have biases; it is only by understanding them that you can best evaluate their advice. Ask yourself, Does this doctor tend to order a lot of tests? Does the doctor favor safer, less invasive tests? Is the doctor an unswerving believer in high technology? Are tests being ordered tests mostly because the doctor's worried about getting sued? Or for profit?

If you perceive that your doctor is ordering tests inappropriately, you can try to negotiate. Ultimately, no test can be

---

Seven Principles of Appropriate Medical Testing

1. Use tests selectively.
2. Results should affect prognosis or therapy.
3. Weigh the risks and benefits.
4. Go where the money is.
5. Start with less invasive tests.
6. Think twice about surprising results.
7. Examine the financial incentives.

done unless you agree to it. Ask why the test is being recommended and if there are alternatives. Find out if it needs to be done immediately or if it would be safe to wait a while. If you decide against a recommended test, decline it politely or tell the doctor you need more time to think about it. For any major intervention that isn't an emergency, it's never a bad idea to go home, do some reading, talk with your friends or family, and try to decide how you feel about the test, removed from the glare of the doctor's office.

A good doctor should be willing to negotiate. If the doctor thinks you're making a mistake by refusing a test, he or she should explain why. If you nevertheless decide against the test, the doctor should accept your decision. It's your body, after all, and your life. If a doctor orders tests inappropriately and is inflexible to boot, my advice is to find a new one.

If, on the other hand, your doctor doesn't want to order a test you feel you need, the situation is more difficult. Few tests can be done without a doctor's order. In a private practice or other fee-for-service setting, where doctors profit from ordering tests, if the doctor opposes a test, the odds are you don't need it. Doctors do make mistakes, though, so you may want to consider seeking a second opinion. In an HMO or other managed care setting, where doctors are pressed to minimize test ordering and specialist referrals, the situation is tougher still. We'll discuss how to get good care in an HMO in more detail in chapter 7, but the basic principle is that the squeaky wheel gets the grease. Ask for a test enough times and back up your request with good reasons, and most doctors even in an HMO will acquiesce.

Remember, though, that in general American physicians—spurred sometimes by greed, sometimes by a fear of lawsuits, sometimes by an overreliance on technology, and probably most often by their genuine desire to help patients—order too many tests. There is a delicate balance between doing too much and thereby raising costs and risking side effects, and doing too little and thereby missing diagnoses. As an alert consumer, taking an active role in medical decisions, you can help steer your doctor down the prudent middle road.

4

IS YOUR DOCTOR PRESCRIBING THE RIGHT DRUGS?

VOLTAIRE WROTE, "DOCTORS POUR DRUGS OF WHICH THEY KNOW little for diseases of which they know less into patients of which they know nothing." While there have been great advances in the science of drugs since his time, the truth endures: many physicians prescribe drugs illogically. They are ignorant of how drugs should be prescribed, use them for conditions for which they were never intended, and even when drugs are advisable, use the wrong ones.

Patients too play a role in inappropriate drug prescribing. We Americans eagerly pop pills we know little about, oblivious to potential risk, hoping for some improvement in our health or well-being, even when there is little evidence the drug will provide it. We have come to expect a prescription whenever we visit the doctor. Many of us view doctors who fail to provide prescriptions as doing nothing—as not taking our problems seriously.

Doctors know it's good business to keep the customers happy. Many are only too willing to prescribe drugs when expected to do so, whether needed or not. Doctors also want to help their patients, of course, and drugs often do help. Some physicians, though, resort almost reflexively to their prescription pads, prescribing drugs when there is only a remote chance the patient will benefit. Others prescribe drugs because they don't know what else to do and they want to do something.

Case History: The Highest
Court in the Land

In 1981 lawyers appearing before the United States Supreme Court noticed that Justice William Rehnquist was behaving peculiarly. His speech was slurred, he stuttered, and he sometimes seemed unable to finish a sentence.[1]

His problems, it turned out, were side effects of the drug Placidyl, prescribed by his doctor for chronic lower back pain. According to reports, he'd been on the medicine for nine years, at times taking three times the recommended dose.[2] *According to the* Physician's Drug Reference (PDR), *the drug reference book doctors most often use, Placidyl should only be used to treat severe insomnia not helped by milder sedatives. The drug is not recommended for back pain. The* PDR *advises that Placidyl should be used for a maximum of one week. The following warning is printed in bold type: "Prolonged use of Placidyl may result in tolerance and psychological and physical dependence. Prolonged administration of the drug is not recommended."*

Despite the drug, Rehnquist's back pain worsened. Just after Christmas of 1981 he was admitted to the George Washington University Hospital in Washington, D.C. Doctors there stopped the drug. Three days later Rehnquist began "seeing things and hearing things that other people didn't see or hear," according to hospital doctors. He had become temporarily psychotic—a known withdrawal reaction to Placidyl. After ten days in the hospital, Rehnquist was over his addiction and was discharged.

TEN PRINCIPLES OF APPROPRIATE
DRUG PRESCRIBING

Doctors vary enormously in how they prescribe drugs. Some prescribe drugs sparingly. Others give them out like candy at Halloween. My medical training allows me to examine a list of a patient's medications and surmise a lot about the prescribing physician. I can often guess if a doctor is out-of-date, overly influenced by drug companies, or oblivious to the cost of drugs. Even without any medical background, you can learn to make similar determinations. All you need is a basic understanding of how drugs should and should not be prescribed.

Drug Principle 1. Understand the Drug

In order to prescribe a drug appropriately, a doctor must understand how it's supposed to be used. Justice Rehnquist's doctor had prescribed a powerful drug in an utterly illogical manner: Placidyl was used for a condition for which it is not intended, at up to three times the recommended dose, and for more than 450 times as long as recommended. The doctor either had little knowledge of the drug he prescribed or chose to ignore what he did know.

Before writing a prescription, doctors should ask themselves a few questions. Is the drug appropriate for the condition in question? What dose should be used? How many times per day should it be taken? For how long? What side effects are possible? Will the drug interact with other drugs the patient's taking?

With the multitude of drugs available these days, no doctor can know them all. Good doctors know a lot about the drugs they frequently prescribe, and they read about unfamiliar ones before prescribing them. Obviously, not all doctors take the time to do so.

The Most Common Prescribing Errors

The Physician Insurers Association of America analyzed almost four hundred recent malpractice claims due to medication errors. In most cases the doctor involved had made more than one error. The most common errors made and their frequency were:

Types of Error	Frequency by percent
Incorrect dose	27.2
Inappropriate drug for the condition	24.9
Failure to monitor for side effects	20.6
Poor communication by doctor	18.1
Failure to monitor drug levels	13.2
Lack of knowledge about drug	13.2
Failure to use most appropriate drug	13.0
Inappropriate length of treatment	12.7
Failure to monitor drug's effectiveness	12.5

Inadequate medical history (interview)	12.2
Inadequate notes in the patient's chart	9.9
Failure to notice patient was allergic to drug	9.7

While some of the errors involved drugs the doctors were not very familiar with, the vast majority involved the drugs the doctors used most. Almost all the errors were completely avoidable.[3]

Although prescribing drugs is one of the main duties of the physician, medical students receive remarkably little training in pharmacology, the science of drugs. In fact, many drug company promotional representatives have more training in pharmacology than the average doctor. Since new drugs are being introduced all the time, a doctor who has been out in practice for ten years may be prescribing dozens of drugs for which he or she has no formal training. Many doctors will, of course, educate themselves about any new drug they prescribe. Others rely on information they read in advertisements or hear from drug company representatives. Still others prescribe drugs they know little about.

For example, since its introduction in the 1980s, nicotine gum has been shown to be effective in helping some smokers quit. In order for the gum to work, however, it has to be used properly. You must stop smoking completely before starting the gum; you are not supposed to use it just to cut down. Nicotine gum must be chewed slowly and the juice should be left in the mouth, not swallowed, otherwise you may absorb too much and risk side effects. Surveys show that most prescriptions are given with little or no instructions about how to use the gum.

Doctors' Knowledge of Nicotine Gum

A survey of doctors in the San Francisco Bay area found that almost 40 percent believed that patients should be advised to use the gum to help them cut down the number of cigarettes they were smoking. Another 20 percent thought patients should be told to swallow the juices so that the nicotine could be absorbed through the stomach. Those doctors who held mistaken beliefs about nicotine gum were just as likely to prescribe it as doctors who understood its proper use. The researchers also discovered that almost a quarter of the doctors prescribed tranquilizers to help people quit smoking, even though tranquilizers are neither approved nor recommended for this use.[4]

Is the Drug Appropriate for the Condition in Question?

When a drug is approved by the FDA, it's approved only for certain conditions, but once it's approved, doctors may prescribe it as they see fit. Rehnquist's case is just one example of a drug's being prescribed for a condition for which there is no evidence it works.

Inappropriate Tagamet in Nursing Home Patients

Harvard researchers reviewed the records of nursing home residents to see how often doctors prescribed the ulcer drug Tagamet (cimetidine)* appropriately. In 90 percent of the patients receiving the drug, the researchers judged that the prescription was unjustified. When prescribed appropriately, the drug is usually given for eight weeks or less. In this study 81 percent of the patients received the drug for more than a year and a half. To make matters worse, doctors rarely reduced the dose for older patients, an oversight which greatly increased the risk of side effects.[5]

The *PDR* and the package insert (which you can ask the pharmacist for) list the approved *indications* for each drug, that is, the conditions for which it is an appropriate treatment. If your doctor recommends a drug for a condition for which it is not officially indicated, ask if there is good evidence to support its use for your problem. Sometimes after a drug has been around for a while, new uses for it will be recognized. Studies may appear in medical journals demonstrating a drug's effectiveness in some area that wasn't initially appreciated. When there is good evidence that a drug is effective for a different

---

* When discussing a drug by its brand name, I'll usually also give the generic name in parentheses.

condition than initially approved, it can be appropriate for the doctor to prescribe it. Many drugs end up being prescribed, however, when they don't work or are overkill.

How Frequently Should the Drug Be Taken?

Some drugs stay in the blood for a long period of time and so only need to be taken once per day. Others are excreted within a few hours and must be taken four or more times per day in order to be effective. I've seen hundreds of instances in my career in which doctors have instructed patients to take a drug either not often enough for it to be effective or too often, risking an overdose.

While doctors generally prescribe too many drugs, there is one huge exception. When it comes to pain relief, doctors tend to give far too little medication.

For severe pain, such as that following surgery, narcotics like morphine or codeine are usually the best and safest drugs to prescribe. Doctors, though, are often reluctant to prescribe narcotics. When they do, the doses are usually too small. I had a five-year-old cousin who died many years ago of cancer. In the last weeks of her life she was in nearly constant pain because her doctors feared that if they gave her enough morphine to relieve the pain, she might become an addict. This fear is irrational. Patients who take narcotics for acute pain or for cancer pain rarely get high or become addicted.

There is another basic principle in pain relief that many physicians don't seem to understand: it is easier to prevent pain than to treat it once it appears. For this reason, experts in pain relief recommend against prescribing pain medicines to be taken "as needed." Instead they advise doctors to prescribe pain medicines to be taken around the clock to prevent pain from gaining a foothold. When pain relievers are given by the clock, the total daily dose is often reduced, superior pain relief is achieved, and side effects are reduced.

Relieving pain is more than just a matter of making patients more comfortable. In patients coming out of surgery, for example, inadequate pain relief can cause them to avoid coughing and breathing deeply, which can lead to pneumonia. Surgery patients whose pain is adequately relieved get out of bed sooner after their operations, walk more, and are able to go home sooner.[6]

Drug Principle 2. Diagnose, Then Treat

Whenever possible, the doctor should attempt to make a diagnosis before prescribing drugs. A thorough interview and exam should therefore almost always precede drug therapy. Lab tests may also be necessary.

A Prescription Instead of an Interview

Researchers at Harvard Medical School presented over five hundred doctors with the hypothetical case of a man with sharp pain in the stomach area, relieved by eating but worse on an empty stomach. They were told the man had had a test a month earlier which showed some irritation of the stomach lining but no ulcer. The doctors were asked if they would choose a therapy at this point or whether they would like additional information. Without asking any further questions, more than a third of the doctors were ready to start drug therapy, usually with such ulcer drugs as Tagamet (cimetidine) or Zantac (ranitidine). Had they asked more questions, these doctors would have learned that every day the man took eight aspirin for stomach pain, drank five cups of coffee, smoked two packs of cigarettes, and drank two cocktails at lunch and two glasses of wine in the evening—all of which contributed to his stomach problems. Had the doctors asked about stress, they would have learned that the man's son had been killed in a car crash two months earlier. On average the doctors asked fewer than two questions. Only one in six doctors asked about stress. An inadequate interview by the doctor correlated strongly with the recommendation of a prescription drug.[7]

Be concerned if your doctor turns too quickly to the prescription pad. If your doctor seems to be simply treating a symptom, rather than looking for an underlying cause, ask what could be causing your symptom. Would any further questions, exams, or tests help sort it out? The risk of not looking for a cause and merely suppressing a symptom is that you could delay the diagnosis of a serious condition like cancer.

Before starting a medicine, particularly when therapy will be prolonged or when side effects are likely, try to determine how certain the diagnosis is. Find out how confidant your doctor feels about the diagnosis and on what basis it was made. When the diagnosis is unclear, sometimes drug therapy only serves to muddy the water. If your condition improves, did the drug do it or was it going to happen anyway? What do you do if the symptoms recur? If the diagnosis is in doubt and the situation is not critical, it's often best to hold off on drug therapy and see what happens. Many doctors seem to have the opposite attitude: the drug won't hurt and might help, so why not use it?

The Misdiagnosis of High Blood Pressure

High blood pressure—hypertension in medical parlance—if unchecked can strain the heart and the arteries and lead to premature heart attacks and strokes. Because hypertension often has no symptoms and treatment can lower the risk, it's important to periodically monitor your blood pressure. A blood pressure of 120/80 or less is considered normal. When the second number—the diastolic blood pressure—is greater than 90, many doctors recommend treatment.

Blood pressure is quite variable; it changes minute to minute and day to day. To be sure of the diagnosis of hypertension, it's always necessary to take multiple readings. If a doctor wants to start you on medicine on the basis of one or two readings—unless they're sky-high—watch out. There's a strong possibility you don't need it.

Many of the following factors can lead to an incorrect diagnosis of hypertension:

- *Pain.* If you go into the clinic with a broken arm or painful arthritis, your blood pressure readings may be higher than usual. It's best to recheck your readings after your pain has been controlled.

- *Alcohol.* Alcohol directly raises blood pressure. If you have a few drinks the night before your visit to the clinic, you might end up with a higher-than-usual reading.
- *Medications.* Even many over-the-counter medications, from Advil (ibuprofen) to Sudafed (pseudoephedrine), can raise blood pressure.
- *Stiff blood vessels.* Some elderly people have such stiff arteries that the blood pressure cuff gives falsely elevated readings. If treated for hypertension, these people are at high risk of developing dangerously *low* blood pressure.
- *Large arms.* People with large arms need to have their blood pressure measured with a large cuff. If a normal-sized blood pressure cuff is used, the readings will be too high. People with thin arms, by the way, will get falsely low readings if normal-sized cuffs are used.
- *Stress.* If your job or home life is more stressful than usual, your pressure can rise. The stress of simply walking into a medical clinic is enough to bump some people's reading 20 points, a phenomenon known as white coat hypertension.

White Coat Hypertension

Doctors at New York Hospital wondered how many people with elevated blood pressure readings in their doctors' offices actually had hypertension. Almost three hundred patients who had been referred to their hypertension clinic had their pressures checked repeatedly in the clinic and at home. The researchers found that 21 percent of the people with diastolic readings persistently elevated, in the 90–104 range in the clinic, had normal blood pressure readings at home. These people do not need blood pressure medicine.[8]

Sixty million Americans carry the diagnosis of hypertension. Millions of them, particularly those whose readings are only moderately elevated, may be under treatment for a condition they don't have.

Drug Principle 3. Use Drugs Sparingly

Writing a prescription is one of the easiest and most natural things a doctor can do. Studies show that 75 percent of visits to the doctor result in a prescription for at least one drug. Some doctors give at least one prescription to virtually every patient who walks into their office. If a patient develops a new symptom, their first instinct is to reach for the prescription pad. Modern medicine is, unfortunately, powerless to treat many medical problems. Perhaps doctors don't want to admit this to themselves or to their patients, so they try drugs to see if they'll help.

All this might be fine if drugs were perfectly safe. They're not. There has yet to be a drug invented that doesn't cause side effects. This fact applies equally to prescription and over-the-counter drugs. One of the most common reasons for hospitalization is a reaction to a prescribed medicine.[9] Drug reactions in the hospital are also common.

Drugs' Side Effects in the Hospital

When researchers at the Montreal General Hospital investigated all patients admitted to their hospital for a year, they determined that 18 percent suffered drug reactions in the hospital. They judged 27 percent of the reactions as minor, 38 percent as moderate, and 35 percent as severe. One quarter of the people who suffered severe reactions died from them.[10]

Given their potential for harm, drugs are probably best viewed as selective poisons: they fight pain, cancer, and infections but also attack you. This is not to say you should never take medicine, only that you carefully consider whether it's a good idea before you proceed.

As Franz Kafka wrote, "It is easier to write a prescription than to come to an understanding with the patient." It takes a doctor perhaps thirty seconds to write a prescription, ten minutes or longer to explain why one is not needed. Handing you a prescription is a shorthand way of saying, Your appointment is over. It's also a way for the doctor to get you out of his or her hair—by answering the question, "What are you going to do for me, doc?" **Given time constraints, it's often the best and most concerned physicians who take the time *not* to write a prescription.**

The Marketing of Drugs

Many doctors consider themselves immune to the power of drug advertising. They are scientists, not influenced by marketing techniques, or so they believe. Yet again and again, a new drug—often presenting little advantage over previously available drugs along with a whopping price tag—comes on the market, accompanied by an advertising blitz, and within months becomes one of the top selling drugs.

Where Do Doctors Get Their Information on Drugs?

Harvard researchers quizzed doctors in the Boston area about two types of drugs that, although heavily promoted at the time of the study, were considered ineffective by most experts. One was the narcotic Darvon (propoxyphene), which despite its high price tag and addictive qualities has been repeatedly shown to less effective as a pain reliever than aspirin. The other was a group of drugs that dilate blood vessels in the brain. Despite overwhelming evidence to the contrary, they were being advertised as helpful in treating senility. To encourage doctors to prescribe these drugs, the drug companies had been promoting the misconception that mental failure in the elderly was due to low blood flow to the brain.

Asked to rate the importance of drug ads in influencing their prescribing habits, 68 percent of the doctors surveyed claimed the ads were of "minimal importance," while only 3 percent believed them "very important." Almost two-thirds of the doctors believed that scientific papers were very important in influencing their choice of drugs. When asked, however, if decreased blood flow to the brain was a major cause of senility, 71 percent of the physicians responded yes. Only 14 percent disagreed. Similarly, 49 percent of the doctors believed that Darvon was more effective than aspirin, and only 20 percent believed it less effective. Doctors whose beliefs were highly influenced by drug company advertising were generally unaware of the influence. And the evidence is that doctors act on these beliefs: at the time of the study, Darvon and drugs to dilate blood vessels to the brain were among the most commonly prescribed drugs in the United States.[11]

Pharmaceutical manufacturers are shrewd at their business. Their profit margins are three times those of other companies on the Fortune 500. Drug companies spend the money they do promoting drugs to doctors—and increasingly of late, directly to patients—for one reason: it works.

Drug companies will do just about anything to influence which drugs a doctor prescribes. They give doctors books and videotapes, free dinners, tickets to Celtics games, trips to the Caribbean. Some of the gifts are ostensibly educational, others little more than bribes. One drug company, Ayerst Laboratories, offered a frequent flyer program that awarded doctors free airline tickets if they started more than fifty patients on the blood pressure medicine Inderal LA (propranolol).[12] Some promotional efforts are even made to look like science.

Drug Study or Marketing Ploy?

A bright yellow envelope on top of the stack of mail proclaimed: "Urgent Info-Gram Express." Inside was my invitation "to join approximately 200 other physicians in a nationwide post-marketing study of Maxzide," a drug for high blood pressure. To participate in this "study," I would need to start ten patients from my practice, at least half of whom were already taking other blood pressure medicines, on Maxzide.

According to the letter, "The honorariunm [sic] for participating in the study and providing ten patients who complete the four-week study will be $750.00. This amount includes $125.00 for attending each of two meetings and $50.00 for each completed patient." The meetings included free dinner.

Usually when doctors take part in scientific studies, they do so to further science or their careers, not for monetary compensation. You might wonder, What kind of study was this going to be? The researchers were going to take two hundred doctors, most of whom had no particular training in performing studies, and have them put ten of their patients on Maxzide.

The study's design was flawed in that there was no control group that would take a placebo. Even if it had been well designed, the study would have provided little new information. There are already plenty of well-controlled studies demonstrating that the ingredients in Maxzide (triamterene and hydrochlorothiazide, known as HCTZ) effectively lower blood pressure. Why else, you might ask, would the drug company be running the study? Do they even care about the results? Is this study nothing more than a cleverly disguised marketing ploy?

Even without any meaningful results, the study provides enormous benefit to Lederle Laboratories, the company that makes Maxzide. Two hundred doctors, many of whom may never have prescribed Maxzide before, will get a chance to use it. By having participated in the study, they may even develop brand loyalty. At the very minimum, two thousand new patients around the country will have been placed on Maxzide. At the conclusion of the study, many of them will continue on the drug. The company will have effectively increased their market share and probably in a more cost-effective manner than with their usual journal ads.

What about the patients? At my local discount pharmacy, a year's supply of Maxzide costs $156. Generic HCTZ costs less than $14 a year. Besides, if a patient has tolerated another drug and his or her blood pressure was well controlled, why switch? Patients starting blood pressure medicine for the first time might be well controlled on generic HCTZ for less than a tenth the price.

Drug promotions are akin to political ads. They hype their product and are one-sided. They point out their product's advantages and minimize any disadvantages. Price is seldom mentioned. Drug company representatives may not legally lie to doctors, but they aren't required to tell the whole truth. Doctors who rely on drug companies for information do their patients a disservice. **If the drug your doctor prescribes is the same as the one advertised on the posters, pens, and note pads in the office, you should be concerned that the doctor is overly influenced by the ads.**

You might say advertising is part of our society. What's

wrong with drug companies doing it? There is one key difference between the advertising of prescription drugs to doctors and normal advertising. With prescription drugs, the person who makes the decision is not the person who pays the bill.[13] Any money spent on lavish promotional efforts comes out of your pocket, directly through higher prices or indirectly through higher insurance premiums and taxes. Do you think you should be paying to have your doctor wined and dined or taken to the World Series?

When evaluating whether your doctor is prescribing more drugs than necessary, or the wrong dosage, keep the following in mind:

- *The best drug may be no drug.* Many conditions routinely treated with drugs can be successfully managed without them. High blood pressure, elevated cholesterol levels, and adult-onset diabetes, for example, can all sometimes be treated with safer, nondrug therapies.

- *The marketing of drugs promotes unnecessary prescribing.* As we've seen, drug companies spend billions of dollars to influence the prescribing habits of physicians, and these efforts are remarkably successful. They want doctors to prescribe new drugs when they've got no advantage over old ones, to prescribe name-brands when there are good generic equivalents, and to prescribe drugs when no drug is really necessary.

- *Consumer demand promotes unnecessary prescribing.* In many patients' minds, a prescription shows them that the doctor is both competent and concerned. Drug companies are learning how to manipulate consumer demand by aiming promotional efforts directly at patients. Prominent ads in magazines and on TV urge you to "ask your doctor." Like the ones directed at doctors, these ads invariably promote new and highly profitable drugs. The drug companies hope you'll request the drugs from your doctor. Consumer advertising also indirectly influences doctors who may not have paid attention to the ads for the same drugs in medical journals.

• *Doctors overestimate the effectiveness of drugs.* Other factors besides drug promotions lead doctors to overestimate the effectiveness of drugs When they prescribe a drug and the patient gets better, doctors tend to assume cause and effect. The fact is that many of their patients would have improved without drug therapy.

Even medical journals tend to present data in a way that exaggerates the effectiveness of therapy. Researchers are often enthusiastic about the benefits of a drug they are studying. Rather than tell us that one hundred people took drug X and two got better, compared with only one improvement with Y, we're told that drug X is twice as effective as Y. Technically, of course, this statement is true, but in reality neither drug seems terribly effective. Be careful when you see results of a study reported in terms of the percentage of improvement, rather than in terms of the actual number of people who improved. When the numbers are small, percentages can be highly misleading. Drug company advertisements, by the way, use similar techniques to make drugs appear effective. Remember what Mark Twain said about there being three types of lies: "lies, damned lies, and statistics."

To illustrate, a recent, widely publicized study showed that men over fifty who took an aspirin every other day had a 45 percent lower rate of heart attacks than men who didn't.[14] Thousands of people swarmed to their doctors' offices in the weeks following the report to see if they should start taking aspirin. Many others just started taking it on their own.

A 45 percent reduction in the rate of heart attacks sounds pretty impressive, but let's look at the numbers more closely. After five years, 2.2 percent of the men who didn't take aspirin had suffered heart attacks, compared with only 1.2 percent among those who did—a 1 percent difference. Stated differently, one hundred men would have to take aspirin for five years to prevent one heart attack. Ninety-nine out of a hundred men would be taking aspirin—which though fairly safe, can lead to intestinal bleeding and other problems—without any benefit.

Now it may be that the risk and inconvenience of aspirin therapy are justified to lower the incidence of heart attacks. How the results of the study are framed, however, can affect the judgment. The statement that "aspirin can lower your risk of heart attack by 45 percent" is technically correct but feels very different from "aspirin can lower your risk from 2 percent to 1 percent." If doctors and the public had the data presented the second way—in the context of the overall incidence of heart attacks—they might make a different judgment about whether drug therapy is justified.

The important question to ask your doctor is "How many people like me would have to take this drug, and for how long, to have the desired effect in one person?" Remember too that the goal should be an improvement in your symptoms or in your life expectancy. If a medicine lowers your cholesterol, for example, but doesn't make you live longer, why bother?

- *Doctors underestimate the risks of drugs.* If your doctor tells you a medicine doesn't have any side effects, be skeptical. It may just mean that the drug is too new for side effects to have been recognized yet. It's only as time goes on and the reports trickle in that many side effects come to light.

  If you look in the *PDR*, you will see that most drugs have dozens, if not hundreds, of potential side effects. Many of these side effects are fairly rare, but when you add them all up, the overall total may be larger than you'd expect. Many less common side effects may not be recognized by either doctors or their patients as side effects, especially if they occur weeks or months after the start of therapy.

- *Doctors sometimes prescribe unnecessary drugs out of a fear of lawsuits.* Many doctors prescribe drugs even when they think there isn't much chance they'll help you, because they worry that if they don't, they may later be charged with negligence. There may be circumstances when such behavior is warranted, as when the drug is cheap and safe or when the situation is grave, but in general, "just in case" drugs aren't a good idea. Given the litigious atmosphere in American medicine, when a doctor says "just in case," he or she may mean *just in case you sue me.*

When there is only a small chance a drug will help you, you may or may not want to try it. At the very least, you have the right to be involved in the decision. If a doctor thinks you have only a small chance of benefiting, that doctor should tell you, so that together you can weigh the risks and benefits and make a decision. If you decide to forgo the drug, the doctor can warn you which symptoms might indicate that you're getting worse and need to be seen again.

• *Once a drug is started, doctors may continue to prescribe it, whether you need to remain on it or not.* Many doctors automatically renew prescriptions without reassessing the need. Many doctors seeing patients for the first time will automatically continue all the drugs a former doctor had prescribed without evaluating whether the drugs are necessary or appropriate. I have seen instances where people have remained on drugs for thirty or forty years—sometimes prescribed by a series of doctors—that were never needed in the first place.

Drug Principle 4. Weigh the Risks and Benefits

Before taking a drug, carefully consider what the potential benefits are, how likely they are, what side effects are likely, and whether the likelihood of benefit justifies the risk. Ask your doctor about side effects, but don't stop there. Consider consulting one of the prescription drug references aimed at consumers.

When weighing the risks and benefits of a drug, consider that:

• *The most effective drug is not always the best drug.* The best drug is the one that balances likely effectiveness against the risk of serious side effects. A small risk of a very serious complication should be given a lot of weight.

• *The less severe your symptoms, the less risk you should be willing to accept.* Say a new pain reliever is extremely effective, but one out of every ten thousand people who use it dies from a side effect. Most people wouldn't want to take that chance when there are other pain relievers out there, even if they aren't quite as effective. A cancer patient, racked with pain that hasn't responded fully to other drugs, might decide the risk was worth it.

The more life-threatening a disease, the greater the risk that can be justified. Chemotherapy itself may be deadly, but if that's your only chance of beating cancer, that risk may be worth taking. In fact, even when there is only a small chance for cure, most people opt for chemotherapy.

• *There may be alternatives.* You can't fully evaluate the risks and benefits of a drug unless you understand the risks and benefits of the alternatives. Ask the doctor, "What are the risks of not taking the drug? Are there nondrug therapies that could work? Could my condition improve without treatment? Are there other drugs that could be tried? What are their risks and benefits?"

• *Your values count the most.* Different people will examine the same information and come to different conclusions. Many rational people with cancer believe that the prospect of living a few extra months or even years is not worth spending several months in the hospital tethered to IVs, getting poked and prodded and feeling sick from chemotherapy most of the time. Others feel that the chance at longer life makes almost anything worth enduring. Your physician's advice can help you make the decision about whether to take a drug but since ultimately it's a matter of values, you want *your* values to be considered. The question should not be How much risk and discomfort is your doctor willing to accept? but rather How much are you willing to accept?

Drug Principle 5. Try Safer Drugs First

Drugs vary in their safety. When given a choice between two drugs with similar effectiveness, it makes sense to use the drug that's safer. If a problem isn't immediately life-threatening, it often makes sense to start with a somewhat less effective but safer drug, to see how well it works. Particularly if a drug is going to be taken long-term, it may be worth trading a little effectiveness for greater safety or fewer side effects.

Pain relievers for arthritis are a case in point. Many older Americans have chronic discomfort from simple degenerative arthritis. Osteoarthritis, as it's known, often affects the fingers, neck, knees, and hips. Since there's no cure other than replacing the affected joint surgically—a procedure so far usually reserved for knees and hips—doctors rely on pain relievers.

In recent years drugs like Motrin (ibuprofen), Naprosyn (naproxen) and Feldene (piroxicam) have been used more and more for degenerative arthritis. These drugs are all part of a class called nonsteroidal anti-inflammatory drugs, or nonsteroidals for short. The table on the following page lists several different nonsteroidals by brand name and by generic name. (All drugs, by the way, have a generic name whether they are available generically or not. A generic equivalent can only be manufactured after the patent on the brand name version expires.) For each drug, the table lists the cost at my local discount pharmacy for a one month's supply at the lowest usual dose.

These drugs are effective pain relievers, but they frequently cause side effects, especially in the elderly—the people most likely to suffer from arthritis. It has been estimated that ten thousand Americans are hospitalized every year due to intestinal bleeding caused by nonsteroidals and that one thousand of them die of it.[15] Nonsteroidals also can cause kidney problems.

Because of the huge market, these drugs are heavily promoted by drug companies. Partly in response to these promotional efforts, doctors prescribe nonsteroidals at times when they may not be the best choice. Nonsteroidals are now the most frequently prescribed drugs in the United States, with some 70 million prescriptions per year.[16] But how much more effective are they than the much cheaper and safer acetaminophen?

Acetaminophen Versus Ibuprofen for Arthritis Pain

Researchers at the Indiana University School of Medicine compared the effectiveness of Tylenol (acetaminophen) with the nonsteroidal ibuprofen in treating people with knee pain from degenerative arthritis. One group of patients was given Tylenol at an extra-strength dose, another group ibuprofen at a low dose, and the third group ibuprofen at a high dose, all

Selected Nonsteroidal Pain-Relieving Drugs

Brand Name	Generic Name	Monthly Cost of Brand Name	Monthly Cost of Generic (if generic is available)
Clinoril	sulindac	$59	$42
Daypro	oxaprozin	$80	...
Dolobid	diflunisal	$69	...
Feldene	piroxicam	$75	$49
Indocin	indomethacin	$43	$16
Lodine	etodolac	$72	...
Motrin*	ibuprofen	$20	$14
Naprosyn**	naproxen	$51	$42
Orudis	ketoprofen	$116	$90
Relafen	nambumetone	$70	...
Toradol	ketorolac	$74	...
Voltaran	diclofenac	$77	...

* Also sold over-the-counter as Advil, Nuprin, etc.
** Also sold over the counter as Aleve.

taken four times per day. The researchers found that all three groups benefited from the medicine but that there was no difference among the groups in how well their pain was relieved or in how much their functioning improved.[17]

Because of its safety, effectiveness, and low cost, many experts recommend that acetaminophen be tried first in degenerative arthritis. Only if it doesn't work should the riskier and more expensive nonsteroidals be tried, starting first with a low dose.

Use the Smallest Effective Dose

It is sometimes possible to increase the safety of a drug by taking it at a lower dose. When deciding on the dose of a drug, consider the following:

- *For most drugs, there is a trade-off between effectiveness and side effects.* If you take too small a dose, they won't work. Higher doses are more effective, but the risk of side effects rises. The effectiveness of some drugs plateaus with increasing doses, while side effects continue to increase. For non-life-threatening situations, it often makes sense to start with a small dose of a drug and see how you do. If you are tolerating its side effects and the drug is working, fine. If you're tolerating it and it's not as working as well as you'd like, the dose can be increased. If you're not tolerating it, you can get off it and be thankful that you weren't taking a higher dose from the start.

- *Doses of drugs once recommended are now considered too high.* The sleeping pill Halcion, for example, was once commonly prescribed at the dose of half a milligram (mg). The company no longer even manufactures pills that big. The largest pill currently available is half that dose, and most experts feel that even that's too much for many people. Not long ago many doctors prescribed a 50 mg dose of the blood pressure medicine hydrochlorothiazide (HCTZ) once or even twice per day. Today many patients are successfully treated with 12.5 mg per day, some with only 6.25 mg. One study found that a lower dose was equally effective in reducing blood pressure but didn't cause a drop in the blood potassium level, a common and potentially dangerous side effect.[18]

- *Resist increasing the dose of a drug until you've given it enough time to work.* It often takes a week or two for a drug to reach its full effectiveness. This is especially true for pain-relieving nonsteroidals and for drugs for high blood pressure. In the study just mentioned, the drugs were increasingly lowering the blood pressure eight weeks after they were started. The rule, particularly with the elderly, is to start low and go slow.

- *By using nondrug therapy along with drugs, it is sometimes possible to reduce the dose even further.* Arthritis, for example, can be helped by exercise, weight loss, hot packs before activity, ice packs afterward, and the use of canes and walkers. High blood pressure may respond to exercise, weight loss, less salt in the diet, and stress reduction. Some people can get off drugs entirely when they make changes in their lifestyle.

Use Drugs for the Shortest Effective Duration

The longer you're on a drug, the more likely it is to cause side effects. Consider the example of bladder infections. As recently as a few years ago, women with uncomplicated bladder infections were usually treated for ten to fourteen days with antibiotics. This treatment was quite effective, but a significant number of women developed diarrhea, yeast infections, and other side effects from the antibiotic. About ten years ago, in an effort to reduce the rate of side effects, single-dose therapy became popular, but there have since been concerns that a single dose of antibiotic is not as effective a cure.

How Long Should Women Be Treated for Bladder Infections?

A doctor from the University of Lund in Sweden examined dozens of studies to compare single-dose treatment for bladder infections, with three days of treatment, with five days or greater of treatment. For sulfa drugs, for example, he found the following results:

	percentage of cures	percentage suffering side effects
single dose	89.0	7.4
three days	94.6	6.7
five days or more	95.5	24.9

From these results he concluded that for sulfa drugs, three days of treatment optimally balanced effectiveness with side effects.[19]

Be particularly careful when the doctor wants to put you on medicine for what may be the rest of your life, as is common for high blood pressure or elevated cholesterol. In these instances you want to be especially sure you need the drug and have pursued nondrug options fully.

Local versus Systemic Drugs

When a drug is taken by mouth, it is absorbed into the system and distributed throughout the body. That's why a medicine you take to relieve knee pain can affect your kidneys, liver, or brain. To get around the problem of a side effects in a distant area of the body, it is sometimes possible to apply medicine directly to the area of the problem. If you suffer a rash from poison ivy, for example, you can apply a lotion directly to it. While oral medicine for poison ivy is more effective, the risk of side effects is higher, so doctors generally only prescribe pills for more extensive cases. Since systemic side effects can often be avoided by applying a medicine locally, in less serious situations an effective local medicine, if available, should probably be tried first.

As an example, consider the treatment of asthma. In the past the mainstay in asthma treatment was the oral drug theophylline, sold under such names as Theo-dur and Slo-phyllin. Theophylline, a chemical cousin of caffeine, dilates bronchial tubes and can relieve the obstruction to the flow of air that asthmatics suffer. Theophylline, however, causes lots of side effects. People who take it often feel hyper, as if they'd drunk too much espresso. They may have difficulty sleeping. Their hearts may pound. Their hands may shake. In order to get enough of the drug to effectively dilate the breathing tubes, you risk these side effects.

In the last few years, the thinking on asthma has changed radically. Theophylline has fallen out of favor due to its prominent side effects and only moderate effectiveness. Now inhaled medicines—some of which fight the inflammation of bronchial tissues and others of which directly dilate the tubes—are the preferred therapy, with the systemic oral medications used only in the more extreme cases.

Remember, though, that local medicines do cause side effects. They can irritate the area to which they're applied. More importantly, many local medicines are partially absorbed into the general circulation and can cause side effects similar to those of oral medicines. Many asthmatics who take inhaled medicines to dilate their bronchial tubes, still notice their heart pounding or a mild tremor in their hands, although not usually to the degree they would with theophylline.

Drug Principle 6. Avoid New Drugs

When a drug is introduced for a condition for which there is no good therapy, it's often appropriate that the drug be widely prescribed early on, especially when the disease is life-threatening. This was the case when AZT was introduced as a treatment for AIDS. The drug may or may not turn out to be everything that it's initially hoped to be, but when the situation is dire, it may be worth a shot.

Because many drugs become widely prescribed in their first year or two on the market, their side effects may not be fully appreciated at that time. This is one reason that doctors underestimate the risk of drug side effects: at the time they begin to prescribe a drug, many side effects may be unrecognized. If a doctor is going to do some reading about a drug, it's most likely to occur when the drug is new and the doctor is unfamiliar with it. Once the doctor has been prescribing a drug for a few years, he or she is less likely to pick up the *PDR* or other drug reference, even if new side effects and warnings have appeared.

Occasionally it can take much longer for a drug's side effects to be recognized. Aspirin had been around for more than one hundred years before the connection between its use and Reye's syndrome was appreciated. Reye's syndrome causes liver and brain abnormalities and can lead to coma and death. It usually strikes children who are already sick with influenza, a time when parents might naturally give their children aspirin to lower fever and relieve pain. Because of this potentially fatal disorder, it's now recommended that children *never* take aspirin. Yet how many of us grew up sucking on orange-flavored children's aspirin whenever we got sick?

In order to obtain approval from the Food and Drug Administration (FDA) to market a new drug, the manufacturer is required to perform studies demonstrating the drug's safety and effectiveness. There are limitations to these studies that make their usefulness in predicting side effects less than optimal:

- *The people studied are young and healthy.* Most of the studies are performed on young, healthy people, who have more resiliency in their systems and who are far less likely to suffer side effects. In the real world, of course, most drugs are taken by people who are old and infirm.

- *Women have often been excluded from premarketing studies.* If a woman in a drug study were to become pregnant, the drug could damage the fetus. Rather than deal with this possibility and the lawsuits that might ensue, drug companies have found it easier to exclude women of child-bearing age. Companies have also feared that monthly hormonal changes could complicate interpreting test results in women. Since men and women react to some drugs differently, important information may be lost by excluding women.

- *The people studied aren't taking other medications.* Medicines interact with each other in unanticipated, even dangerous ways. Some medicines may be safe by themselves but when prescribed with another drug, pose a problem. Drug interactions among three or more drugs taken together can be even more complex. The more drugs you're on, the greater the likelihood of an unfavorable interaction, whether they're prescription or nonprescription. Since there are thousands of medicines, it isn't possible to test each new drug before its release to see if it reacts with every other drug and every other combination of drugs. Since interactions aren't systematically looked for in the studies, some are only recognized years after a drug's been on the market. People already on medicines who add new drugs are, in effect, acting as guinea pigs.

  For example, Seldane (terfenadine) is an antihistamine that has become wildly popular since its introduction a few years ago. Both doctors and patients like it because it doesn't cause the sedation and dry mouth common with previously available antihistamines. Within a short time of its introduction in 1985, it became the top-prescribed antihistamine in the country, despite its steep price. In 1988, for example, almost 13 million Seldane prescriptions were written in the United States.

It wasn't until 1990 that the first reports of a potentially life-threatening interaction between Seldane and the anti-fungal drug Nizoral (ketoconazole) trickled in.[20] In 1992 the FDA issued a warning that Seldane when taken with Nizoral could cause heart rhythm problems, cardiac arrest, and death. The FDA also warned that Seldane could prove fatal if taken by itself in higher-than-recommended doses or when taken with the drug erythromycin, one of the most commonly prescribed antibiotics.

- *Most drug studies last only a few weeks or a few months,* meaning that side effects that take longer to develop won't be seen. If a drug causes cancer in people who've been taking it for twenty years, it's only after people have been taking it for twenty years that this fact will come to light.
- *The number of people studied is small.* Rare side effects may not be apparent. If one out of a thousand people die from a drug, but only a few hundred people are involved in the premarketing studies, the fatal side effect may not be discovered until after the drug is on the market and pre-scribed to thousands of people.

When a drug has been on the market for many years, most of the side effects it causes will have come to light. Doctors and their patients are less likely to be in for nasty surprises. It's rare for an older drug to be suddenly with-drawn from the market because of side effects—a relatively common occurrence with new drugs. **Execpt in the most desperate cases, new drugs should only be used when they promise to be much safer or much more effective than previously available therapy.** This principle is routinely violated by thousands of doctors who prescribe new drugs almost as soon as they are introduced.

The Rise and Fall of Zomax

When I was a third-year medical student, the drug Zomax was all the buzz around the university hospital where I was working. This pain reliever drug—yet another nonsteroidal—

had just been introduced and was being promoted by its manufacturer, McNeil Pharmaceutical, with one of the most vigorous sales campaigns in history. Within four months of its introduction, Zomax had captured 11 percent of the market for prescription pain relievers.[21] McNeil was touting studies suggesting that Zomax pills were as effective in relieving pain as a shot of morphine but nonaddictive and that the drug had fewer side effects than aspirin.[22]

Free samples were given out by the so-called detail men, promotional representatives who swarm hospital corridors and medical clinics trying to pitch whatever their company happens to be pushing that month to any doctor who will listen. Medical students and residents were using Zomax on their patients and on themselves and extolling its effectiveness. Doctors were writing out prescriptions for Zomax with pens emblazoned with the Zomax logo—free gifts from the drug company. I never had cause to try the drug, but at the time I was swept up in the enthusiasm all around me. I thought it was a great drug.

Twenty-nine months after its introduction, Zomax was suddenly pulled from the market. Doctors had reported hundreds of cases in which patients had suffered life-threatening allergic reactions. At least thirty-two people died from Zomax. Experts estimated that the risk of a severe allergic reaction to Zomax was five-hundred to a thousand times more likely than with other nonsteroidals. The possibility of severe allergic reactions was not even mentioned in the original package insert and was not generally known to doctors until after the drug was pulled from the market.[23]

The history of another nonsteroidal was similar: the drug Oraflex was introduced in 1982 with a $12 million promotional blitz by its manufacturer, Eli Lilly. Within six weeks half a million Americans were taking it every day. Within three months, after some sixty deaths were reported, the drug was pulled from the market.[24]

Drug company promotions work. Doctors prescribe new drugs not because they have a callous disregard for their patients' safety but because they believe the drugs are safe and effective. They'd take these drugs themselves and often do.

Mixed Messages From the Drug Companies

In June of 1992 I received letters from two different drug companies on the same day. The first, from Abbott Laboratories, announced that they were voluntarily withdrawing their recently introduced quinolone antibiotic Omniflox (temafloxacin) from the market due to reports of serious side effects and deaths. Quinolones, by the way, are the latest hot stuff broad-spectrum antibiotics being hyped by the drug companies. The second letter, from the pharmaceutical company Searle, heralded the introduction of yet another quinolone antibiotic called Maxaquin (lomefloxacin). The letter highlighted Maxaquin's effectiveness and safety.

In July of 1993 I received another letter from Searle regarding Maxaquin. This letter warned that since the drug's introduction, "increasing numbers of reports of phototoxicity," serious skin reactions caused by sunlight, had been reported. The letter went on to say that the reaction occurred in people exposed to shaded or diffuse light, including people exposed through glass. It advised that "exposure to direct or indirect sunlight (even when using sunscreens or sunblocks) should be avoided" while taking the drug and for several days thereafter. In other words, it's probably safe to take the drug as long as you stay in your closet—at least until the next letter arrives advising us otherwise.

Genuinely New Versus Me-Too Drugs

Many new drugs aren't truly innovative. They are, instead, chemical cousins of drugs already on the market, often not any more different from their competition than a new brand of cigarettes is from its. Rather than inventing drugs for rare diseases for which the market is small, drug companies spend most of their energy researching these so-called me-too drugs. Me-too drugs don't so much fill a need as vie for a share of a lucrative market.

Among the me-too drugs aimed at huge markets are Zantac (ranitidine), Pepcid (famotidine), and Axid (nizatidine) for ulcers, Vasotec and Zestril for high blood pressure, and a slew of nonsteroidals. Most of these are probably good drugs, but it's only thanks to the promotional efforts of their manufacturers that they often become widely prescribed within months of their debut. Their early popularity belies the fact that they usually don't present much if any advantage over the drugs already on the market; they also tend to be more expensive, and their long-term safety is unknown.

Drug Principle 7. Favor Generic and Less Expensive Drugs

Studies have shown that **doctors often have little clue how much their patients pay for drugs.** If doctors knew that their patients were going to have to pay a small fortune for a drug, they might think twice before they prescribed it. In fact, many patients in effect veto their doctors' recommendations by not filling their prescription when they learn how much it costs. The American Association of Retired Persons (AARP), for example, found that one elderly person in seven had failed to take prescribed medicine because it was too expensive.

Generic Drugs

One simple way doctors can save their patients money is by prescribing generic equivalents to name brand drugs. Name-brand Motrin costs $20 for a one-month supply. The same amount of generic ibuprofen costs $14. If you don't mind the inconvenience of taking two small pills at a time instead of one larger pill, you can buy the same amount of store-brand ibuprofen over the counter for as little as five or six dollars. The name-brand antibiotic Keflex costs almost $50 for ten days' worth. Generic cephalexin costs less than $20 for a ten-day supply. You'll notice, by the way, that even the naming of drugs favors the use of name brands. *Keflex* is catchy, easy for both doctors and patients to remember. *Cephalexin* is a bit of a mouthful.

The very existence of a generic drug can keep the price of the name brand down. Once a generic drug is introduced, the manufacturers of the name brand often lower its price. As we saw, Motrin, for which there is a generic equivalent, costs about $20 for a month's worth. Daypro, a similar drug that is still under patent and is currently being heavily promoted, costs $80 for a one-month supply.

Drug companies naturally encourage physicians to prescribe expensive drugs. They promote name-brand loyalty and discourage generic substitution. An ad which appeared a few years ago in many medical journals proclaimed, "For the money saved with generic chlorpropamide, your patient couldn't even call your office." It explained that the name-brand equivalent, Diabinese, costs twenty to twenty-five cents more a day than the generic version, less than the cost of most pay-phone calls. That may not sound like much to doctors, but a twenty-five-cent difference a day means almost one hundred dollars per year.

New and expensive drugs are advertised extensively; generics are not. Drug companies provide doctors with a seemingly endless stream of information about the drugs they are currently promoting. Doctors receive free handouts, copies of journal articles, and videotapes. They are invited to all-expense-paid seminars and symposia, some held in tropical locations. The *PDR* is paid for by the drug companies and is provided to doctors free of charge. Since the book is in essence a series of paid advertisements, it contains almost no information on generic drugs. If doctors want objective information about drugs—generic or name-brand—they usually have to go out of their way to get it and must pay for it themselves. **It's a good sign if your doctor is willing to prescribe generically. It means that doctor is more likely to have independently investigated which therapy is best, rather than having simply relied on information provided by the drug companies.**

Keep the following in mind when making the decision between a generic and a name-brand drug:

- *Not all drugs are available generically.* Pharmaceutical companies that develop a drug are generally granted a patent for its exclusive production for seventeen years. Allowing several years for testing and approval, they often have about ten years to market the drug exclusively before it comes off patent, at which time any other firm can manufacture a generic equivalent.

Several years ago I briefly worked in a number of walk-in medical clinics. I noticed that many of the doctors in these clinics prescribed the antibiotic Keflex for just about everything from skin infections to the common cold. I'd also noticed all the Keflex pens and notepads and assorted trinkets scattered around the clinic. In my training I'd been taught that when antibiotics were necessary, it was best to choose drugs like penicillin and sulfa drugs, which, as it turned out, were usually available generically. According to my professors, an antibiotic like Keflex was only rarely the drug of choice.

Just about that time Keflex was due to come off patent; and a generic equivalent was going to be available soon. In anticipation, I presume, the drug company that made Keflex stopped promoting it. Instead, pens and other promotional material for a new drug called Keflet started to appear. Keflet was the same drug as Kelfex but was formulated as a caplet instead a pill, supposedly making it easier to swallow (I never once heard a patient complain of difficulty swallowing Keflex). Because of this slight difference, at least initially, there would be no generic equivalent of Keflet available. I noticed that within weeks several clinic doctors had stopped writing prescriptions for Keflex and were now instead specifying Keflet.

- *Even when no generic equivalent is available, it's often possible to save money by substituting another similar drug.* Even though there are no generic equivalents for the arthritis drug Voltaren, for most people generic ibuprofen works just as well. As we've seen, for some people Tylenol or its generic equivalent, acetaminophen, may be as effective. Generic acetaminophen costs pennies a pill.

- *The quality of most generic drugs is good.* By law, generic drugs must be exactly the same drug as the name-brand and must be absorbed in a similar fashion by the body. Minor differences in absorption don't alter the effectiveness of most drugs. Drug companies have spent millions of dollars to try to convince doctors that generic drugs are inferior. Ads in medical journals implore doctors to write the words "no substitutions" or "dispense as written" on their prescriptions, which prevent pharmacists from substituting a generic drug for the name brand. Except for the few exceptions listed below, the appearance of these words on your prescriptions may indicate that your doctor is unduly influenced by the pharmaceutical industry.

- *Most side effects of generic drugs are likely to be known.* Because drugs that are available generically have been around longer, they generally have longer track records than newer drugs still on patent.

- *Not all generics are cheaper.* Some pharmacists purchase generic drugs at a discount price and then mark them up so they're almost as expensive as the name-brand. Sometimes the generic is even priced higher than the name-brand.[25] It pays to shop comparatively. Most pharmacies will give their prices over the phone, so you can compare not only the price of the generic to the name-brand drug but also one pharmacy's prices to another's.

- *Name-brands may be better for those few drugs whose effectiveness depends on having a precise amount in your system.* Examples include the heart drug Lanoxin (digoxin), the blood thinner Coumadin (warfarin), the epilepsy medicine Dilantin (phenytoin), and the thyroid medication Synthroid (levothyroxine). With these drugs doctors typically will start you on a certain dose and then check your blood a few days later to make sure you're getting the right amount. Depending on the result of the test, they may instruct you to raise or lower your dose. Once the medication in the blood stabilizes at the right level, no further adjustment of the dose may be needed, although the doctor may want to get a blood test periodically to recheck the level.

Epilepsy is one condition that requires precise drug levels to control. Too little medication can lead to seizures. Too much can cause a toxic side effect. Although the active ingredients are exactly the same in the generics as in the name-brand product, some generics, because of the way they're formulated, will be absorbed at a different rate.

Generic epilepsy drugs manufactured by different companies may also differ from each other. Dozens of companies may manufacture the same antiseizure medicine and each different generic brand may be absorbed differently. The important thing, then, may not be to choose the name-brand over a generic but rather to continue the brand you started on and on which your blood levels were checked. If it's a generic equivalent, you need to be sure you get the generic manufactured by the same company each time. Since pharmacists may change which company's generic they purchase, you need to be careful. It's sometimes easier just to stick with the name-brand, because that way you know you'll be getting the same thing every time. You will, however, pay a premium.

Drug Principle 8. Personalize the Prescription

The dose of a drug that is appropriate for a twenty-five-year-old linebacker may be overkill for an eighty-year-old dowager. In order for doctors to prescribe a drug correctly, they should consider:

* *Your age.* The elderly are extraordinarily sensitive to drug side effects. A drug that a younger person could handle without difficulty could send an elderly person into the hospital with kidney failure, confusion, or intestinal bleeding. The kidney and the liver are the two main organs responsible for eliminating drugs from the body, and the function of both is compromised in the elderly. Elderly livers may not deactivate drugs, such as sleeping pills, as effectively as they once did, allowing a buildup of the drug. Similarly, even a minor disruption in blood flow to the kidneys, as happens with many drugs, can tip an older person into kidney failure.

Case History: The Cure Was Worse Than the Disease

Harry Vronsky was an eighty-four-year-old retired hardware salesman who emigrated from Russia as a boy. Since his wife died, he'd been living in a boarding house. Harry had numerous medical problems including angina, swollen legs from congestive heart failure, and arthritis. Years earlier he'd undergone an operation for ulcers.Harry had various aches and pains for which his doctor prescribed the nonsteroidal Naprosyn. He'd been taking 500 milligrams three times per day, which is a huge dose even for a younger man. In addition he was on eight other medicines, including a strong diuretic (a water pill), potassium, and several medicines for his heart.

A few months after starting Naprosyn, he was brought into an emergency room complaining of weakness, poor appetite, and an inability to urinate. Lab tests showed that he had gone into kidney failure—a well-known side effect of nonsteroidals, especially in elderly patients with his medical problems. It was so severe that he almost died. Harry required repeated dialysis, and after two miserable months in the hospital, he eventually recovered enough to go home. He died a few months later.

It's possible that Harry Vronsky needed to be on Naprosyn, but there is little justification for the huge dose he was given. Given his age and chronic medical problems, his risk for side effects was huge. The most common side effect of the nonsteroidals is bleeding from the stomach. Considering he'd already had ulcer surgery, this risk alone should have ruled out Naprosyn.

The elderly are also more susceptible to drug interactions. Since they tend to be taking more drugs than younger people, their risk is increased even further. Elderly people should regularly review all of their medications—prescription and over-the-counter—with their doctors, to make sure they're not taking anything they don't need.

- *Your weight.* Experts recommend that doctors adjust the dose of many drugs based on your size. Out of habit, though, doctors usually prescribe standard doses for all patients, with little adjustment for weight.

Heavy Drugs for Light-Weights

Looking at how well doctors prescribed medications to eighteen hundred elderly patients, researchers at Harvard Medical School found no trend toward lowering doses either for advancing age or for weight. Pound for pound, the thinnest patients received 46 percent higher doses. Because elderly patients tend to lose weight as they age, those patients who were receiving the highest doses pound for pound were also the oldest, already at the greatest risk for side effects. Also, because their doctors failed to adjust for weight, heavier patients were sometimes receiving doses that were too low to be effective.[26]

- *Your medical history.* Some people have medical conditions, such as kidney or liver disease, that affect how quickly their bodies excrete certain drugs. People who drink large quantities of alcohol may need to receive higher doses than average of some drugs but lower doses of others. A doctor should also be aware of any allergies you've had before prescribing a drug. Two drugs that have different-sounding names or that are used for different conditions may be chemically related. If you've had a reaction to one, you may react to the other.

- *Your race.* Although people of different races handle most drugs similarly, there are important exceptions. Studies have shown, for example, that blacks with high blood pressure tend to respond better to water pills than to other types of blood pressure medicine.[27]

- *Your gender.* It's assumed that men and women have similar reactions to most drugs, but our knowledge is incomplete. Until recently most studies were done predominantly on men. When treating women of childbearing age, doctors also need to consider the possibility of pregnancy, since fetuses are extremely susceptible to the effects of drugs.

- *What side effects you're more likely to tolerate.* When choosing among drugs, the doctor can sometimes opt for the one whose side effects are least likely to interfere with your life. Say a doctor is going to prescribe a drug for depression. Some antidepressants are sedating, some are not. For a person who has a lot of difficulty sleeping, a more sedating drug to be taken at night might be a good choice. For patients who can't seem to drag themselves out of bed, a less sedating drug would be better.

Drug Principle 9. The Doctor Should Teach You About Your Medications

For every drug prescribed, it's the doctor's duty to explain what the drug is and how it should be taken. Many doctors, either because they're busy or because they themselves don't know, fail to do so. If a patient isn't told how to take a drug correctly, the treatment may fail. The antibiotic tetracycline, for example, must to be taken on an empty stomach. It isn't absorbed if taken with food. If a patient on tetracycline has failed to improve after a week, the doctor who has not instructed the patient adequately may wrongly conclude that the diagnosis was incorrect or that a different drug is needed. In the meantime the patient may have gotten worse.

Patients, similarly, must be warned about possible side effects. If you know to be on guard for a certain symptom, you are much more likely to recognize it early. Some side effects aren't even recognized as such, because it never occurs to the patient (or even sometimes to the doctor) that the drug could be causing the problem. **If you develop a new symptom while on medicine, always consider the possibility of its being a drug side effect.**

According to Dr. David Kessler, the head of the FDA, inadequate communication about drugs is one of the main reasons that somewhere between 30 and 55 percent of people take their medicines incorrectly. Poor communication, he believes, also contributes to many side effects.[28]

Giving Patients Information About Drugs

Researchers from the University of Washington and Manchester University questioned patients about how often they received information about fifteen commonly prescribed drugs, the effectiveness of which depends on their being taken correctly. The researchers found that doctors provided information to their patients as shown below:

Information Provided by the Doctor	Percentage of Time Provided
how often to take the drug	59
how much to take each time	58

how long to take the drug	40
best way to take the drug	17
possible side effects	27

Doctors asked only 29 percent of patients about drug allergies. Despite their lack of information, less than one-third of patients asked either the doctor or the pharmacist any questions about the prescribed medicine.[29]

Drug Principle 10. Keep It Simple

Doctors sometimes prescribe needlessly complex regimens of drugs. One drug is taken four times a day. Another three times a day with food. Another every Monday, Wednesday, and Friday. Another at bedtime. Another every fours for pain, as needed. These regimens are particularly ill-advised in people with chronic medical conditions who sometimes take more than a dozen medicines per day. The more complex the drug regimen, the harder it will be for patients to follow the doctor's recommendations.

How Many Pills Per Day?

A Yale University study measured how often patients take their medicine as prescribed. Patients were given their pills in special bottles with a computer chip in the cap that measured how many times per day the bottle was opened. The researchers found that when a pill was prescribed once per day, patients took it 87 percent of the time. The rate dropped to 81 percent when the pill was taken twice daily, 77 percent when taken three times per day, and to only 39 percent when the pill was prescribed four times per day.[30]

In order to be maximally effective, drugs should be taken at the correct times and in the correct manner. When people are confused about how they are supposed to take their medications, the possibility of a side effect or an accidental overdose increases.

Adding to the Confusion

A study of patients at the University of North Carolina taking medicines for either diabetes or heart failure found that when only one drug was prescribed, 15 percent of patients made errors taking the medicine. The error rate increased to 25 percent when two or three drugs were prescribed and to 35 percent when five or more drugs were prescribed. Patients in this study had been prescribed as many as fourteen different drugs. Overall, only 27 percent of the heart patients and 40 percent of the diabetics were taking all their medicines as prescribed.[31]

I remember hearing of an elderly widow who was admitted to the hospital with a toxic level of the heart medicine digoxin in her body. Emergency measures were required to stabilize her condition. Once she started to improve, her doctors asked her how she'd been taking her pills. She told them she was on so many medications that she couldn't keep them all straight. To simplify matters, she'd emptied all her medications into a big bowl on her kitchen table. A few times a day, when she happened to be walking past, she'd dip her hand in the bowl and swallow whatever pills she came up with. Not exactly what the doctor ordered.

Seven Warning Signs of Inappropriate Drug Prescribing

Several signs can tip you off that a doctor may be prescribing drugs inappropriately. Think of the following warning signs as rules of thumb, not absolutes. Even though most prescriptions for tranquilizers are inappropriate, for instance, there are occasions when prescribing these drugs is justified. A pattern of warning signs, on the other hand, is far more worrisome.

Drug Warning Sign 1. Tranquilizers and Sleeping Pills

In the 1960s millions of Americans, particularly women, got hooked on Valium. At one time it was the most commonly prescribed drug in the United States. We now know that there are only a few good reasons to use drugs like Valium.

Valium belongs to a class of drugs called benzodiazepines.

These drugs are used for anxiety, for muscle spasms, and as sleeping pills. The table lists several benzodiazepines by generic and brand names.

Consider the following when evaluating a recommendation to use a benzodiazepine:

- *Benzodiazepines, like Halcion, Xanax, and Valium are tranquilizers.* They smooth life's rough edges, making people happy—or at least sedate—in the short term and easing the burden on busy physicians. In the long term, though, these drugs can be dangerous.

- *Except in rare instances, experts advise against long-term use of benzodiazepines.* When these drugs are necessary—and in most cases they aren't—they generally should be taken for a week or two at most. Benzodiazepines are highly promoted by the drug companies, however, and continue to be among the most commonly prescribed drugs in the United States. Doctors continue to prescribe them routinely for long-term use.

Selected Benzodiazepine Tranquilizers and Sleeping Pills

Brand Name	*Generic Name*
Ativan	lorazepam
Dalmane	flurazapam
Doral	quazapam
Halcion	triazolam
Klonopin	clonazapam
Librium	chlordiazepoxide
Prosom	estazolam
Restoril	temazepam
Serax	oxazepam
Tranxene	clorazepate
Valium	diazapam
Xanax	alprazolam

- *It takes the body weeks to excrete some benzodiazepines, such as the sleeping pill Dalmane.* If a person takes Dalmane regularly, the levels of drug in their system can build up, leading to drowsiness and coordination problems during the day. This problem is especially worrisome in the elderly, who are at risk of falling and breaking a hip. Hip fractures are one of the leading causes of death in elderly Americans.

Tranquilizers and Falls in the Elderly

Researchers from Vanderbilt University who examined hospital records to look for a correlation between the use of benzodiazepines and hip fractures in people over sixty-five found that patients taking such long-acting benzodiazepines as Dalmane, Valium, and Librium had 70 percent more hip fractures than those in the control group.[32] This study and others also show that about one-third of elderly patients prescribed a benzodiazepine are given the more dangerous long-acting ones.

- *Benzodiazepines are addictive: people who discontinue them suddenly may experience withdrawal reactions, even seizures.* These drugs are particularly dangerous when combined with alcohol. Xanax (alprazolam), the most addictive (some people get hooked after just a few weeks on it), is also the most popular. Xanax is the number-one selling psychiatric drug and the fifth most frequently prescribed drug is the United States.[33]

Drug Warning Sign 2. Unnecessary Antibiotics

Antibiotics, one of the most commonly prescribed "just in case" drugs, are frequently given for conditions in which they're useless. When used properly, antibiotics work wonders. Certain bacterial pneumonia and bladder infections respond to antibiotics within hours. Perhaps because antibiotics are so effective for some problems, many doctors use them for conditions where they won't help or where there's only the slightest chance of benefit.

Remember the saying, There's no cure for the common cold?

It's still true, even if many people, including lots of doctors, don't seem to believe it. To illustrate, let's return to the case of Mathra Samuels, described in the last chapter.

Case History: Treating Martha's Cold

Martha, a generally healthy thirty-four-year-old woman, visited a walk-in clinic with typical cold symptoms. There was nothing to suggest she had anything other than a common cold. After performing a series of tests, the doctor prescribed two drugs, the antibiotic Ceclor and an antihistamine-decongestant combination called Bromfed. Both drugs were being heavily promoted at the time by the drug companies that manufactured them. The walk-in clinic desk was littered with pens and notepads with the Ceclor logo. The sample bin was overflowing with Bromfed, Ceclor, and several other drugs. Martha took the medicines and, within a few days, was feeling much better.

Ceclor (cefaclor), like other antibiotics, is effective against bacterial infections but worthless against viral infections like colds. Considering that most people with colds start to feel better within a few days anyway, Martha was probably feeling better in spite of the Ceclor, rather than because of it. While an antibiotic can be useful to treat some of the bacterial infections that can complicate a common cold, such as an ear or sinus infection, taking one won't prevent these complications.

A ten-day prescription for Ceclor cost Martha $70. It couldn't have helped, might have caused side effects, and was at the very least inconvenient to take three times a day. There are other important downsides to the unnecessary prescribing of drugs like Ceclor. Powerful antibiotics kill most of the bacteria in the intestines, allowing yeast to take over. After using antibiotics, many women end up with vaginal yeast infections, which are uncomfortable and may require treatment. Many people are allergic to antibiotics and some have life-threatening reactions. Finally, the overuse of antibiotics leads to drug-resistant bacteria, which are becoming a very serious problem.

Antibiotics for the Common Cold

Before New Mexico began a program to try to improve antibiotic prescribing by doctors, researchers from the Rand Corporation examined the records of thousands of patients treated for colds and other common respiratory infections. The researchers measured how often doctors treated the infections properly, using criteria intentionally set up to give doctors the benefit of the doubt. The researchers found that some doctors gave antibiotics to virtually every patient. Almost two out of three patients with common colds, for example, received antibiotics. Only 29 percent of people with another viral infection, influenza, were judged to have been treated appropriately.[34]

Asthma is another condition for which antibiotics are often used without good reason. In young patients asthma attacks are almost never caused by bacterial infections. Here again, antibiotics won't help, but doctors routinely prescribe them "just in case."

Drug Warning Sign 3. Shotgun Therapy

Sometimes the doctor is not at all sure what's causing your symptoms. Rather than do what's necessary to find out, the doctor gives you drugs to cover all the likely possibilities and hopes for the best. The Ceclor Martha Samuels received is an example of a typical shotgun. The same antibiotic would work on strep throats and most cases of bronchitis, some pneumonias, and most sinus and ear infections. By choosing a drug that covers just about everything, the doctor isn't required to think. Simple tests that might differentiate one type of infection from another are never done. Whatever infection you've got, you get Ceclor. The shotgun antibiotic that's currently popular with doctors is called Biaxin (clarithromycin). If someone is dying and there is no time to make an exact diagnosis, a shotgun approach may be justified, but in most cases it's not.

Bromfed, the prescription cold remedy given to Martha, is another example of a shotgun. As anyone who watches commercial TV knows, cold remedies fight numerous cold symptoms.

What most people don't know is that medical experts recommend you not take multisymptom cold remedies. When you use these combination drugs, you usually end up taking medicine for symptoms you don't have and therefore risk side effects from drugs you don't need.

Many of the ingredients in leading cold formulas are ineffective. Others can relieve some symptoms but aren't necessarily advisable to take. Almost all of them contain antihistamines, for example, which can make a cold worse. By slowing down running noses and reducing sneezing, antihistamines actually inhibit the body's natural way to clear mucus. These drugs also tend to be sedating. The decongestants contained in cold remedies can help unclog stuffy noses and sinuses—assuming you have those symptoms. Decongestants, however, have side effects; they can raise blood pressure. Some people have difficulty sleeping when they take them. And while generic pseudoephedrine (the active ingredient in Sudafed) can cost as little as a few cents per pill, Martha paid almost a buck a pill for hers.

The shotgun approach with cold remedies—whether prescription or over-the-counter—is both expensive and generally misguided. The best, cheapest, and safest approach is to take single-ingredient drugs to fight only the symptom or symptoms that bother you. Millions of dollars in advertising would have you and your doctor believe otherwise.

Drug Warning Sign 4. One Drug to Counteract Another

When a patient develops a side effect to one drug, some doctors will prescribe a second drug to fight the first drug's side effects. This course of action may be appropriate when the first drug is essential. Ask yourself if you really need to be on the first drug. Perhaps your problem can be treated with nondrug therapies. Or maybe an alternative drug can be found that doesn't cause the same side effects.

The most common side effect of the nonsteroidal pain relievers like Motrin is stomach problems, including bleeding ulcers. To prevent stomach problems or to treat them after they develop, many doctors will prescribe an ulcer medicine. One drug, called Cytotec (misoprostol), is currently being promoted specifically to prevent stomach problems induced by nonsteroidals. In patients who truly need to be on a nonsteroidal and who are at high risk of an ulcer, Cytotec's high price (almost $50 per month) and its risk of side effects may be justified. Many patients, however, can instead be successfully treated with the pain reliever acetaminophen, which essentially never causes stomach problems.

Sometimes neither the patient nor the doctor is aware that one drug is interfering with another. I saw a patient recently who had been started on a large dose of the sleeping pill Halcion by his primary care doctor. Within weeks the man had become so dependent on Halcion that if he didn't take it, he couldn't get to sleep at all. During the interview I learned that he drinks a large cup of coffee after dinner each night—less than three hours before he goes to bed. He was in effect taking Halcion to counteract the effects of another drug, caffeine. His doctor had never asked him about his habits and it had never occurred to the man that his insomnia could be related to the coffee.

Another common example involves the effect of nonsteroidal pain relievers on blood pressure. It's estimated that one-third of the 60 million Americans with high blood pressure are prescribed nonsteroidals for pain or arthritis. Since ibuprofen and naproxen are available over the counter, millions of others take them without a prescription. Studies have shown that nonsteroidals like Motrin can lead to a five- to twenty-point increase in blood pressure by interfering with the action of blood pressure medicines.

Nonsteroidals and Blood Pressure Medication

Researchers at Harvard Medical School reviewed records of over nine thousand people in New Jersey over the age of sixty-five who had been started on blood pressure medications in the 1980s. They discovered that recent use of a nonsteroidal drug increased the likelihood of being started on blood pressure medication by 66 percent. The higher the dose of the nonsteroidal, the greater the likelihood of a prescription for blood pressure drugs.[35]

If your blood pressure goes up after starting a nonsteroidal, many doctors will either start you on blood pressure medication or increase your dose. Simply discontinuing the nonsteroidal, on the other hand, would return your blood pressure to its previous lower level.

Drug Warning Sign 5. Combination Drugs

Two or more drugs are often combined in one pill. The ostensible reason is to increase patient convenience and to make things easier for forgetful patients. Consumers, though, pay for these advantages. Before starting treatment with a combination drug, consider the following:

- *Combination drugs are often far more expensive than if the individual components were bought separately.* Before accepting a combination drug, find out from the pharmacy how expensive the drugs are individually. If you think the added convenience of one pill is worth the price difference, go ahead and get it.

- *Only take a combination drug when it contains the exact drugs at the exact doses you would be taking separately.* Otherwise you'll be risking side effects unnecessarily. As with cold remedies, many combination drugs contain ingredients you may not need. Combination drugs may also combine drugs in ways that make no sense medically or contain ingredients that are simply ineffective.

- *Drugs companies sometimes market combination drugs as a way to fight generic substitution.* Two drugs available generically are combined, given a new name, and advertised. In many cases there is no generic equivalent for the combination, so the manufacturer can charge a name-brand price.

- *Combination drugs make it more difficult to adjust the dose properly.* Say you are taking the combination pill for high blood pressure called Inderide. Inderide contains two drugs, propranolol, a so-called beta blocker which slows the heart, and HCTZ, a diuretic. If the doctor wishes to double the dose of the beta blocker but keep the same dose of HCTZ, you have to stop the combination drug and go back to individual pills. In the real world many doctors will simply tell you to take twice as much of the combination drug, even though this means doubling the dose of HCTZ too, with the attendant increased risk of side effects.

Because it's so difficult to personalize the dose with combination drugs, the FDA requires many of them to carry a warning in the *PDR*. The following appears in bold type under Inderide: "This fixed combination drug is not indicated for initial therapy of hypertension. Hypertension requires therapy titrated [adjusted] to the individual patient. If the fixed combination represents the dosage so determined, its use may be more convenient in patient management. The treatment of hypertension is not static but must be reevaluated as conditions in each patient warrant." In other words, doctors shouldn't be prescribing this combination drug at the start of therapy or when adjusting the dose.

• *A few combination drugs are exceptions to the above rules.* The drug Bactrim (also sold under the name Septra) combines two different antibiotics, trimethoprin and sulfametroxazole, which work synergistically. The combination makes sense and is available generically.

Drug Warning Sign 6. Outmoded Drugs

Many once popular drugs are now considered outmoded. When they initially appeared on the market, some of these drugs were considered safe and effective. As better, safer drugs have come along, however, these older ones have fallen from favor. Other drugs that were initially well regarded have been proven ineffective. Some now discredited drugs have serious side effects which took years to come to light. Because many physicians have a hard time staying up-to-date with advances in the practice of medicine, they continue to prescribe these outmoded medications. As we've discussed, the longer the time that's elapsed since the doctor finished his or her training, the more likely that the doctor's prescribing habits are behind-the-times.

An example of an outdated treatment still in use is one used for an underactive thyroid. As many as one American in one hundred suffers from this disorder, known as hypothyroidism. Luckily, if the condition is recognized, the missing hormones can be replaced. Historically, thyroid hormones have been obtained from animal thyroids, usually pigs', ground down and formulated into pills. In recent years synthetic hormones have come along and largely supplanted the older, animal preparations.

The problem with the animal preparations is that the amount of thyroid hormone they contain ranges from 15 to 120 percent of the expected quantity. Too little can lead to a recurrence of the symptoms of hypothyroidism, including weight gain, fatigue, and a constant sensation of cold. Too much can be a problem too. In someone with blockages in the coronary arteries, for example, too much thyroid hormone can precipitate angina or even a heart attack. Some doctors, nevertheless, persist in prescribing such out-of-date preparations as Armour, S-P-T, Proloid and thyroid tablets U.S.P. The synthetic hormone, levothyroxine—sold under the brand names Synthroid and Levothroid—is chemically identical to the naturally occurring hormone. Thyroid hormone, by the way, because of the variability in the amount of hormone in the various generics, is another case where one of the name-brands may be worth the higher price.

Other outmoded or otherwise discredited drugs include amphetamines for weight loss, barbiturates for insomnia, and the pain reliever Darvon (propoxyphene), either alone or combined with other medicines. The antinausea drug Tigan (trimethobenzamide) has fallen from favor because it's not terribly effective and has significant side effects. Theophylline preparations for asthma, as mentioned earlier, have largely, but not entirely, been supplanted by inhaled medicines. There is little rationale, however, for doctors' continuing to prescribe several older theophylline preparations that also contain sedatives, including Marax and Quibron. Medicines to treat spastic colon or irritable bowel syndrome that include sedatives, such as Donnatal Extentabs or Librax similarly have little to recommend them.[36]

If a patient has tolerated an old-fashioned drug well, it may sometimes make sense to continue it. Due to side effects like dizziness, the blood pressure medicine Aldomet (methyldopa) has fallen from favor in the elderly, even though it effectively lowers pressure. In some elderly patients who don't experience the drug's side effects, it may be riskier to change to a different drug. It's generally considered inappropriate, however, to start an elderly patient on the drug, since doctors now have many better choices.

Drug Warning Sign 7. Free Samples With a Prescription to Match

Patients love drug samples. Doctors want to please their patients, so they gladly accept samples from drug company representatives and pass them on to patients. The free samples are usually given a few at a time in so-called starter kits. In other words, you get enough to last a few days. After that if you want to keep taking the drug, you have to buy it.

Even though samples may seem like something for nothing, they may end up costing you money. Say you need ten days' worth of antibiotics. If you are given a three-day supply of some expensive new drug, you still have to buy seven days' worth. Since the doctor probably has no samples of generic drugs, you will almost always end up with a name-brand drug, even when a cheaper alternative exists. In most cases it would be much cheaper to purchase a ten-day supply of a less expensive drug.

Since samples are usually for brand-new drugs that haven't yet stood the test of time, they could end up costing you even more in the long run. You end up using a new medication that may turn out to have dangerous side effects. Many doctors will give patients samples of a drug that they would otherwise never prescribe. **If you need a drug, you want the one that is best for you, not the one the doctor happens to have free samples of.** In general, my advice is to just say no to drug samples.

The one exception is when a doctor gives a patient who otherwise could not afford to fill a needed prescription all the medicine he or she will need. Some doctors, for example, will give a needy patient ten three-day starter kits to last them an entire month. This may not be an ideal situation, but even samples of a drug that's not the doctor's first choice may be better than the patient's not getting treated at all.

Ten Principles of Appropriate Drug Prescribing

1. Understand the drug.
2. Diagnose then treat.
3. Use drugs sparingly.
4. Weigh the risks and benefits.
5. Try safer drugs first.
6. Avoid new drugs.
7. Favor generic and less expensive drugs.
8. Personalize the prescription.
9. The doctor should teach you about your medications.
10. Keep it simple.

Putting It Together

Using the ten principles of appropriate drug prescribing and the seven warning signs of inappropriate drug prescribing, you can begin to assess how competently your doctor prescribes drugs. By examining how a doctor prescribes drugs, you garner clues to the doctor's competence, agenda, and overall philosophy of medical practice. Ask yourself, Is the doctor prone to intervene? Worried about getting sued? Does the doctor rely on

Seven Warning Signs of Inappropriate Drug Prescribing

1. Tranquilizers and sleeping pills.
2. Unnecessary antibiotics.
3. Shotgun therapy.
4. One drug to counteract another.
5. Combination drugs.
6. Outmoded drugs.
7. Free samples with a prescription to match.

unproved therapies? By speaking with the pharmacist or looking up each drug in one of the consumer guides to prescription
drugs, you can double-check what the doctor told you and gauge
that doctor's knowledge of drug side effects and interactions.
The better you understand your doctor, the better you'll be able
to evaluate his or her suggestions.

What you learn about your doctor may be either reassuring
or disturbing. Remember, though, that even if your philosophy
of using medications is different from your doctor's, if the
doctor shows flexibility and a willingness to involve you in
decisions, you can usually work together. If you absolutely can't
agree or if your physician can't abide your involvement in
decision making, then you may need to look elsewhere.

5

DOES YOUR DOCTOR KNOW WHEN TO INTERVENE (AND WHEN NOT TO)?

IN THE EARLY TWENTIETH CENTURY DOCTORS HAD LITTLE TO OFFER patients other than sympathy and morphine. In recent decades we've become accustomed to miracles. We have witnessed the development of open heart surgery, cures for childhood leukemias, vaccines for once-deadly diseases. As a result doctors are increasingly expected to provide answers and effective therapies for every problem that comes along. The fact remains, however, that about 90 percent of the time patients visit doctors with conditions that will either improve on their own without treatment or that are out of reach of modern medicine's powers.[1]

Many interventions employed by physicians over the years have proven to be utterly worthless, some even dangerous. We don't need to think back to the age of leeches and blood lettings to find examples. In the 1950s and '60s millions of children had their tonsils removed for no good reason; hundreds of babies were born without arms and legs because of the drug Thalidomide; thousands of people who received X-ray therapy for acne or unwanted facial hair and are now turning up with thyroid cancer. The list goes on and on.

These horror stories are not just historical curiosities. Many of the interventions commonly employed today are similarly suspect. The cesarean section (C-section) rate has skyrocketed, without a corresponding improvement in the health of mothers or their infants. Dozens of common surgical procedures have never been proven effective. Chemotherapy saves many lives but is also given to patients with no realistic hope of improvement. The terminally ill are hooked up to tubes and wires and breathing machines only to prolong the process of dying.

In medical school physicians are taught the maxim articluated by the ancient Greek physician Hippocrates, First do no harm. It is the physician's duty to try to help patients, but they shouldn't be made worse by the doctor's efforts. Since every drug, test, or procedure entails some risk, the burden on physicians is to avoid harming patients unless the prospect of helping them seems good. That's the theory, anyway. In reality a new maxim seems to have taken hold among physicians: When in doubt, do something.

Case History: "Standard Procedure"— The Medicalization of Childbirth

Claire Brooke was pregnant for the first time and terrified. Everything had gone fine during her pregnancy, but she was late for her due date and the doctor suggested they "break her water" to induce labor. Actually, he'd been talking about inducing her for weeks. He told her it would be easier to plan that way. When she needed to get to the hospital, she "wouldn't get stuck in traffic."

Never having won the approval of her parents or of the distant man she married, Claire hoped to get it from her obstectrician. Even though she was vaguely informed about natural childbirth, her strongest impulse was to avoid acting out as a patient and alienating this avuncular man. Her whole life she'd been given the message that she was "too much." As a child, her mother had even paid her to not speak during dinner.

She checked into the hospital that day. Since she wasn't allowed to eat, the nurse put an IV in her arm to run in some sugar water to "give her some energy." Her husband was asked to leave the room while the nurse gave her an enema and shaved her pubic hair. A few hours later the doctor started an infusion of the drug Pitocin (oxytocin) intravenously to start contractions. The pain from the contractions became so strong that Claire was given a shot of the narcotic Demerol. To monitor the baby's progress, the doctor screwed a tiny electrode into the baby's head—an internal fetal heart monitor. Whenever she asked why they were doing something, she was told it was "standard procedure."

Claire was brought into the delivery room and laid down flat on her back with her legs up in stirrups. The light in the delivery room was so bright that Claire's husband didn't need a flash on his camera. To avoid tearing her tissues, the doctor performed a "routine" episiotomy—a surgical incision to widen the vaginal opening. After the baby was born, the child was placed on the other side of the room in a bassinet and given a bottle. Claire lay there, wanting nothing more than to hold her new daughter and let the child feed from her breast. She wondered if there was something wrong with the way her body worked that made the whole process so complicated.

Let's consider the advisability of each intervention.

- *To "break her water"* or artificially rupture the membranes of the amniotic sac effectively induces labor, but not without risk. Rupturing the membranes increases the risk of infection and occasionally leads to the umbilical cord getting wrapped around the baby's neck. It is sometimes appropriate and necessary to induce labor artificially. If the doctor's estimate of Claire's due date was off—a common mistake— he may have intervened when simply waiting a little longer was all that was necessary. We'll never know whether Claire needed to be induced or not, but of all the reasons for inducing labor, avoiding traffic has got to be one of the worst.

- *Withholding food and giving intravenous fluid.* In the 1940s doctors began withholding food from women in labor, in case general anesthesia was needed for a C-section. Studies have shown that the risk of eating is minimal and that there are risks to intravenous fluids. Once a woman is tethered to an IV, she can't move as much, which can slow down labor and make her feel more pain.[2]

- *Enemas* are often given routinely to women admitted to the hospital in labor. The ostensible reasons are to speed up delivery and to reduce the rate of infections, but studies suggest that enemas make no difference.[3] There is little justification for performing this embarrassing and uncomfortable intervention.

- *Shaving the pubic hair,* done to reduce the risk of infection, may have the opposite effect. Shaving irritates sensitive tissues and can increase the woman's discomfort after the birth. There is no good reason for this practice.

- *The drug Pitocin* can increase the contractions and speed up labor. The drug is appropriate in cases where labor is not progressing satisfactorily, but it's overused. I have seen cases where Pitocin was given so that the delivery would not happen in the middle of the night—primarily for the convenience of the obstetrician. I've observed doctors on the obstetrical service turning the Pitocin down at night to "let the woman sleep." I've always suspected it was more to let the doctors themselves sleep. It may not have been coincidence that Claire's Pitocin was started at four in the afternoon and that she gave birth at 9:30 P.M. I once saw an obstetrician give the order to start Pitocin, bragging to me and the nurses that "that kid will be out by 5 P.M.," just before he was scheduled to leave for vacation. It was.

- *Electronic fetal monitoring (EFM)* can detect a drop in the baby's heart rate, which might indicate problems such as the baby's not getting enough oxygen. The rationale for the use of EFM is that if the doctor detects a problem, an emergency C-section can be done and the baby will have a better chance of surviving and developing normally. Eight separate randomized studies have shown that EFM does not reduce the mortality rate; another shows that EFM does not result in improved neurologic development of the newborns.[4] One thing is certain, EFM greatly increases the risk of having a C-section.

Doctors often cite their concern about malpractice suits as the reason they continue to use EFM despite the risk and its lack of effectiveness. It may be appropriate to use EFM in some complicated cases, but there is no good reason to use it on someone like Claire at low risk of problems. With a low probability of a problem, a minor abnormality on EFM is likely to be a false positive. Doctors worried about getting sued are likely to respond by recommending a C-section.

- *The lithotomy position,* where the woman lies flat on her back with her legs up in stirrups, is designed for the doctor's convenience. Women traditionally gave birth in a squatting position, which uses gravity to advantage and which enlarges the birth canal by about 25 percent. Modern birthing tables simulate this position, allowing the woman to remain more vertical. Several studies suggest that a vertical position leads to better contractions and a shorter duration of labor.

- *The drug Demerol,* like other narcotics, can relieve the mother's pain but causes side effects. Nausea is common, blood pressure can drop, and more importantly, the drug can affect the baby. Several other interventions—artificially inducing labor, keeping her in bed, and using the lithotomy position for delivery—made Claire more likely to need pain relievers.

- *The routine episiotomy.* About two-thirds of women in labor are given an episiotomy, a surgical incision to widen the birth canal. There is no evidence that episiotomies prevent injury to the baby or that women who undergo them have fewer problems with urinary incontinence, sexual pleasure, or pelvic relaxation in later years, as is sometimes maintained. Because the risk of infection, bleeding, and pain, women should only have episiotomies when absolutely necessary. Using alternate birth positions and avoiding stirrups can reduce the rate.

- *Giving the child a bottle with sugar water or formula* makes little sense. Nature intended a baby's first food to be mother's milk, which is nutritious and provides antibodies against infection. Under normal circumstances mothers should be encouraged to begin breast feeding as soon as possible.

Seven Principles of Appropriate Medical Intervention

Intervention Principle 1. Intervene Sparingly

Medical interventions have the power to save lives but also to kill. When deciding whether to consent to a proposed intervention, keep the following in mind:

- *Medical interventions can cascade out of control.* In *Poor Richard's Almanac,* Ben Franklin wrote the following lines:

  > For the want of a nail the shoe was lost,
  > For the want of a shoe the horse was lost,
  > For the want of a horse the rider was lost,
  > For the want of a rider the battle was lost,
  > For the want of a battle a kingdom was lost—
  > And all for the want of a horseshoe nail.

  This so-called cascade effect[5] is one of the primary risks of medical intervention: one intervention leads to a second intervention, which leads to a third intervention, and so on.

  Claire Brooke received Pitocin to speed up her labor. This intervention necessitated the use of the fetal monitor. Although Claire didn't require a C-section, the use of the monitor increased her likelihood of having one. The lithotomy position and stirrups made an episiotomy more likely. Several interventions may have increased her pain: she was on Pitocin, which makes contractions stronger, she couldn't move around because of the IV and the fetal monitor, and she gave birth in the lithotomy position. Because of the pain she was given the narcotic Demerol, which might have led to further problems. Luckily, Claire and her baby girl did fine, but intervention cascades can sometimes spiral out of control.

  I have seen numerous cases in which a patient suffered a side effect from an intervention, which then initiated a cascade that only ended when the patient died. One middle-aged woman complained to her doctors of chest pain. No one thought the pain was coming from her heart, but the decision was made to do a cardiac catheterization. The test showed no evidence of heart disease, but as the catheter was being removed, it nicked one of her heart's arteries. She suffered an immediate heart attack. In the intensive care unit, complaining of severe pain, she was treated with high doses of morphine. The morphine contributed a leakage of fluid into her lungs, necessitating the use of a breathing machine. On the breathing machine she developed pneumonia and other infections. One organ after another started to malfunction. She spent over a year in intensive care, tortured by the machinery of modern medicine, before finally dying. All for a test she never needed.

- *Many common interventions are either completely unnecessary or performed at rates much higher than can be medically justified.* Shaving her pubic hair couldn't have benefited Claire Brooke or her baby and might have brought harm. The use of a fetal monitor is appropriate in some cases but wasn't in hers. Given the way things went in the hospital, Claire was lucky to have avoided an even more extreme intervention, a C-section.

- *There are major differences in rates of intervention among doctors.* We now know that the vast majority of tonsillectomies done in the 1940s, '50s, and '60s were unnecessary. One major factor that led to this recognition was the observation that the rates of tonsillectomy varied markedly from one geographical area to the next. Similar regional variations in surgery rates are found today. In general, the more controversial a procedure, the greater the variation in how often it's done.

Variations in the Rates of Intervention

Researchers from the RAND Corporation studied geographic variations in the rates of various procedures in thirteen different regions of the country. Measuring the rate of each procedure per ten thousand people, they calculated the areas with the highest and lowest rate.[6]

Procedure	Highest Rate	Lowest Rate	Ratio of Highest to Lowest
injection of hemorrhoids	17	0.7	26.0
knee replacement surgery	20	3	6.0
carotid endarterectomy	23	6	4.0
bypass surgery	23	7	3.1
heart catheterization	51	22	2.3
hip replacement surgery	24	8	3.0
appendix removal	5	2	2.2
hernia repair	53	38	1.4

Because there is little disagreement within the medical community about when it's appropriate to remove someone's appendix, there are only minor geographic differences in the rates. In some areas of the country, though, you're more than twenty-five times as likely to have a hemorrhoid operation than in other areas.

• *The biggest variable in the rate of intervention is the individual physician.* It all goes back to the doctor's philosophy of practice.

The Individual Doctor's Role in Unnecessary C-sections

Researchers at Wayne State University in Detroit investigated the role of differences in the practice styles of physicians on the rate of cesarean sections. They studied over fifteen hundred affluent women at low risk of birth complications. Overall, 26.9 percent of the women had C-sections, but the rate varied from 19 to 42 percent, depending on the doctor. For women who had never before had a C-section, the C-section rates for different doctors ranged from 9.6 to 31.8 percent. Variation in the rate of C-sections was not attributable to the degree of risk of the pregnancy. Babies delivered by doctors who did lots of C-sections were not any healthier than those delivered by doctors who did few.[7]

Consider the opinion of one doctor who believes all women should give birth by cesarean. "Why should the modern woman," he writes in a letter to the *Journal of the American Medical Association,* "undergo the sweaty, gut-wrenching ordeal of labor that may last 12 to 24 hours or more?" He continues, "And let's face it—the female perineum [pelvic tissues including the vagina and anus] never returns to its original state after two or more vaginal deliveries."[8]

- *The best intervention may be no intervention.* According to the proverb, the three greatest physicians are nature, time, and patience. Many problems are what doctors call self-limiting, meaning that if they are left alone, they'll improve by themselves. Claire Brooke's doctor assumed she was late based on the date of her last menstrual period, a method of estimating the due date that's often inaccurate. If he'd given her a few more days, things might have progressed naturally.

Sometimes, as in an emergency situation, an intervention must be performed without delay. When the situation isn't urgent, watchful waiting or tincture of time may be a better course of action. Many people who decide against back surgery, for instance, get better anyway. If their symptoms don't improve or worsen, they can often still have the surgery. If their symptoms go away, they've saved themselves the money, pain, and risk of surgery.

Delaying Heart Catheterization

Cardiac catheterization, in which dye is injected into the heart's arteries, is the most accurate method to look for blockages. It's also often a step on the road that leads to bypass surgery. A group of Harvard cardiologists studied patients who came to them for a second opinion on catheterization, to determine how often the test was needed. They judged that 80 percent of the patients didn't need the test, that 4 percent should have it, and that the remaining 16 percent needed further, less-invasive testing before the decision could be made. Once that testing was completed, a few more were recommended catheterization, bringing the total to 6 percent. Over the next four years, about 15 percent of the patients went on to get either an angioplasty or bypass surgery, but 66 percent remained well and did not require hospitalization.

The authors conclude that half the catheterizations performed in the United States are either unnecessary or could be safely delayed.[9]

If your doctor proposes an intervention, you might ask, "Why now? What would happen if I waited a month? A year?" If the problem is acute appendicitis, you can't afford to wait a few hours. If it's a small hernia, you might be able to wait years.

- *An incorrect diagnosis can lead to inappropriate intervention.* If the doctor has misdiagnosed your condition, an intervention carries all its usual risks without any commensurate benefits. There is little chance that you'd benefit from an intervention aimed at something you don't have. Proper diagnosis is based on the doctor's performing a thorough interview and physical examination and confirming or ruling out hypotheses with a judicious use of diagnostic tests. As time goes on, the physician needs continually to reassess your condition, making sure the initial diagnosis was correct and that nothing new has cropped up.

- *Just because an intervention is appropriate and effective for one medical condition does not ensure that it will help others.* Antibiotics are appropriate for certain pneumonias but not for the common cold. Likewise, doctors perform C-sections for both appropriate and inappropriate reasons. Before you sign on, be sure you know your diagnosis and the track record of the proposed intervention *for your specific problem.*

- *Doctors believe in intervention.* Probably the biggest reason doctors recommend interventions is that they believe in them. They'd recommend the same thing to their families and often do.

Rates of Surgery for Doctors and Their Spouses

Researchers at Stanford University hypothesized that doctors, as informed consumers aware of both the risks and benefits of surgery, would undergo fewer operations than other groups. Contrary to their expectations, male physicians had rates of surgery similar to or higher than businessmen, lawyers, and ministers. Female physicians had their gallbladders removed twice as often as female lawyers. Perhaps more interestingly, the spouses of physicians tended to have higher rates of operations than the spouses of other professionals. For hysterectomy—an operation frequently performed unnecessarily—over 50 percent of physicians' wives had one by the age of sixty-five, compared with the national rate of about 33 percent.[10]

- *Many interventions become popular despite a lack of evidence that they are beneficial.* When a surgical technique is invented, it often becomes popular rapidly. Millions of operations may be performed before the scientific evidence of effectiveness (or of ineffectiveness) trickles in. Even when studies come along showing a procedure is ineffective, doctors may cling to it. Doctors became so accustomed to performing the disfiguring radical mastectomy for breast cancer that it took almost fifty years to reevaluate and modify their approach. These days less-invasive breast cancer surgery is done with no loss in cure rates and fewer complications for patients.

- *Studies tend to overestimate the effectiveness of interventions and underestimate the risks.* Most published studies are conducted under ideal circumstances that bear little resemblance to the real world. A study of surgery will examine the effectiveness of an operation when performed by the best surgeons in the best hospitals. Older and sicker patients are excluded from the analysis. The study's results are usually more favorable than what the average patient in an average hospital with an average doctor will experience.

    Consider, for instance, the complication rate of radical prostate surgery. When proposing the surgery as a treatment for cancer, doctors must inform patients of the potential risks and benefits. One risk is incontinence, the inability to control urination. Based on published studies conducted at prestigious medical centers, doctors often quote a 1–5 percent rate of total incontinence and a 10–20 percent rate of partial incontinence caused by the operation. A recent survey of patients' actual experience, however, showed markedly higher levels. Only 37 percent of patients reported no problems. Almost half said they drip every day. Almost a third wear pads, adult diapers, or clamps on their penises.[11]

- *Patient demand is a major cause of unnecessary interventions.* A patient may have read an enthusiastic report in a magazine or have seen a story on TV about some "breakthrough." Someone who is suffering may be willing to try just about anything, even when the likelihood of benefit is exceedingly small. I've seen cases where patients have browbeaten surgeons into performing unnecessary surgery that only made them worse. Since people with insurance don't pay directly for most interventions, normal cost-benefit analysis often doesn't sway the patient.

- *Your race, gender, sexual orientation, and age can affect what the doctor recommends.* Ideally your medical condition would be the biggest determinant of what medical interventions were employed, but in reality subtle and sometimes not-so-subtle bias can affect a doctor's recommendations.

Racial Differences in Interventions

Researchers from the University of Pennsylvania examined whether there were differences in the rates of various medical procedures in blacks and whites. The rates show the number of operations per ten thousand people.

Procedure	White Rate	Black Rate
bypass surgery	30.6	8.1
balloon angioplasty	9.9	3.2
carotid endarterectomy	17.3	5.8
heart catheterization	85.6	43.1
hip replacement surgery	22.5	9.5
knee replacement surgery	18.2	8.9
hernia repair	33.7	16.5
glaucoma surgery	8.0	17.9

Whites were more likely than blacks to receive twenty-three of the thirty-two procedures studied. Whites had especially greater use of newer, higher-technology services. Rural blacks, almost all of whom live in the South, were much less likely than urban blacks or rural whites to receive services. Urban whites, for example, were 2.5 times as likely as urban blacks to have an angioplasty, but rural whites were more than twenty times as likely to have one than rural blacks. Racial differences were found in all areas of the country but were greatest in the South.[12]

Part of the racial difference in intervention rates may be due to the fact that more whites are well-off and have private insurance, which reimburses doctors well for procedures. But money isn't the whole story.

Racial Differences in Treatment at V.A. Hospitals

Researchers from the Veterans Administration examined the number of heart procedures done on black and white heart attack victims. The VA is in some ways the perfect place to look for racial differences in care because treatment does not depend on the ability to pay. The researchers found that blacks were 33 percent less likely to have a heart catheterization, 42 percent less likely to have an angioplasty, and 54 percent less likely to undergo bypass surgery. Despite having fewer procedures, a significantly higher percentage of blacks were alive one month after their heart attack. There were no differences in survival rates one and two years later.[13]

More intervention doesn't necessarily mean better care. Procedures in which physician discretion plays a big role may be precisely those that are often unnecessary or inappropriate. Blacks may have benefited by avoiding procedures they didn't need.

The elderly, too, may be discriminated against when it comes to medical interventions.

Age Differences in Treating Breast Cancer

The appropriate treatment of breast cancer, for instance, involves various combinations of surgery, hormones, chemotherapy, and radiation therapy, depending on the cancer. Researchers from UCLA looked at how women of different ages with breast cancer were treated in seven southern California hospitals, they found that the care was inappropriate 16.6 percent of the time in women aged fifty to sixty-nine but 32.6 percent of the time in women over seventy. Even when elderly patients were vigorous and healthy, their doctors were less likely to provide optimal treatment.[14]

The situation for women is especially complex. Overall, women receive more medical care than men. They visit doctors more often, have more lab tests done, and receive more drug prescriptions. They have lower rates, however, of heart catheterizations, kidney transplants, and certain other procedures that cannot be explained by a lower incidence of disease.[15]

There are few good studies documenting discrimination against gays and lesbians in medical intervention, but every reason to suspect a problem. I have personally come across dozens of openly homophobic physicians in my career.

Intervention Principle 2. Examine the Financial Incentives

Financial considerations can affect a doctor's recommendations either for or against an intervention. When evaluating the potential influence of money, consider the following:

- *Whether or not a doctor recommends an intervention could depend on what kind of insurance you have.* Doctors typically bill for every procedure they do, but these days insurers will pay only part of the bill. Doctors may be less likely to perform a procedure when the reimbursement rates aren't as good. Since people without insurance and the indigent may have difficulty paying their bills, doctors may attempt to cut their losses by offering them a lower-cost alternative.

Financial Incentives for C-sections

A researcher at the University of California assessed the relationship between the amount of payment a doctor gets for a caserean section and the rate at which the doctor performs it. Doctors' fees (exclusive of hospital charges) for C-sections are more than two thousand dollars, compared with under fifteen hundred dollars for vaginal deliveries, but physicians may only receive partial payment, depending on who pays the bill. Here's what the researchers found:[16]

Source of Payment	C-section Rate, By Percent
Private Insurance	29.1
Medicaid	22.9
Kaiser HMO	19.7
Indigent Patients	15.6

At the time this study was conducted, most private insurers tended to pay most or all of the doctor's fee, whereas Medicaid, the government program for the poor, paid a lower percentage of it. These days in some states Medicaid reimbursement is actually better than that of many managed care plans. We might therefore expect the C-section rates seen above to have changed. The principle that doctors respond to financial incentives—whatever they are—has not.

- *Financial incentives are less likely to play a role in your doctor's recommendation when the proper course of action is obvious.* Some people definitely need or do not need a particular operation, and in those instances only a few particularly unscrupulous physicians will be influenced by the profit motive. In a case where the proper course of action is less clear, financial incentives are more likely to influence a doctor's recommendation.

- *In an HMO the less the doctor does, the more profit the HMO makes.* HMOs achieve much of their cost savings by decreasing the rate of elective surgery and other pricey interventions. Their doctors' salaries and bonuses often depend on how effectively services are denied. Conscientious doctors in HMOs will still recommend needed interventions, but clearly their judgment may be influenced by the reimbursement system.

HMO doctors may not have the same incentives as doctors in private practice, but that doesn't mean that they won't recommend intervention when it's inappropriate. These doctors were trained in our intervention-oriented medical system, a system that developed its norms of practice under fee-for-service reimbursement. Over the years what doctors consider appropriate intervention may have been subtly influenced by the financial rewards for intervening. Keep in mind that even within tightly controlled HMOs, individual doctors vary in their practice styles.

• *If a hospital or clinic buys equipment, it has an incentive to use it.* Hospitals often invest millions of dollars to buy MRI machines, dialysis units, and heart catheterization labs. To pay off their loans, hospitals encourage their staff to use the facilities.

A case in point: It has become common for patients to undergo heart catheterization in the first few days after suffering a heart attack. If a hospital has a catheterization lab, it can do the procedure right there. Otherwise the hospital must transfer the patient to a hospital that has a lab.

Because It's There

Researchers from the University of Washington wondered whether the presence of an on-site cath lab would result in more catheterizations. They discovered that 66 percent of heart attack victims in hospitals with labs had a catheterization, compared with 36 percent of patients in the other hospitals. When the researchers adjusted the numbers to account for the patients' ages, symptoms, and other factors that affect the rate of catheterization, they found that patients in the hospitals with cath labs were more than three times as likely to have the procedure. The presence of a cath lab increased the likelihood of catheterization more than any other factor, including the patient's medical condition. The presence of an on-site cath lab had no discernible affect on death rates.[17]

In order to be competitive, many hospitals feel they must offer on-site catheterization or risk losing business to their competition. Several hospitals in a small area will offer on-site catheterizations, even though there isn't a sufficient need in the community to justify it.

Like superpowers acquiring warheads, competing hospitals fight a battle of one-upmanship, acquiring on-site MRI machines, bypass surgery programs, and radiation therapy centers. With the pressure to recoup investments, the result is more intervention, both appropriate and inappropriate. We've seen that for hospitals performing interventions like heart surgery, the more they do, the better they get. When too many hospitals offer a procedure, there aren't enough patients to go around. As a result, some hospitals may be performing too few operations for the optimal safety of their patients.

Intervention Principle 3. Favor Less Invasive Interventions

Doctors use the word *invasive* when referring to medical procedures that invade the body. A urinalysis, for example, is considered a noninvasive test (unless they need to stick a catheter into your bladder to remove urine). A blood test is considered minimally invasive. Since X-rays invade the body, even if the invasion can't be seen, they are considered more invasive. Bypass surgery is obviously highly invasive.

Whenever possible, if a noninvasive or less invasive alternative exists, it should be tried first. The more invasive an intervention, the greater the likelihood of side effects. Not so many years ago, if you had a benign growth in your intestines called a polyp, it could only be removed by undergoing a major abdominal operation. You would have to be hospitalized. The operation would require general anesthesia, which itself causes death a small percentage of the time. The operation frequently caused such problems as bleeding and infections. Recovery took weeks. These days a polyp can usually be removed via an endoscope—a fiberoptic tube inserted via the mouth or anus—in a simple and much safer outpatient procedure. The recovery time is measured in hours. The invasiveness of many other interventions, including operations for enlarged prostates, cysts on the ovaries, and more recently, diseased gallbladders, has been reduced using similar techniques.

Reducing Intervention in Childbirth

The bright-light, high-tech, intervention-oriented world of modern obstetrics isn't the most conducive environment for the normal progression of labor. Recently there has been a counter-current toward a lower-tech alternative. A study in the *New England Journal of Medicine* has shown that if nurses or doctors regularly listen to the baby's heartbeat by placing their stethoscopes on the mother's stomach rather than using the invasive fetal monitor, the babies do just as well.[18] More importantly, when the fetal monitor isn't used, false positive readings of fetal distress that may scare the doctor into performing an unnecessary C-section are never obtained. The cascade that ends with a C-section can be stopped before it starts.

Doctors Versus Midwives

Researchers at Johns Hopkins University compared the rate of obstetric interventions at a large Philadelphia teaching hospital with the rate at a family-oriented maternity center staffed by midwives, backed by on-site physicians. The mothers in the two institutions were similar in age, race, and education. The following table shows the percentage of time each intervention was employed:

Procedure	Maternity Center	Teaching Hospital
induction of labor	9.7	12.1
pitocin administration	22.2	32.1
electronic fetal monitoring	42.7	63.3
anesthesia (e.g. an epidural)	24.5	78.6
episiotomy	62.2	86.4
forceps delivery	9.7	27.0
C-section	5.3	18.2
normal vaginal delivery	83.0	53.9

Both institutions tended to intervene with high-risk pregnancies. Low-risk women at the teaching hospital were twelve times more likely to have an invasive delivery (C-section or forceps) and twenty-two times more likely to receive an anesthetic. Despite all the intervention, infants born at the university hospital fared no better than infants born at the maternity center.[19]

Lower-tech care, care less driven by technology, can be more human. One difference between midwives and obstetricians is that midwives attend more to the women and better meet their emotional needs. The result can be better-quality care.

Emotional Support During Labor

Two studies from Guatemala suggest that the presence of a supportive companion, a *doula*, during labor reduces the need for C-sections and other interventions. Researchers from Case Western Reserve University studied whether *doulas* would be effective in the environment of a modern American hospital. The *doula* stayed at the woman's bedside throughout labor, soothing and touching her, explaining what was happening and giving encouragement. In every other sense the childbirth experience was typically American: the women were confined to bed as soon as they were admitted to the hospital to allow for electronic monitoring, an IV was started, and the woman's membranes were routinely artificially ruptured. Pitocin was started if labor didn't progress fast enough; drugs and epidural anesthesia were given as deemed necessary by the doctors to relieve pain.

Marked differences were noted between the women who had *doulas* and those who didn't. For the women with *doulas*, the total duration of labor was two hours shorter. Overall, 8 percent of women with *doulas* needed an epidural, compared with over 55 percent of the women in the control groups. The risk of an epidural, by the way, is that it tends to prolong labor, increases the use of forceps for delivery, and makes C-sections more likely (another potential cascade). Only 17 percent of the women with *doulas* needed Pitocin, compared with 44 percent of the control group. Only 8 percent had C-sections, compared with 18 percent of the control group. Forceps were used on 8.2 percent of the women versus 26.3 percent of those without. Even the babies of supported mothers did better: 10 percent of them had to stay in the hospital for a medical complication, compared with 24 percent in the control group.[20]

Intervention Principle 4.
Weigh the Risks and Benefits

For any intervention you are contemplating, you should weigh the possible advantages and disadvantages. Some possible advantages of an intervention include:

- increased life expectancy
- reduction in pain or other symptoms
- reduction in anxiety about your diagnosis or prognosis
- better ability to function

Some of the possible disadvantages of an intervention include:

- suffering a side effect that makes you feel worse or less able to function
- initiating an intervention cascade
- pain during and after the procedure
- time lost from work
- cost
- death

Is the Intervention What You Want?

Remember, it's how you view the relative importance of the various risks and benefits that matters, not how your doctor views them. For you the inconvenience of missing several weeks of work after an elective operation could tip the balance against having it. In another situation you might feel that you simply need to find out whether you have a certain condition or not and want to proceed to the invasive procedure that will give you the answer. It's your life and your decision.

People vary in how much risk they are willing to undergo in order to feel better or live longer. Studies suggest that in order to give their patients a greater chance at long-term survival, doctors may be willing to accept a higher risk of death in the short-term than many of their patients would be willing to accept, if they were asked.

Cancer doctors typically refer to the five-year survival rate when evaluating treatment, but the likelihood of surviving five years may not be the patient's most important concern. To some patients, an improved chance of surviving the first year is more important. For some types of lung cancer, for example, the choice of treatment is between surgery and X-ray therapy. Doctors usually favor surgery because the five-year survival rate is better. In the short term, however, there is a high death rate from the surgery itself. If you compare the survival rates after surgery and after X-ray therapy, you find that a higher percentage of people who opt for X-ray therapy are alive one year after treatment. By the end of the second year the survival rates for surgery and radiation are similar. Five years later a significantly higher number of patients who underwent surgery are alive.

The Choice Between Radiation and Surgery for Lung Cancer

Boston researchers quizzed a group of lung cancer patients to see which was more important, the chance of long-term survival or a greater likelihood of surviving in the short-term. They found that most lung cancer patients were averse to risk: they preferred treatment with a lower five-year survival rate but a smaller chance of immediate death. There was no difference in preference between those who had been treated with surgery and those who had received radiation. If the patients' preferences had been followed, the majority of both groups would have been treated with X-ray therapy.[21]

For any proposed intervention, be sure you understand what the doctor hopes to accomplish by doing it. Cure you? Lengthen your life by a few months? Make you more comfortable? If your doctor has one goal and you have another, the doctor may consider the intervention a success when you view it as a failure. Not communicating about the goals of treatment can not only lead to great disappointment; it is a common cause of lawsuits.

Consider the example of the use of chemotherapy to shrink tumors. For some cancers, doctors may recommend chemotherapy to shrink the size of a tumor even when the chance of cure is remote. You might conclude that doing so would improve your life expectancy or make you feel better, but it doesn't always follow. In some instances the intermediate goal—in this case shrinking the size of the tumor—may have little impact on the ultimate goal.[22] Ask the doctor what impact shrinking the tumor would have on your life expectancy and quality of life. For some cancers, shrinking the size of the tumor reduces symptoms, but this benefit needs to be weighed against the side effects and hassle of chemotherapy. If the chance of cure is minimal and you feel worse because of the chemotherapy, you may want to decide against it. There is no right answer. It's a matter of what's most important to you.

Remember, **as a competent adult, you have the right to refuse any medical intervention, no matter how much your doctor or anyone else thinks you should have it. Doctors are legally bound to respect your wishes.**

More Than Survival: Quality of Life

Some treatments may increase your life expectancy but lower the quality of your life. The treatment of prostate cancer, the most common cancer among American men, presents this dilemma. When we read about the deaths of men in the prime of their careers, such as the musician and composer Frank Zappa, it's natural to feel that aggressive therapy is called for. In reality, the decision whether to treat prostate cancer is a very personal one, fraught with uncertainty. Consider the following:

- *At the time prostate cancer is diagnosed, most men have no symptoms.* At diagnosis most men have localized tumors, that is, tumors confined to the prostate gland. Since they have no symptoms, the goal of treatment is to prevent or to delay spread of the cancer to other parts of the body.

- *Most men with prostate cancer never get symptoms.* Since prostate cancer often affects older men, many of them will die from other causes before the prostate cancer gives them any problems. When autopsies are done on eighty-year-old men who die of unrelated causes, small areas of prostate cancer are found in two-thirds of them.[23]

- *Treatment for prostate cancer has never been proved effective.* Treatment with either surgery or radiation therapy *theoretically* reduces the likelihood of the cancer's spreading to other parts of the body, but the theory has never been proved. We simply do not know whether radical prostate surgery or radiation therapy will increase life expectancy. It will be years until studies currently under way will give us the answer. For the majority of men who were never destined to get symptoms, treatment definitely decreases their life expectancy and the quality of their lives.

- *Any benefit of treating localized prostate cancer may not be realized for years.* When prostate cancer is treated, doctors are betting that by preventing the later spread of the cancer, they can add years on to the end of their patients' lives. Many men die of other causes before they ever have a chance to realize this benefit. Many develop other conditions such as Alzheimer's disease or debilitating heart conditions, that lower the quality of the extra years provided by the prostate cancer treatment. In other words, when you treat prostate cancer you trade an immediate risk for the possibility of gain later on. Some men are unwilling to give up several more years of high-quality life for the possibility of adding time of uncertain quality on to the end of their life. Experts believe that men over seventy-five are unlikely to live long enough to realize the benefits of treatment.[24]

- *The complications of treatment begin immediately.* Prostate cancer tends to grow slowly. If prostate cancer is going to spread to other parts of the body, it often does so years later. The average time between the diagnosis and the spread of the cancer is fourteen years.[25] Prostate cancer surgery, the so-called radical prostatectomy, is a major operation with a significant recovery period. Impotence and incontinence are common side effects. In a recent survey of men two to four years after the operation, only 11 percent reported any erections sufficient for intercourse in the prior month.[26]

Major complications in the first month after surgery, such as heart attack or a blood clot in the lung, strike 7 percent of men over seventy-five and 10 percent of men over eighty. For men over seventy-five, one in seventy-one dies within one month of the operation. For men over eighty, one in twenty-two is dead within a month.[27]

Treatment Versus Watchful Waiting for Prostate Cancer

Investigators reporting in the *Journal of the American Medical Association* analyzed the advantages and disadvantages of treating localized prostate cancer. Ignoring quality and looking only at life expectancy, they found that treatment provided some benefit to men under seventy. But when quality of life was factored in, the benefits of treatment were modest. Even though treatment is more effective for less malignant tumors, because these tumors are less likely to spread, the benefits of treatment are less likely to offset the impact of complications, like impotence and incontinence, on the quality of life. For men with less malignant tumors, treatment offers little advantage over watchful waiting. On the other hand, even though treatment is less effective for more malignant tumors, these tumors tend to spread, and treatment is more likely to benefit the patient.[28]

• *Prostate surgery rates are going up.* Despite the lack of evidence that most men benefit from radical prostate surgery, the operation is being performed more and more, especially in some regions of the country.

Increasing Use of Radical Prostate Surgery

Researchers from Dartmouth Medical School discovered that radical prostate surgery was performed almost six times more often in 1990 as in 1984. Doctors in the Pacific and Mountain states perform radical prostate surgery more than twice as often as doctors in New England and the Mid-Atlantic states. In Alaska, the state with the highest rate, the operation is done twenty times as often as in Rhode Island. More than 10 percent of the operations were done on men over seventy-five and 1.5 percent on men over eighty. Despite the increasing efforts at early detection and aggressive treatment, death rates from prostate cancer have not decreased, not even in the states with high rates of radical prostate surgery.[29]

Urologists, the surgeons who perform prostate operations, believe strongly in the effectiveness of radical prostate surgery. Two factors may color their assessment, consciously or unconsciously. First, they see some men die painful prostate cancer deaths and the experience is so powerful that they want to avoid it in the future. The treatment they have to offer may not be effective in preventing such deaths, but they feel the need to do something. Second are the financial considerations. The average urologist makes tens of thousands of dollars per year performing radical prostate operations.

Intangible Factors

When contemplating surgery or other major interventions, you need to consider a number of intangible factors. A long period of convalescence can disrupt work and family life. After an intervention you may need to return to the hospital or doctor for frequent checkups. Dealing with insurance companies and doctors' bills is at best a hassle. These are not necessarily reasons to avoid intervention, just factors to contemplate before agreeing.

Trendy Treatments

As regularly as hairstyles, new medical and surgical procedures come into vogue. Their popularity is warranted when the fashionable procedures represent real advances over existing therapies. Sometimes, however, a procedure catches on when there is little evidence it's superior to the traditional treatment. New does not necessarily mean improved. In general, **newer interventions are appropriate only when they promise significant advantages over previously available treatments. They should either be safer, more effective, or less invasive.**

New treatments become popular for many reasons. The companies that manufacture the required equipment stand to reap huge profits if the procedure catches on. The investigator who invents a new technique is usually extremely enthusiastic and more than happy to fuel any media hype. His or her career may rise or fall with the popularity of the technique.[30] The media, of course, love stories about medical breakthroughs. When the evidence starts to accumulate that last year's breakthrough hasn't panned out, they usually aren't as interested.

Unlike the situation with new drugs, the proponents of a new intervention don't have to prove to the government that it's safe and effective before putting it on the market. Only a small fraction of new medical devices are formally reviewed by the FDA prior to their introduction.[31] Unanticipated side effects may only come to light years after the introduction of a new intervention. Vasectomy has been used as a birth control method on men for decades, yet only recently have studies suggested it may cause prostate cancer.[32] More studies will be necessary to determine whether this connection is real. The point is that with any new intervention there are unknowns.

Intervention Principle 5. Assess the Doctor's Track Record

Doctors vary in how technically competent they are. This should come as no surprise, since hairdressers and second basemen vary in their abilities too. For certain operations, like bypass surgery, a good outcome depends on, among other things, the manual dexterity of the surgeon. Other operations, like traditional gallbladder surgery, are easy enough that most surgeons can do them well.

The Death Rate From Bypass Surgery by Different Doctors

A study in the *Journal of the American Medical Association* looked at the variation in death rates of all surgeons performing heart bypass surgery in Maine, New Hampshire, and Vermont. The death rate ranged from 3.1 percent to 6.3 percent, depending on the hospital. The death rates for individual surgeons varied even more. The best surgeons had a death rate of 1.9 percent. The worst surgeons had a death rate of 9.2 percent, almost five times as high.[33]

A doctor needs to perform a procedure a minimum number of times to gain competence. He or she must continue to perform the procedure with some regularity to continue to do it well. Practice may not make perfect, but it helps. Ask the doctor, "How many of these have you done? How often do you do them now? How have your patients done? What complications have you seen? How common are they?" Keep in mind when assessing a doctor's track record, however, that some excellent surgeons have high complication records because they are willing to operate on patients that no other surgeons will touch.

In the past few years a technique has become popular which allows doctors to remove diseased gallbladders with the help of a laparoscope, a fiberoptic tube inserted through a small incision in the abdomen. Other tubes inserted through small incisions allow the doctors to clamp, cut, and staple while watching the video image transmitted by the laparoscope. When done well, the new procedure can reduce the patient's pain after surgery and cut the recovery time from weeks to days. When news of this revolutionary technique spread in the popular media, patients were soon clamoring for it.

When the technique was introduced, many surgeons worried that if they didn't learn it, they'd lose business. Normally surgeons learn how to perform operations during residency, a several-year apprenticeship they complete after medical school. If a new technique comes along after they've completed their training, surgeons need to learn it on their own.

Laparoscopic gallbladder surgery is very different from what most surgeons have been doing for their entire careers. Rather than cutting the patient open and locating the gallbladder and the various blood vessels by looking at them and feeling them, the surgeon watches a mirror image of the proceedings on a TV monitor. Depth perception may be difficult. Until you get used to it, navigating with the remote control instruments may be awkward. There is a definite learning curve to mastering the operation, and especially early on, many doctors performing it weren't that proficient.[34]

To learn the technique, most doctors take intensive one- or two-day courses usually given in hotels. They hear lectures, watch demonstrations, practice on models, and finally try out the technique on dogs or pigs. Approximately ten thousand surgeons have taken these courses since the late eighties.

According to the *New York Times,* some doctors did their first cases on a human a few days after practicing on a pig.[35] It's perhaps not surprising then that early on there were reports about high rates of complications.

Complications of Laparoscopic Surgery

Operations performed by doctors who had taken an intensive two-day course in laparoscopic surgery were reviewed for common complications like bleeding and infection. Researchers at the University of Iowa discovered that almost one-third of doctors performed the operations without further training. These doctors had a 22 percent rate of complications in the first three months. Doctors who underwent further training had a complication rate of only 5 percent. In general, the more procedures a doctor performed, the lower the complication rate. Doctors in solo private practice were almost eight times as likely to have had a complication in the first year as doctors in group practice.[36]

Remember, though, that a doctor who performs a procedure often may also be recommending it often—perhaps inappropriately. Technical competence at performing a procedure does not ensure good judgment in recommending it.

The Hospital's Track Record

Where you have a procedure done will often depend on what doctor you choose to do it. Some doctors have privileges at more than one hospital, in which case you may have a choice. Consider the hospital when you choose your surgeon. The quality of the nursing staff, physical therapists, and laboratories, all of which affect your care, varies greatly from hospital to hospital. In general, a hospital that performs a lot of operations is a better bet.

High-Volume Versus Low-Volume Hospitals

A *New England Journal of Medicine* study found that hospitals performing more than two hundred heart bypass operations per year had a death rate of 3.4 percent, compared with 5.7 percent in hospitals that performed fewer than two hundred. The death rates in hospitals performing only a few bypasses per year are often several times higher than expected. For a few simple operations, like traditional gallbladder surgery, volume had no effect. According to the authors, the greater the difference in death rates for an operation between high- and low-volume hospitals, the greater distance you should be willing to travel to find the right hospital and surgeon.[37]

By telephoning, it's sometimes possible to determine how often a hospital does a particular operation. Hospitals want your business, so they have an incentive to cooperate. Although hospital death rates are occasionally published, it's usually difficult to get useful, up-to-date information.

Intervention Principle 6. Get a Second Opinion

Except in an emergency situation, a second opinion is almost always a good idea before any major intervention. Whenever possible, the second opinion should come from a doctor unaffiliated with the doctor recommending the intervention. Mount Sinai Hospital in Chicago implemented a program to lower the C-section rate. One of the primary aspects of the program was a stringent requirement for a second opinion which could not be obtained from the doctor's associates in practice. During the first two years of the program, the rate of C-sections dropped from 17.5 percent, already well below the national average, to 11.5 percent, without any apparent adverse effects on either the mothers or the babies.[38]

Many insurance companies now require patients to get a second opinion before undergoing elective surgery. They figure the small cost of the second opinion is outweighed by the money saved by cutting down on unnecessary operations. As a patient you stand to benefit from getting a second opinion because at the very least you'll end up better informed about your treatment options. Perhaps more importantly, when surgeons know a colleague will be looking over their shoulders, so to speak, they tend to recommend fewer operations of dubious value.

The Impact of Mandatory Second-Opinions on Surgery Rates

Researchers from Boston University examined the effects of a mandatory second opinion program instituted by the state of Massachusetts for Medicaid patients recommended to have elective surgery. The doctor offering the second opinion found the surgery to be unnecessary 14.5 percent of the time. The numbers were the worst for back surgery, hysterectomies, and knee operations, all of which were judged unnecessary about a quarter of the time. The patients' decisions were greatly influenced by the second opinions: 85.5 percent of those patients for whom the second doctor concurred with the need for surgery had the operation, compared with only 31 percent of patients for whom the second doctor disagreed.[39]

For more details on how to obtain a second opinion, please see the section "Trust But Verify" in the final chapter.

Intervention Principle 7. Stay Out of the Hospital, If Possible

When you are seriously ill and in need of medical intervention, the hospital is often the best place to be. But before you agree to an elective admission, consider the following:

- *The hospital can be a dangerous place.* Among the most common complications of hospitalization are hospital-acquired infections. As mentioned earlier, each year in the United States these infections cause nineteen thousand deaths and contribute to another fifty-eight thousand. Hospital-acquired infections strike people who are already in a weakened state, and the bacteria that cause them tend to be more virulent than those found in the community. The bacteria that colonize hospitals are often resistant to many antibiotics. As discussed, infections tend to be spread by nurses, by X-ray technicians, and especially by doctors.

    One hospital-acquired infection of the past is making a resurgence: tuberculosis. TB, partly because of flagging control efforts in the seventies and eighties and partly because of the AIDS epidemic, is coming back strong. Of particular concern is that the recent outbreaks of TB have increasingly involved strains resistant to the usually effective drugs. In the past few years at least a dozen outbreaks of multidrug-resistant TB have occurred in hospitals, often spread through the hospitals' ventilation systems.[40] The resurgence in TB will in all likelihood get worse before it gets better.

Other common complications of hospitalization are drug reactions and side effects of medical tests.

• *The elderly are at especially great risk in the hospital.* Hospitalization often results in decreased ability of elderly people to function, even if the problem that brought them to the hospital is remedied. People who spend a week or more in bed lose muscle strength; some patients who walk into the hospital may not be able to walk out. Falls from bed are a common hospital complication that can cause fractures and other injuries.

Loss of Function During Hospitalization

A report in the *Journal of the American Geriatrics Society* looked at elderly patients admitted to a community hospital in California to see how hospitalization affected their functioning. The researchers found that 75 percent of independent people over the age of seventy-five were no longer independent when they left the hospital. Fifteen percent of them were discharged to nursing homes.[41]

• *Routine practices make the hospital more dangerous than it needs to be.* Beds are set high for the convenience of the doctors and nurses, increasing the risk of injury if the patient falls. Patients routinely are given IVs even if they aren't taking any intravenous medications.[42] Catheters to drain urine are put in when they're not really needed or left in when they're no longer necessary. Many patients are needlessly restricted to bed, which leads to dehydration, loss of muscle strength, and weakening of bones. Medicines, the unfamiliar environment, and the lack of stimulation can all lead to confusion.

All of these routine hospital practices can initiate dangerous cascades, especially in the elderly. Patients who have a catheter put in to drain urine may be left incontinent when it's removed. Urinary catheters and IVs can lead to infections; the longer they're left in, the greater the risk. Confusion, dehydration, and loss of muscle strength make falls more likely. If the patient falls, weakened bones and high beds make fractures more likely. Infections and falls lead to prolonged hospitalizations, increasing the risk of more complications. Confusion, incontinence, infections, and fractures can all lead to nursing home admission. Once admitted to a nursing home, most people never return home.[43]

• *Many hospitalizations are unnecessary.* Under traditional government and private insurance plans, the more a hospital admitted patients and the longer they stayed, the greater the hospital's revenue. The result was many inappropriate admissions and inappropriately long stays.

Inappropriate Hospitalization

Researchers from the Rand Corporation and UCLA found that 23 percent of hospital admissions were inappropriate. Another 17 percent could have been avoided if patients had surgery on an outpatient basis. The rate of inappropriate admissions varied from site to site: in Seattle only 10 percent were judged inappropriate; in a rural area of South Carolina 35 percent were inappropriate. Overall, more than one-third of the days spent in the hospital were inappropriate—an average of more than two days per admission. Women were much more likely than men to be admitted inappropriately: 27 versus 18 percent. Patients whose health insurance paid the entire cost of the admission were hospitalized 31 percent more often, both for appropriate and inappropriate reasons.[44]

In recent years the financial incentives have changed. Rather than reimbursing hospitals for each service rendered, the traditional method, the government and some insurance companies now pay a flat fee based on the patient's diagnosis. Since hospitals receive the same amount of money if they do a lot or if they do a little, these incentives favor doing less. It can therefore be in a hospital's financial interest to admit people who aren't that sick, because they require fewer services and can usually go home earlier. The same incentives can lead hospitals to prematurely discharge some seriously ill patients.

* *Even when patients are admitted to the hospital for appropriate reasons, they may be kept there too long.* In general, the longer you stay in the hospital, the more drugs you'll be given, the more tests you'll have, and the greater the chance that you'll suffer a complication. Once the juggernaut of modern medicine gets rolling, it can be hard for you as a patient to apply the brakes. Consider the following example.

Case History: Got to Get Back to the Garden

Henry Santini never eats breakfast. He usually throws down a cup of black coffee and goes to work in his garden. At the age of seventy-six, he is known to work for hours without interruption, weeding and planting, hoeing and shoveling.

Even a mid-summer heat wave failed to deter him. It was 95 degrees and cloudless as he toiled all morning with his plants. By 1 P.M. he still hadn't eaten anything. Sweat rolled down his face. The back of his shirt was damp. He was thirsty, so he walked up to the corner store and bought a six-pack.

He had already drunk a couple of beers when he started to feel lightheaded. He fell to his knees and softly lowered his head to the ground of his garden but never lost consciousness. He called for help, but his wife couldn't hear him from inside the house. His neighbor found him a short time later, stood him up, and helped him into the house.

As they walked in his front door, Henry started feeling dizzy again. He started to fall, and his neighbor helped lower him to the ground. This time Henry did briefly pass out. The neighbor called the paramedics, and a short time later an ambulance whisked Henry away. Henry had regained consciousness before the paramedics arrived, though, and was able to answer their questions lucidly.

In the emergency room of the nearby university medical center, Henry was alert. Lying down, his blood pressure was normal at

120/76. But when the doctor stood him up, his pressure fell to 80/50, a sign of profound dehydration. The doctor decided to admit Henry to the hospital for observation and for intravenous fluids.

Henry did well overnight. After several bags of IV fluids, he felt much better. His blood pressure no longer dropped when he stood up. Henry felt he was ready to go home, but his doctors had other ideas. Even though dehydration, from the combined effects of the heat and the alcohol, had almost certainly caused Henry's black-out, his doctors wanted to be sure that he hadn't had a seizure or heart rhythm problem. They asked the heart specialists and the neurologists to see him.

The cardiologists recommended several tests. They wanted a twenty-four-hour tape recording of his heart rhythm, an ultrasound of his heart, and a MUGA scan, a test in which radioactive dye is injected into the blood to measure how well the heart pumps. The neurologists recommended more tests. They wanted a CAT scan of the head, an electroencephalogram (EEG), and an ultrasound of his carotid arteries to look for blockages.

The twenty-four-hour heart rhythm showed loads of extra beats but no serious rhythm problems and nothing that might have caused him to black out. Still, the result concerned the cardiologists enough to recommend repeating the twenty-four-hour monitoring. They also suggested Henry undergo an exercise stress test to look for blockages in the coronary arteries. The ultrasound of the heart showed normal valves and good pumping action of the heart. The MUGA scan was normal, except that the right side of the heart was mildly thickened.

The cardiologists thought that the thickening was probably due to emphysema from Henry's long-time smoking. They recommended the lung specialists see Henry. The lung specialists recommended several blood tests, as well as breathing tests to measure lung function. The results showed that Henry indeed has mild emphysema. Henry is not terribly bothered by his lung problems and plans to continue smoking.

In the meantime Henry was going stir-crazy. He had been feeling fine for five days, yet he was still in the hospital undergoing tests. He badgered the intern to please let him go home, but the intern felt he shouldn't go until all the recommended tests were completed. Henry finally decided he'd had enough. The next morning he left the hospital against the doctor's advice.

Henry reportedly did well at home—no doubt back in his garden, working even harder to make up for the week of neglect his plants had suffered.

- *If possible, avoid hospitals on weekends.* One thing which can lead to unnecessarily long hospital stays is being there on a weekend when hospital staffing is reduced. Many tests and therapies that are easy to obtain Monday through Friday are either unavailable or harder to come by on Saturday and Sunday. You may end up risking the complications of hospitalization while not much is happening on your case. In an emergency, of course, you shouldn't wait, but for an elective admission, try to arrange it so you won't be there over a weekend.

  It's also probably safer to avoid hospitals on weekends. Your regular doctors may not be available, and if not, you'll be stuck with whoever happens to be covering. The covering doctors won't know your case as well and may be responsible for more patients than is usually the case during the week. Things can fall through the cracks. It's a common experience for doctors to return on Monday morning only to find their patients in much worse condition.

- *Many hospitalizations continue to be unnecessary, but inappropriate denial of hospital admission is becoming a big problem.* HMOs require preapproval of anything other than emergency admissions. Since HMOs have a financial incentive to keep costs down and hospital stays are extremely costly, we would expect them to have much lower rates of inappropriate hospitalization. The risk is that they will deny hospital admission to some people who need it. **A recent trend is for private insurers, who are feeling increasingly pressured to lower their costs, to apply HMO-like tactics to lower hospitalization rates. They too may be preventing necessary hospitalizations.**

  People without insurance are particularly likely to be denied needed services if they can't afford to pay for them up front. While it's illegal for a hospital to refuse to treat a patient in an emergency, what constitutes an emergency can be a judgment call. To avoid losing money, private hospitals sometimes transfer medically unstable patients who lack insurance to city or county hospitals that treat anyone regardless of their ability to pay. This practice, known as "patient dumping," has resulted in patients dying or suffering complications en route to the other hospital; pregnant women have lost their babies.

• *HMOs and now many insurance companies pressure hospitals and doctors to discharge patients as soon as possible.* Henry Santini's hospitalization was more than five years ago. These days, his insurance company and the hospital's utilization reviewers might have been breathing down his doctors' necks to get him out of the hospital sooner.

Many insurance companies now apply best-case scenarios to estimate how long you should stay in the hospital. Depending on your diagnosis, they will approve a certain numbers of days—two days for a C-section, for example, or four days for a heart bypass operation.[45] If you stay longer and they haven't approved the extra days, they will refuse to pay for them. The new guidelines can result in drastic reductions in the number of days in the hospital. In the past, for example, patients who underwent a leg amputation averaged over two weeks in the hospital. Under the new guidelines, the optimal length of stay is set at two days.[46]

Pressure to discharge you early can be to your advantage if it cuts down on inappropriate days in the hospital, but the risk is that you'll be sent home too soon. Another downside is that your entire hospital stay will be compressed. You many undergo three or four tests per day instead of one or two. Little time to recover between procedures may leave you exhausted, which is hardly therapeutic if you're already in a weakened state. If your doctor thinks you need more time in the hospital, he or she may have to fight the HMO, your insurance company, or the hospital's utilization reviewers to have the extra days allowed. Not all doctors are willing to do so.

* *Home health care can be a viable alternative to hospitalization or to extra days of hospitalization.* Most people who are admitted to hospitals inappropriately need medical care, but they don't need to get it in the expensive and potentially dangerous environment of the hospital. Other patients may need to be stabilized in the hospital but then can complete their therapy elsewhere.

In recent years there has been a return to the concept of medical care in the home. With the use of visiting nurses and house visits by doctors, treatments that were once only provided in the hospital such as chemotherapy and blood transfusions, can be given at home. **If quality nursing, physical therapy, and other services are not available in the home, discharging patients from the hospital can be inappropriate—especially in light of the current tendency to send patients home earlier and sicker.**

Home health care has several advantages. Most older people and people with such chronic diseases as AIDS greatly prefer treatment at home. The environment is familiar. They can continue to live independently in the face of serious disease. Supportive friends and family members are around. And most of all, outside the disorienting, intervention-prone world of the modern hospital, the likelihood of a complication that could result in death or a nursing home admission goes way down.

SEVEN COMMONLY INAPPROPRIATE INTERVENTIONS

The seven commonly inappropriate interventions described below are not the only ones that could have appeared on the list. Casarean sections may be the most commonly performed unnecessary procedure in this country, but since it was discussed earlier, we won't cover it again. Other procedures, including cataract operations, back surgery, gallbladder removals, and hemorrhoid surgery, are also performed more often than can be medically justified.

Inappropriate Intervention 1.
Blood Transfusions

In the late 1970s no one new that the AIDS epidemic was coming and no one knew that the blood supply had already been contaminated with the deadly HIV virus. Scores of people, including tennis great Arthur Ashe, were infected by blood transfusions, his given during a hospitalization for bypass surgery.

Rates of Blood Transfusion During Bypass Surgery

In a study in the *Journal of the American Medical Association* that examined the transfusion records of patients hospitalized for bypass surgery, researchers found marked differences between different hospitals in how often they gave transfusions. On average, 68 percent of bypass patients received blood transfusions, but the percentages varied tremendously. One hospital transfused only 17 percent of patients, while three others transfused 100 percent of patients. The hospitals that transfused more often also tended to give more units (pints) of blood. The more units you get, the higher the risk of infection. Of the patients who received transfusions, 41 percent had blood counts on being discharged that suggested they'd received inappropriate transfusions.[47]

At more than 11 million per year in the United States, blood transfusions are one of the most common major interventions. When contemplating a blood transfusion, keep the following in mind:

- *When needed, blood transfusions can be life-saving.* Someone who is hemorrhaging from an ulcer and going into shock clearly needs an immediate transfusion. Operations sometimes cause so much bleeding that one or more transfusions are necessary for recovery.

- *The blood supply seems to be safe, but you can never be absolutely sure.* Since 1985 we have had a blood test to screen for HIV, the AIDS virus. While the test is not perfect, it is very good, and as far as we know, the blood supply is currently safer than it's ever been. The point is that we don't know. There is a window, a period of time after a person becomes infected with HIV but before the blood test becomes positive. If a person donates blood during this period, the virus can be transmitted to the recipient of the blood. In addition, some types of hepatitis are still not detectable with blood tests. We have tests to detect most of the known infectious hazards of transfusion, but if there is another, as yet unrecognized, virus contaminating blood, it may be years until we find out. Given the risks, blood transfusions should be given only when absolutely necessary.

- *Infection is not the only risk of blood transfusion.* More and more evidence suggests that blood transfusions suppress the body's immune system. There is evidence that people who get transfused are more likely to get wound infections after surgery. Studies also suggest that people who receive transfusions while hospitalized for colon cancer surgery are more likely to have recurrences of the cancer. The same may be true for other cancers.[48]

- *Donating your own blood prior to elective surgery is safe and completely eliminates the risk of infection by contaminated blood.* In the above study of blood transfusion during bypass surgery, only 8 percent of the patients had donated their own blood. Blood donated by friends and family members, by the way, has never been shown to be safer than blood from the blood bank and is not recommended.

- *Many transfusions are inappropriate.* Surgeons aren't the only doctors transfusing unnecessarily. One study of patients on medical wards showed that 18 percent of transfusions were unjustifiable and another 18 percent doubtfully justifiable. The researchers noted that even in justifiable cases, many of the patients received an excessive number of units of blood.[49] It only takes one tainted unit to give you an infection, and it's as likely to happen during the fourth as the first.

- *Physicians' lack of knowledge leads to inappropriate transfusions.* One reason that physicians may transfuse blood inappropriately is that they aren't knowledgeable enough about when transfusions are appropriate and when they're not.

Doctors' Knowledge About Blood Transfusions

Researchers from Harvard University surveyed 122 general surgeons, orthopedic surgeons, and anesthesiologists to determine their knowledge and attitudes about transfusion. Less than one-third correctly answered four questions about when transfusions were appropriate. Physicians tended to overestimate both the risks of transfusing and the risks of not transfusing. Almost one quarter of doctors thought the risk of a transfusion's causing AIDS was more than ten times as likely as it really is (about one in forty thousand). Doctors who transfuse inappropriately may be more concerned with harm coming to the patient because they didn't order a transfusion, than with harm caused by the transfusion.[50]

A common, inappropriate reason that doctors transfuse blood is a blood count that is low but not dangerously low. Many doctors will automatically transfuse anyone whose blood count, or hematocrit, drops below 30. Many surgeons will not consider elective surgery on anemic patients unless they are first transfused to raise their blood counts to this level. A panel of experts from the National Institutes of Health, however, concluded that this standard was too high and would lead to inappropriate transfusion.

Experts recommend that instead of merely looking at the numbers, doctors look at the patients. Are their vital signs stable? Are they short of breath? Are they bleeding? A careful interview and examination of the patient is more likely to result in an appropriate decision than simply relying on the blood count.

- *Under normal circumstances the human body has a remarkable ability to tolerate anemia.* Many people with low blood counts experience no symptoms. In others who do have symptoms, transfusions don't bring relief. For many patients with anemia, experts recommend watchful waiting.[51]

- *A transfusion can be the result of too many blood tests.* In the hospital patients have many tubes of blood drawn every day, much of it for unnecessary routine tests. The more tests you have, the greater the chance you'll become anemic and be given a transfusion. This is another example of a potentially harmful cascade started by seemingly harmless tests.

Inappropriate Intervention 2. Hysterectomy

If a blood transfusion sounds like overkill for mild anemia, what would you think of a hysterectomy? Yet mild anemia was precisely the rationale my mother's doctor gave when he proposed taking out her uterus several years before I was born. Lucky for me, she refused.

Although down from its peak in the mid-seventies, the rate of hysterectomies in the United States is still about 650,000 per year, making it the second most common surgery after cesarean sections. Approximately 200,000 of these procedures are done to treat cancer, which no one disputes as an appropriate reason for the operation. The remaining operations are usually done for symptoms. While the rate of inappropriate hysterectomies is probably dropping, many gynecologists continue to have the mentality, You don't need that thing anymore, why don't we just take it out?

This mentality might make some sense if the operation were completely benign. It's not. The chance of dying from the operation is about one in five hundred and increases as women age. About 10 percent of women require a blood transfusion with its attendant risk. Infection is a common complication, as is damage to surrounding organs. Repeat surgery for complications is a common occurrence.

There are several commonly invoked rationales for unnecessary hysterectomies. The operation is often performed to treat benign growths, known as fibroids, even when they cause no symptoms. Such treatment is rarely appropriate. Hysterectomies are also often performed to relieve pain or bleeding. Before proceeding to the operation, however, tests should be done to determine the cause of the symptoms. You don't want to undergo a hysterectomy for pain when you are really suffering

from arthritis of the lower back that the doctor hasn't diagnosed. Even when symptoms are coming from the uterus, they
can often be relieved with medications, making the operation
unnecessary. Preventing cancer is an inappropriate reason for a
hysterectomy.[52]

We saw earlier that even in HMOs, where the financial
incentives militate against unnecessary operations, that only
around 65 percent of hysterectomies performed were appropriate. We would expect that doctors in private practice, who
receive a fee for every procedure, would have an even lower rate
of appropriate operations.

Inappropriate Intervention 3. Bypass Surgery

In bypass surgery, known in medical parlance as coronary
artery bypass grafting, blocked arteries in the heart are literally
bypassed with veins removed from the leg. One end of the vein
is sewn above a blockage, one below, allowing blood an alternate path. In order to do the operation, surgeons saw the chest
open and pull the ribs apart. Even in good hospitals more than
3 percent of people die from the operation.

As with many other interventions, bypass surgery caught on
before there were any good studies demonstrating that it
improved life expectancy. It was clear that surgery could reduce
symptoms, at least initially, but many people can have their
symptoms relieved with medication alone. The data now coming in suggest that only certain groups of patients benefit from
the surgery.

Medications Versus Bypass Surgery

Doctors from the Veterans Administration studied over
four hundred men with severe angina randomized to receive
either drug therapy and bypass surgery or drug therapy alone.
Of those assigned to have surgery, 4 percent died from the
operation. In the two years following, there was no significant
difference in the rate of heart attacks between the group
operated on and the group given only drugs. The survival rate
also did not differ. Only those whose hearts functioned poorly
as pumps lived longer if they had the operation.[53]

The fact that studies suggest little benefit and substantial risk and expense for most people undergoing bypass surgery not only hasn't deterred doctors, they are doing the operation even more. Despite a reduction in the rates of heart disease in recent years, the rate of bypass surgery in the United States more than doubled between 1983 and 1990, up to 380,000 per year.

How Often Is Bypass Surgery Appropriate?

When researchers from UCLA and the Rand Corporation examined records from three randomly chosen hospitals in the western United States, they found that overall, 56 percent of bypass surgeries were performed for appropriate reasons, 30 percent for equivocal reasons, and 14 percent for inappropriate reasons. The rates varied a lot, though. One hospital's operations were appropriate 78 percent of the time, while another's were appropriate only 37 percent of the time. As usual with Rand studies, when in doubt, the experts chose to label the surgery appropriate. The actual levels of inappropriate surgery may therefore be even higher.[54]

Inappropriate Intervention 4.
Carotid Endarterecomy

Endarterectomy is a surgical procedure in which the main arteries to the brain, the carotids, are literally reamed out to remove fatty blockages that could cause strokes. The operation is fairly drastic but like bypass surgery became popular despite a lack of evidence of its effectiveness. Doctors who performed the operation were responding to a real need. Stroke is the third leading cause of death, and many people who survive one are permanently disabled.

For people who've had the surgery, however, the cure is sometimes worse than the disease. Almost 5 percent of people over eighty die of the operation and about twice that number suffer a stroke *as a result of the surgery*.[55] This high rate of complications is particularly disturbing when one considers that many of the operations were never needed in the first place.

Inappropriate Endarterectomies

Researchers from the Rand Corporation found that only 36 percent of endarterectomies were done for appropriate reasons. The researchers found these results particularly disturbing because once again, when in doubt, they labeled the procedure as appropriate.[56]

In part because of studies such as this one and greater public scrutiny, fewer endarterectomies are being done in the United States today than were ten years ago, when more than a hundred thousand were done per year. This reduction undoubtedly means that fewer inappropriate procedures are being done as well. Studies are still being conducted to determine which patients are most likely to benefit from endarterectomies.

Evidence so far suggests that the only people likely to benefit from surgery have severe blockages—narrowing the artery more than 70 percent—and recent transient ischemic attacks (TIAs). TIAs are ministrokes that cause strokelike symptoms but that go away within minutes. The predictions of benefit for these patients depend on the operation being done by a surgeon and at a hospital with low death and complication rates. An acceptable death rate is less than 1 percent, a rate achieved only in selected centers, usually university hospitals. People whose symptoms have gone away, those who have already had strokes, and those whose carotid arteries are already 100 percent blocked should not have the operation.

Unless you are at extremely high risk for stroke, you probably want to avoid an endarterectomy until better evidence comes in of its benefit. In the meantime most people are more appropriately treated with low-dose aspirin.

Inappropriate Intervention 5. Angioplasty

Angioplasty, commonly known as the balloon, is a procedure in which fatty blockages in coronary arteries are pulverized by inflating a tiny balloon mounted on a catheter threaded into the heart. The doctor performing the procedure watches on an X-ray monitor and, when the catheter tip is in the area of the blockage, inflates the balloon. Angioplasty is the medical revolution that was supposed to reduce the need for more-invasive bypass surgery, but it hasn't worked that way. During the seven years up to 1990, in which the bypass rate doubled, the number of yearly angioplasties in the United States went from 30,000 to 285,000. As is so often the case with medical innovation, a new procedure doesn't replace an old one, it merely takes its place alongside the old one.

Consider the following before agreeing to an angioplasty:

- *The surge in popularity of angioplasty has been based more on wishful thinking than on science.* Recent studies suggest that angioplasty is helpful when performed immediately after a heart attack, but there have never been controlled experiments comparing angioplasty to bypass surgery or to drug therapy. There are no studies that prove that angioplasty increases life expectancy, although it can reduce symptoms. Nonetheless, the procedure is sold to patients, some of whom have no symptoms, with the implicit promise that if they have it, their chances of living longer will be improved.

- *One reason that angioplasty may not improve life expectancy is that its effects often don't last long.* Many of the blockages recur, leading to frequent repeat angioplasties and sometimes to surgery. Doctors judge an angioplasty to be a success when they reduce the blockage—a judgment they themselves make—but whether this translates into a lower risk for the patient is unclear.

- *Although angioplasty is much less invasive than bypass surgery, it is still a major medical procedure with serious risks.* Heart attacks, bleeding, and infections are possible outcomes. Because of the risks and the uncertainty about long-term benefits, many of the angioplasties done today must be considered of uncertain appropriateness.

- *The financial aspects of angioplasty are particularly troubling.* With bypass surgery you usually consult a cardiologist or internist who recommends the procedure and then refers you to a surgeon. With angioplasty, the same doctor who recommends the procedure stands to make a lot of money if you have one. By performing just one angioplasty per week, a cardiologist can pad his or her yearly income by $100,000 or more. With profit-sharing plans these doctors even stand to make money if other doctors carry out the procedure. Money may not be the primary motivator for most cardiologists, but it may color their judgment.

Inappropriate Intervention 6. Pacemakers

Pacemakers are one of the great technical advances of modern medicine. People with dangerously slow or irregular heart-beats, who would otherwise have debilitating symptoms, can function normally. The devices have saved thousands of lives. Like many other interventions, however, pacemakers are some-times recommended to people who don't need them. Currently about a half million Americans have pacemakers, and about one hundred thousand new ones are implanted each year.

Unnecessary Pacemakers

Researchers who examined how often pacemakers were implanted appropriately in thirty-one Philadelphia hospitals found that 44 percent of the pacemakers were definitely necessary, 36 percent questionable, and 20 percent definitely unnecessary. Ten of the thirty-one hospitals had a rate of more than 30 percent inappropriate implantations. Four hospitals had a rate of more than 40 percent inappropriate. Sur-prisingly perhaps, university medical centers did no better than community hospitals in measures of appropriateness.[57]

There are several common errors that lead to inappropriate pacemaker insertion. Many elderly people have slightly low heart rates or have brief pauses in their heartbeats. If these patients suffer lightheadedness or blackouts, many doctors will simply assume the heart is the problem. Even when a slow heart rate is the cause of the symptoms, the slowdown can be caused by an underactive thyroid, a common and easily remedied condition.

Perhaps the most common reason pacemakers are im-planted inappropriately is that the irregular heart beat is caused by drug therapy. Dozens of medicines lead to rhythm disturbances, including digoxin, quinidine, narcotics, beta blockers like Inderal (propranolol) and Lopressor (metoprolol), calcium blockers like Calan (verapamil) and Procardia (nifedipine). A side effect of drug therapy needs to be ruled out before implanting a pacemaker, but many doctors fail to do so.[58]

The insertion of a pacemaker can have devastating effects on a person's life. The procedure itself is simple and generally safe. Serious medical side effects, though, like infections and blood clots, occasionally occur later. The psychological and economic side effects, however, may be more damaging. Once a pacemaker is implanted, a person can have an extremely difficult time getting life insurance, health insurance, and sometimes even a job. Many people have a hard time adjusting to the idea of a pacemaker, an artificial device that must remain there for life and which might fail. Depression and anxiety are not uncommon.[59] These consequences are worth enduring if you've got significant symptoms or are at risk of dropping dead, but not if you never needed the pacemaker in the first place.

Inappropriate Intervention 7.
Interventions Near the End of Life

As medical technology has advanced, we have often become more successful at keeping people alive than at curing them. I've seen dozens of people spend their final days emaciated from disease, tethered to tubes, wires, and machines of various descriptions, hands tied to bedrails to keep them from ripping those tubes and wires out.

Going Gently

In what is arguably one of the finest poems written in the English language, Irish poet Dylan Thomas beseeched his dying father:

Do not go gentle into that good night.
Rage, rage against the dying of the light.*

---

* "Do Not Go Gentle Into That Good Night," from *The Poems of Dylan Thomas*, New York: New Directions Books, 1971.

Whether to rage against the dying of the light is an exquisitely personal decision. Someone who has lived a full life may not want every available wonder of modern technology to stretch that life a few weeks longer. For others, a chance at longer life is worth any burden.

Doctors work for cures. Death is the enemy, and even when the battle seems hopeless, they fight on. Doctors are trained to muster every weapon in their arsenal to prolong life and, if the patient dies, to consider it a failure. When evaluating a doctor's recommendation about life-prolonging therapy, you need to decide what's most important to you—even if your decision will disappoint the doctor.

Deciding for or against life-sustaining interventions does not have to be an all-or-nothing choice. Some interventions may seem reasonable to you, while others may not. It is also possible at times to give an aggressive intervention a shot for a few days to see if it helps and if it doesn't, to withdraw it.

To take one example, some people refuse to allow themselves to be placed on a breathing machine, a mechanical respirator, fearing that if they agree they might end up spending the rest of their life stuck on it. It shouldn't have to be that way. Say an elderly woman is admitted to the hospital with an overwhelming pneumonia. Without the respirator she may have no chance of surviving the night. With it she may have a one-in-four chance of fully recovering and going home. In that situation most but not all people would opt for the respirator. The idea of the respirator is to support the her breathing long enough to give antibiotics a chance to work. If two weeks later she's still on the respirator, her chance of going home has probably dropped to less than one in a hundred. If she's still on it a month later, her chance is just about zero.

For some reason, though, doctors have a different attitude about withholding a treatment like a respirator than about removing it once it's been started. Some doctors view removing a machine that's keeping someone alive as "playing God." They don't view initiating a therapy to prevent a death that would have otherwise occurred as playing God. This desire by physicians not to "be responsible" for a death when a machine is withdrawn leads some people who otherwise might have survived to refuse intervention that might have saved them. Just as doctors should respect your wishes in withholding treatment, they should respect your wishes to withdraw it if it clearly isn't working. Because some doctors are morally opposed to withdrawing life support, be sure to ask your doctor in advance if he or she would have any problem respecting your wishes.

Miracles do occur. Some people whom no one expects to recover, recover. But in my experience, **when miracles happen they usually happen quickly.** Pulling all the technological stops to try to achieve a miracle means that the great majority of terminally ill people are denied the prospect of a peaceful death.

Sixty years ago the majority of Americans died at home. Today the overwhelming majority die in hospitals. Death at home can afford privacy, dignity, and the opportunity for closeness with loved ones that is simply not possible in the hospital. Home health care services like visiting nurses can help the family cope with caring for a dying relative.

When my father was terminally ill, he was hospitalized for several weeks. His condition only worsened. He developed painful bedsores. He hated the food. We could only visit a few hours each day. We decided to bring him home, where he spent the last two weeks of his life. He died peacefully on a hospital bed we'd set up in our living room, holding my mother's hand.

Do Not Resuscitate (DNR) Orders

Almost all hospitalized patients who do not request otherwise will receive CPR (cardiopulmonary resuscitation) if their heart stops beating. Hospital CPR consists of rhythmically and forcefully compressing the chest to circulate blood, delivering electric shocks to restore the heartbeat, and inserting a breathing tube down the throat to deliver oxygen to the lungs.

Almost two-thirds of hospitalized patients do not survive CPR. The majority of people who survive CPR initially don't live long enough to be discharged from the hospital. About 10 percent of survivors end up so brain-damaged that they are reduced to a permanent vegetative state. The chronically ill, such as people with cancer, pneumonia, or kidney failure are particularly unlikely to survive.[60]

To prevent what is likely to be a futile effort at lifesaving, patients can request that they not be resuscitated by asking their doctor to write a DNR order. Because of DNR orders almost 90 percent of people who die in hospitals are not resuscitated. Not everyone should choose to forego CPR. A previously healthy person who suffers a cardiac arrest in an intensive care unit has a good chance of surviving with CPR. Even some chronically ill people will opt for CPR, just for the chance to live a few more days. It's a personal decision.

A DNR order does not mean you necessarily forsake other medical treatments. People who decline CPR may still be treated with antibiotics, artificial feedings, radiation therapy, and other measures, if they desire.

Living Wills and Other Advance Directives

There are three main ways to have your preferences regarding life-sustaining treatment known. You can:

- *Discuss the matter with your physician, family, or friends.* It's always useful to discuss your wishes about life-sustaining treatments with your physician. The more detailed the discussion, the better. Remember, though, that many physicians are intervention-oriented. It may be hard for some of them to believe you wouldn't want the treatment that gives you the best chance at survival. Others may incorrectly guess that you don't want intervention when in fact you do.

How Well Do Doctors Predict Their Patient's Wishes?

Researchers from the University of California at San Diego compared the predictions doctors made about their patients' preferences for life-sustaining treatment with their patients' actual preferences and with what the doctors would want if they were the patients. The patients were all judged to have less than a fifty-fifty chance of surviving five years. The following table summarizes the percentage of patients who would want the interventions, the percentage of doctors who thought the patients would want the interventions, and the percentage of doctors who would want each intervention for themselves in a similar situation:

Intervention	Patients Who Wanted	Doctors' Predictions	Doctors Preferring for Themselves
CPR if heart stopped	93	61	52
breathing machine indefinitely	42	18	25
IV fluids and artificial feeding through tubes indefinitely	23	75	71

These numbers show that the doctors seem to be more influenced by what they themselves would want than by what their patients would want. Doctors who admitted not knowing what their patients would want were excluded from the study: the ones who participated were the ones who thought they knew their patients. If anything, then, this study probably overestimates how well doctors can predict their patients' wishes.[61]

Many of us don't have a regular physician with whom we can discuss our preferences. Even if we do, we may change jobs or select new health insurance plans that force us to change doctors. In these situations, if you discuss your wishes with friends and family members, they can relate your wishes to your doctors if it ever proves necessary. This plan assumes friends and family are available and can remember and agree on what you said.

Whoever you discuss your preferences with, try to talk about your goals. Do you want to live as long as possible, no matter what? Do you want to be comfortable? Do you want to pursue aggressive intervention only when you have a decent chance at a meaningful survival, however you define that? It's also useful to consider a few common scenarios. What would you want if you were no longer mentally competent? Say, for example, that you had an advanced case of Alzheimer's disease and could no longer feed yourself or recognize your loved ones. What if you had an incurable cancer? If you were in terrible pain, would you want strong pain-relieving drugs, even if using them risked hastening your death? If you have an opinion about a case you've heard discussed on television or read in the paper or an opinion about something that's happened to a dying friend or relative, discuss your feelings. If there's something you would never want to happen to you, say so.

- *Write a living will.* A more formal approach is to write a document, known as a living will, to express your wishes. In a living will you might specify what treatments you would desire if you were in a coma, terminally ill, or had become irreversibly demented. There is simply no way, however, that you can anticipate every situation that might occur and what you would want if it did.[62] Say you fill out a detailed living will stating that if you are terminally ill, you wouldn't want antibiotics. You may have envisioned when you filled out the form that you wouldn't want to be hospitalized for intravenous antibiotics to fight a life-threatening infection. But what if you had a painful foot infection that a few days of oral antibiotics could clear up, leaving you more comfortable in your final days? Would you still not want the antibiotics?

  Another problem with relying on a living will is that it may not be there when you need it. If you stash it away in your safe deposit box or leave it in a desk drawer, it may not go with you if you're rushed to the hospital. Be sure to give copies of your living will to your doctor, to a family member, and possibly to a close friend.

- *Appoint a health care proxy.* When you appoint a health care proxy, you give that person legal authority to make decisions for you if you become incapacitated. If you regain your faculties, the authority reverts to you.

  Choose your health care proxy carefully. Your proxy needs to know you well. Studies have shown that even spouses can be poor predictors of what you'd want. To prepare your proxy, be sure to discuss explicitly your goals and feelings about end-of-life medical interventions. And don't forget to notify the person you've chosen. A surprising number of people don't bother to do so.

  It's best if your proxy has no financial interest in what happens to you or unresolved emotional conflicts with you. I have seen several instances in which I felt family members were unwilling to forgo heroic medical treatment for a loved one because they felt guilty about how they'd treated the person years earlier. If you are worried about this prospect, you might want to choose someone outside the family. Since your proxy could have to fight your doctors and even members of your family to have your wishes respected, it helps to choose someone who is assertive, someone not too easily intimidated by authority figures.

Be advised that there are several synonyms for health care proxy in use. Some states call such a person a health care agent, others an attorney-in-fact. The form many states employ is called the durable power of attorney for health care.

Since all of these methods have pros and cons, some combination of them may be the best solution. The combination of a living will and a health care proxy in particular makes a lot of sense. By leaving written instructions, you lessen the burden on your proxy. If the doctors seem to be ignoring the dictates of your living will—an unfortunately all-too-common event—your proxy can call them on it.

A new law, the Patient Self-Determination Act, requires hospitals and nursing homes to ask all patients if they have prepared an advance directive and to provide information on them to patients who desire it. The law does little, however, to promote these discussions before the patient is hospitalized. I strongly encourage you not to wait until you go to a hospital or nursing home to articulate your views; you risk never getting the chance. Being young and healthy is no guarantee. Think of Karen Ann Quinlan.

For more information on living wills and health care proxies, speak with your doctor or contact Choice in Dying at 200 Varick Street, New York, New York 10014. Their telephone number is (800) 989-WILL.

Putting It Together

Benjamin Franklin once wrote that "nothing is more fatal to health than an overcare of it." In this chapter I've talked mostly about the overuse of medical intervention. Please don't infer that all or even most intervention is bad. Every intervention I've discussed, from C-sections to radical prostate surgery to blood transfusions, can be lifesaving. The trick is to be sure you need the intervention, because if you don't, you'll be risking your time, money, and sometimes even your life with no prospect of benefit.

Not having an intervention can, of course, also entail risk. Refusing surgery or chemotherapy in certain instances could cost you your life. Remember, medical intervention itself is neither good nor bad. The question is whether it's applied appropriately or inappropriately. The answer to that question depends on your condition and on your desires.

These days, with increasing attention being paid to the high cost of medical care, there is a risk that you could be denied an intervention for financial reasons. If you are poor or don't have insurance, the risk goes up. We can only hope this situation changes with reform of our health care system. Even those *with* insurance may be denied needed treatment because the insurance company doesn't want to pay for it. Except for the most prohibitively expensive interventions, however, if you truly need it and your doctor is supportive, you can usually still get it. HMOs sometimes try to deny needed interventions for financial reasons. Usually persistence will work here too.

Use the seven principles of appropriate medical intervention covered in this chapter both to evaluate whether you need a

---

Seven Principles of Appropriate Medical Intervention

1. Intervene sparingly.
2. Examine the financial incentives.
3. Favor less invasive interventions.
4. Weigh the risks and benefits.
5. Assess the doctor's track record.
6. Get a second opinion.
7. Stay out of the hospital, if possible.

proposed intervention and to gain insight into your physician's attitudes about intervention in general. Ask yourself, Is this doctor prone to intervention? An unswerving believer in high technology? Unduly influenced by financial considerations? Willing to respect my wishes?

As with drug therapy and medical testing, there is a middle ground between too much intervention and not enough. By getting actively involved in the decisions, you increase the odds of finding that middle ground.

6

IS YOUR DOCTOR PRACTICING GOOD PREVENTIVE MEDICINE?

MOST OF THE LEADING CAUSES OF DEATH IN THIS COUNTRY ARE preventable. Once many of these conditions have arisen, however, often either there is no effective treatment or the treatment available has little effect on the ultimate outcome. In spite of all the highly publicized cures, most of the time all doctors can do is treat symptoms and hope to keep the inevitable in check for a while.

The Top Ten Causes of Death
in the United States, 1990[1]

Cause of Death	Number of Deaths	Percentage of Total
1. heart disease	720,000	33.5
2. cancer	505,000	23.5
3. strokes	144,000	6.7
4. accidents, e.g. car crashes	92,000	4.3
5. chronic lung disease	87,000	4.1
6. pneumonia and influenza	80,000	3.7
7. diabetes	48,000	2.2
8. suicide	31,000	1.4
9. liver disease, e.g. cirrhosis	26,000	1.2
10. AIDS and HIV infection	25,000	1.2

Prevention doesn't have the cachet of something like balloon angioplasty, which when it works can result in dramatic improvements. When a cardiologist navigates a tortuous coronary artery with the catheter and blows up the balloon to obliterate a blockage in an artery, the patient's symptoms may be relieved instantaneously. A heart attack may be averted. It's not uncommon for applause to break out in the cath lab after a doctor successfully completes a difficult maneuver. The skilled cardiologist revels in adulation from patients, nurses, and colleagues.

A spectacular cure is a lot sexier than preventing that illness in the first place, especially if the illness was prevented with talk. No one slaps you on the back to say, "Great job, getting that guy to quit smoking." But in many patients who undergo angioplasty, if a doctor had spent five minutes—and sometimes that's all it takes—convincing them to quit smoking or to start exercising, their angioplasties would never have been necessary. A doctor, though, can never be sure when a preventive effort has paid off. When something bad doesn't happen, it's impossible to prove it would have if you hadn't intervened.

Prevention is among the most important duties of a physician. Many practicing physicians largely ignore it, however, focusing instead on diagnosis and treatment. These doctors act as if prevention and their traditional duties were mutually exclusive. Office visits, in fact, present the perfect opportunity to practice preventive medicine, especially if the doctor and patient have established a relationship of confidence and trust. More importantly, **if prevention isn't incorporated into routine care, it may never happen, since many people only go to the doctor when they're sick.**

The bias against prevention starts in medical school. Students spend countless hours memorizing facts about diseases they may never see in their entire medical careers. Almost no time is devoted to such important subjects as nutrition, even though a poor diet is a major contributor to the top three causes of death—heart attacks, cancer, and strokes. The full extent of my nutrition training in medical school in the early 1980s consisted of memorizing complex chemical reactions involving vitamins. I once asked a professor giving a lecture on heart disease whether he would advise a low-fat diet for heart patients. No, he replied, he would not because there wasn't enough evidence yet of a connection. There was, in fact, already plenty of evidence linking high-fat diets to heart attacks by then, but the professor was reluctant to believe it.

The bias continues in medical practice, where financial barriers hinder prevention. The traditional fee-for-service reimbursement system favors procedures: a doctor receives little financial reward for counseling a patient to quit smoking but is rewarded handsomely for performing an EKG, an X-ray, or a blood test. In HMOs, where there is theoretically more incentive to keep patients healthy, doctors are pressured to see patients quickly—which limits time for preventive medicine. Regardless of the pressures, good doctors talk to their patients about prevention because prevention is good medicine.

Case History: The New Sam Cohen

When I walked out to the waiting room to bring Sam Cohen in for his appointment, I hardly recognized him. Sitting in the chair was a trim and tanned man who bore little resemblance to the patient I'd last seen a year and a half earlier. Since then Sam had lost more than fifty pounds. At the age of fifty-one, he had returned to his high school weight and had never felt better.

During our previous appointment we'd spent a lot of time talking about his high risk for heart attack. Sam's father had his first heart attack at fifty-eight and died of another at sixty-two. A history of premature heart disease in the family is probably the best single predictor of a person's own risk for a heart attack. Just being male is another risk factor. Sam's cholesterol was sky-high at 270 (we like to see it under 200) and he had too much LDL "bad cholesterol" and too little HDL "good cholesterol." His blood pressure had been so high that he had needed two medicines to control it. He had been also taking a pill for gout, a disease sometimes associated with dietary excess. Sam had been overweight and had never exercised. I explained the synergy among the risk factors for heart attack. Sam had high blood pressure, elevated cholesterol, and a family history of heart attacks. One plus one plus one equal ten.

I stressed that if he could cut down on the fat, particularly the saturated fat, in his diet and start exercising, he could substantially lower his risk for heart attack. These two measures could improve his cholesterol numbers, help him lose weight, lower his blood pressure, and improve his overall level of fitness. Since these two actions could affect four separate risk factors for heart attack, he could cut his risk to a fraction of what it was. I'm not sure I can take any credit for bringing him around, because Sam didn't make the changes I suggested right away. Maybe I planted a seed. More likely it was turning fifty that put him more in touch with his mortality. In any case, a few months after I saw him, he and his wife attended a five-day fitness retreat where the regimen of low-fat eating and regular exercise was preached. He got religion.

Sam began reading fitness books and started a regular exercise program. He gradually starting running. He currently averages thirty miles per week. He cut down on red meat, although he still eats it about once a month. The biggest change he made was eliminating various fatty toppings and condiments from his diet. He cut out butter, mayonnaise, cream cheese, and salad dressing altogether. He still eats low-fat frozen yogurt three or four times a week. The results have been dramatic: his most recent cholesterol was 167, down more than a hundred points from his highest reading. His ratio of total cholesterol to HDL "good cholesterol" is way down, lowering his risk of heart attack further.

Not only has Sam lowered his risk of heart attack and probably several types of cancer as well, but he also feels better. It used to be that whenever Sam got home from work, he'd need a nap; now he's so full of energy that he skips it. He also requires about an hour less sleep each night. When things get stressful at work, it doesn't affect him the way it used to. He no longer takes pills for high blood pressure, and his readings are lower now than they were on the medicine. He no longer takes the pill for gout either and hasn't had a single attack. The final benefit is in his wallet: the medicines he was on cost hundreds of dollars a year.

The changes that Sam Cohen made were dramatic and may seem unattainable to many. But you don't have to exercise as much as he does or make such drastic dietary changes to see significant improvement in your health. In fact, I often encourage people to make more moderate changes, because I suspect most people are more likely to sustain moderate changes than draconian ones. If you hate your diet and hate your exercise, the odds are you won't stick with them. And sticking to them is the key: there are no short-term fixes and little long-term benefit to being an angel for a few months.

SEVEN PRINCIPLES OF PREVENTIVE MEDICINE

Prevention Principle 1. Focus on Personal Health Habits

Of all the preventive measures at a doctor's disposal, the ability to counsel people to change unhealthy habits is probably the most powerful. The reason is that the real power to prevent disease lies with patients, not doctors. The way you live profoundly affects your chance of getting certain diseases. Even so, many people seem to have the attitude that they can lead whatever kind of crazy existence they want—junk food, cigarettes, no exercise, high stress—and when they get sick, simply go to the doctor and get fixed. They may be dead wrong.

Are Your Habits Killing You?

Researchers from the federal government and the Carter Presidential Center analyzed how frequently various factors other than heredity caused death in the United States. In their system of accounting, if a heavy smoker died of lung cancer, tobacco was listed as the cause. If a heroin addict died of AIDS-related pneumonia, drug abuse was the cause. If a drunk driver was killed in an accident, alcohol was the cause. The following table summarizes their results:

Factor That Caused Death	Number of Deaths	Percentage of Total
tobacco	400,000	19
poor diet and lack of exercise	300,000	14
alcohol	100,000	5
infections, excluding AIDS	90,000	4
toxins (pollution, chemicals, lead poisoning, etc.)	60,000	3
guns	35,000	2
sexual behavior	30,000	1
motor vehicles	25,000	1
drug abuse	20,000	1

The study's authors point out that in 1993 the United States spent about $900 billion dollars on medical care, or about $14,000 for each family of four. Most of the money was spent to treat the conditions caused by the factors listed above. Less than 5 percent of our health care dollars go toward prevention.[2]

Despite the financial disincentives, good doctors discuss healthy habits with patients. Physicians should educate patients about proper diet and exercise. The typical American eats too many calories, too much fat, too much salt, and not enough fiber. High-fat diets are linked to heart attacks, diabetes, and cancer. Regular exercise is known to reduce stress, lower the risk of a heart attack, and strengthen bones. Just twenty minutes of walking three times a week can bring benefits.

Perhaps one reason that doctors do such a poor job of advising patients about diet and exercise is that their own habits are unhealthy. According to a survey reported recently in the *Wall Street Journal,* more than half of physicians consider themselves overweight, almost a quarter prefer beef for dinner, and only one in five eats the recommended daily servings of fruit and vegetables.[3] If you have any doubt, walk into a hospital cafeteria and look at what the doctors have on their trays. Of course, hospital cafeterias don't give them much choice: they seem to specialize in high-fat, high-salt, highly processed slop. Back on duty, though, doctors down coffee and doughnuts during conferences, coffee and candy bars during long nights on call.

Counseling Patients to Quit Smoking

The hazards of cigarette smoking are well known: they include heart attacks, strokes, emphysema, chronic bronchitis, and several kinds of cancer. Smoking by pregnant women is tied to both low-birth-weight infants and to sudden infant death syndrome. Smoking causes one-third of all residential fires in this country. Smoking not only cuts five or more years off life expectancy but often also leads to a decade or more of lower-quality life before death in people hampered by chronic disease. All in all, smoking represents the largest single cause of preventable illness in this country.

A simple suggestion by the doctor to stop smoking will lead up to 10 percent of patients to quit. Even if a doctor's suggestion leads only a small percentage of people to quit smoking, the benefit is huge to those individuals and to the society that pays the bills for smoking-related disease. Counseling people to quit smoking is one of the most powerful weapons in a doctor's arsenal against disease. If a drug came along that could affect as many people's health as profoundly as getting them to quit smoking, you can bet it would be all over the cover of *Time* and *Newsweek*. But how often do doctors deploy this powerful weapon?

Do Doctors Advise Smokers to Quit?

Doctors from the Michigan Department of Public Health discovered that only 44 percent of smokers had *ever* been advised to quit smoking by a doctor, despite averaging over four doctors' visits per year. Young men and blacks were the least likely to be counseled about smoking. More than a quarter of people who'd already suffered a heart attack or stroke had never been advised to quit.[4]

A doctor who is practicing good preventive medicine will ask you if you smoke and, if you do and are at all interested in quitting, will counsel you on how to go about it. The easiest but not necessarily the best method doctors have to help smokers quit is to write a prescription. Nicotine gum and more recently nicotine patches can help some smokers quit, but they're expensive and more effective when combined with other interventions. There are two aspects to the tobacco habit: the physical addiction to nicotine and the psychological addiction to smoking. The nicotine patch helps only with the former. People who have tried to quit in the past but have failed in the first few days due to anxiety, irritability, or difficulty concentrating may be the best candidates for nicotine patches. Most people who quit don't need them, though, so first it's worth a try without them.

The best success tends to come from a combination of methods: the doctor's advice, self-help materials, support groups and behavior modification techniques such as those offered by the American Cancer Society, and in the minority of people who need them, nicotine patches or gum. Effective counseling by the doctor includes repeatedly advising the patient to stop smoking, setting up a mutually agreeable quit date, and arranging return visits to monitor progress. If the doctor doesn't have the time to do all the counseling personally, a nurse or other employee can assist.

Doctors should advise you about the health consequences of your habits but not harass you. Some doctors can be punitive. I know one doctor who threatened to stop seeing any patient who continued to smoke. Punishment, guilt trips, and other forms of coercion almost never work. The doctor is your medical advisor, not your parent.

Preventing AIDS

In this day and age doctors practicing prevention should inquire about sexual habits. If you are sexually active in anything other than a long-term monogamous relationship, your doctor should be talking to you about preventing AIDS. Even monogamous relationships are not perfectly safe, if your partner was previously infected or has dangerous habits (whether you're aware of them or not). The doctor should determine how risky your sexual practices are and teach you to minimize that risk. A good doctor will not let shyness or embarrassment get in the way of this vital communication.

Your doctor should also ask about IV drug use, since it's another risk factor for AIDS. Don't feel insulted; many respectable-looking people use drugs. Asking is simply part of a thorough patient interview. If you do use IV drugs and your doctor doesn't ask, you should volunteer the information. IV drug users should be quizzed about their sexual habits too, since it is through sex that they pass the AIDS virus to their spouses and lovers. Their sometimes unsuspecting partners can in turn pass the virus to their offspring during pregnancy or by breastfeeding.

Efforts at preventing AIDS by discouraging high-risk sexual behavior and encouraging condom use should lower the risk of other sexually transmitted diseases. Pelvic infections strike about 1 million American women each year and are the number-one cause of infertility in this country. Cervical cancer, caused by the virus associated with genital warts, kills four thousand American women every year. Another sixteen hundred die from sexually acquired hepatitis B infection.[5]

The AIDS epidemic hammers home the importance of prevention. Until a cure is found, prevention is the only method we have to control the epidemic. Only a small percentage of physicians treat a large number of AIDS patients, but every doctor must be able to educate patients about preventing it.

Prevention Principle 2.
Prevent Disease With Vaccines

Vaccines are one of the great success stories of modern medicine. Many serious diseases, including polio, measles, and tetanus, can be prevented by vaccination.

In 1989 a federally appointed panel of experts, the U.S. Preventive Services Task Force, published a series of guidelines on preventive medicine. The experts evaluated the scientific evidence for and against various preventive measures and made recommendations about which ones were appropriate. The following table lists their advice on vaccines for adults.

Vaccines Recommended for Adults[6]

Vaccine	Frequency
tetanus and diphtheria booster	every 10 years
influenza ("flu shots")	yearly after age 65
pneumococcal (pneumonia vaccine)	once at age 65

Most adults at risk never receive the vaccines of proven value. The table below lists the annual death rate in the United States from the infections preventable with these vaccines. The table also lists the current level of vaccination in the United States among people for whom the vaccine is recommended.

Death Rates and Levels of Vaccination[7]

Infection	Annual Death Rate	Current Level of Vaccination, By Percent
tetanus and diphtheria	<25	40
influenza	20,000	30
pneumococcal	40,000	14

To put these numbers in perspective, fewer than one thousand children die annually in the United States of diseases preventable by vaccinations.

When deciding whether or not to be vaccinated, consider the following:

- *For recommended vaccines, the risk of the disease the vaccine prevents is higher than the risk of the vaccine itself.* Vaccines do have side effects, as the infamous 1976 swine flu vaccine demonstrated, but the diseases they prevent usually pose a greater risk. Influenza is a case in point. Influenza is a serious viral infection that causes severe headaches, high fevers, and awful body aches. It shouldn't be confused with the "flu" which many people use as a synonym for the much milder common cold. Young, healthy influenza victims often end up in bed for a week. For those weakened by chronic disease or old age, influenza can kill. Even though twenty thousand people die of influenza each year in the United States, only about 30 percent of those at high risk are vaccinated.

The benefit of flu shots in the elderly and in other people at high risk from influenza is clear.

Flu Shots Decrease Hospitalizations and Deaths

Researchers reporting in the *Journal of the American Medical Association* examined the effect of flu shots on the elderly. They found that flu shots prevented almost 36 percent of all hospital admissions with pneumonia and influenza and almost 25 percent of admissions for all lung conditions. Vaccination lowered the death rate from these conditions 54 percent. Perhaps most surprisingly, flu shots lowered the death rate from all conditions by more than 28 percent. The reason the overall death rate was improved, the authors postulated, is that many people who die of other conditions like heart attacks were first weakened by influenza.[8]

In my experience, many patients refuse flu shots out of fear of side effects. Several have told me they got sick in a prior year following their flu shot and thought the illness was related to the vaccine.

Few Side Effects From Flu Shots

To test how common side effects of flu shots are, researchers from three hospitals in Minnesota compared the reactions of elderly patients given either real flu shots or fake shots containing saltwater. Except for minor arm soreness at the injection site, there were no differences in the side effects reported by the two groups. The researchers concluded that most symptoms people attribute to flu shots were due either to illnesses that coincidentally occurred at the same time or to people's increased awareness of their body in the period immediately following a flu shot.[9]

• *Some vaccines not recommended for the general public are appropriate for people at increased risk of particular infections.* Experts recommend that the pneumococcal vaccine, which offers protection against the most common type of pneumonia, be given to people with chronic heart or lung ailments, even if they are under sixty-five, and probably to anyone with AIDS. German measles, also known as rubella, is of particular concern for woman in the childbearing years because it can cause severe birth defects. Young women who might become pregnant who have not had the rubella vaccine should have a blood test done. If the test shows no protective antibodies, they should have the vaccine and avoid pregnancy for three months.

One of the newest vaccines is for hepatitis B. IV drug users, sexually active gay men, and anyone exposed to blood, such as health care workers and dialysis patients, should get this safe and effective vaccine. Sexual partners of people with hepatitis B should also get it. Although hepatitis B causes fewer deaths than AIDS—about five thousand per year in the United States—it is almost ten times as easy to catch.[10] I spoke earlier of the need to be open with your doctor about your sexuality and drug habits. The information could affect which vaccines are recommended to you. Only about 10 percent of people at risk for hepatitis B have been vaccinated.

- *By getting vaccinated, you not only protect yourself from infection, you protect others who might have caught the infection from you.* People who because of the perceived risk decline vaccines benefit from the risk others have taken. I am generally healthy and not at high risk even if I get influenza. Some of my patients, though, are. Since the flu shot I give them is only about 70 percent effective, I have one every year myself, mostly to protect them. If you have elderly parents or friends with chronic illnesses, you may want to consider more than just your personal risk when deciding whether to be vaccinated.

Prevention Principle 3. Detect Treatable Diseases Early With Screening Tests

For many medical conditions, early detection can spell the difference between cure (or control of the problem) and death or permanent disability. Screening tests, like Pap smears and mammograms, are designed to detect medical conditions before any symptoms develop. Keep the following in mind when deciding whether to undergo screening tests:

- *Screening tests are worthwhile if the conditions they detect are treatable and if early treatment improves the length and quality of your life.* If a mammogram picks up a breast cancer at a stage where it can be cured, then the test is justified and desirable. Ideally, screening tests should be cheap, reliable, and safe.

  Pap smears, for instance, screen for cervical cancer. Years before cancer develops, Pap smears can detect abnormal cells. The test is not foolproof; it occasionally misses a cancer. There are two main causes for this error: inadequate sampling by the doctor during the exam and incorrect interpretation of the microscope slides in the lab. Despite all the attention given in the last few years to inaccurate readings by labs, several studies suggest that sampling errors by physicians are a bigger problem.[11] When correctly performed and interpreted, the Pap smear appears to be one of the best screening tests available.

  In order to take an adequate specimen, the doctor should take at least two specimens and place them on a slide immediately. The slide must be immersed in alcohol or sprayed with fixative within the first few seconds or the specimen deteriorates, lowering the quality. When your doctor gives you the results of a Pap, be sure to ask about the adequacy of the specimen, which should be stated right on the report from the lab.

  The misreading of an abnormal Pap smear, a so-called false negative reading, appears to be an especially common problem in large labs, which churn out thousands of Paps per year. Some of these labs have been faulted for not allowing technicians adequate time to analyze the slides, in their desire to increase profits. Recent improvements in federal law should improve the situation by limiting the number that can be read per day. In no case should a technician read more than ninety per day, and seventy or fewer is optimal.[12] Ask your doctor where your Pap smear will be sent and why that lab was chosen.

The Pap test can also be abnormal even though no cancer is developing. These false positive results may lead to unnecessary biopsies and even surgery. If the Pap result is mildly abnormal, the best course of action is simply to repeat the test.

Most authorities recommend women start getting Pap smears at age eighteen or when they start sexual activity, although the benefit of starting at eighteen instead of, say, twenty-three, appears to be small. The most important risk factors for cervical cancer are starting sex at an early age and having had multiple sex partners. Smokers have a 50 percent greater chance of getting the cancer than nonsmokers. Race is also a factor: African Americans, Latinos and Native Americans are twice as likely as whites or Asians to get it.[13] As long as a woman has previously been screened regularly and had negative smears, the benefit of continuing Pap smears beyond age sixty-five appears to be minimal.

Ironically, the Pap smear may be one preventive test some doctors have embraced too wholeheartedly. The suggestion that all women get a Pap every year seems excessive, although that's what most gynecologists recommend. I know an elderly woman who is a virgin—and therefore doesn't need Pap smears at all—whose gynecologist was bringing her in every six months for the exam, something pretty traumatic for her.

Women who have Pap smears every three years instead of annually get about 96 percent of the benefit with considerably less hassle and expense.[14] Whether the added security of a more frequent test is worth it is a personal choice that should be made by the woman herself and not by the doctor. Women with risk factors for cervical cancer may want to opt for more frequent smears.

- *There is major disagreement among different organizations about which and how many screening tests are appropriate.*

The table below lists the screening tests recommended for adults by the U.S. Preventive Services Task Force.

Screening Tests Recommended for Adults by the U.S. Preventive Services Task Force[15]

Test	Frequency
measurement of height and weight	periodically
blood pressure check	regularly
cholesterol level	periodically (most important for middle-aged men)
Pap smear	every 1–3 years until age 65
breast exam (by a doctor)	yearly after age 40
mammogram	every 1–2 years after age 50 (after age 35, if at high risk) until age 75
vision test	after age 65
hearing test	after age 65
urinalysis	after age 65
thyroid function	after age sixty-five in women only
glaucoma (by an eye specialist)	after age 65

The task force felt there was insufficient evidence to make a recommendation either for or against a few other screening tests. In this category fell regular rectal exams to screen for prostate cancer and screening tests for colon cancer, including checks for hidden blood in the stool and sigmoidoscopy, a test in which the colon is viewed through a tube inserted in the rectum. The task force concluded that these tests may be worthwhile but couldn't make a definitive recommendation until more studies are done.

The American Cancer Society recommends many tests

that the U.S. Preventive Services Task Force felt were either unproven or of no benefit. The following summarizes the society's recommendations for routine screening for various cancers.

Screening Tests Recommended for Adults by the American Cancer Society[16]

Test	Frequency
examination of the skin, mouth, thyroid, testicles, ovaries, and lymph nodes	every 3 years until 40, then yearly
breast exam (by a doctor)	every 3 years until 40, then yearly
Pap smear	yearly if 3 consecutive yearly smears are negative, then less often, at the discretion of the physician
mammogram	at age 40, then every 1–2 years until 50, then yearly
rectal exam	yearly after age 40
stool test for hidden blood	yearly after age 50
sigmoidoscopy, preferably flexible	every 3–5 years after age 50
prostate specific antigen (PSA)	yearly after age 50

Many doctors, including me, find some of the American Cancer Society's recommendations excessive. In fact, the cancer society's most recent guidelines eliminate some recommendations they've been making for years. Until recently they advised screening mammograms for all women starting at thirty-five instead of forty. There never was proof that routine mammograms at thirty-five saved lives. Unfortunately, their changed recommendations got little publicity, and many women continue to think they're supposed to get a baseline mammogram at thirty-five.

Unlike the U.S. Preventive Services Task Force, the American Cancer Society makes its recommendations based on the opinions of advisors rather than strictly on scientific evidence. If a preventive test has clearly been shown to lack value, the society won't recommend it, but when in doubt, it tends to. You may decide you want to follow the American Cancer Society's guidelines, but remember that most experts don't agree with all its recommendations.

To understand the differences in recommendations of the various groups, let's examine the issue of mammograms for women in their forties in more detail. The major controversy over mammography involves when to start having them done. The American College of Physicians and the U.S. Preventive Services Task Force both recommend mammography before age fifty only for women at increased risk of breast cancer. The American Cancer Society recommends them for all women starting at forty.

Hearing the cancer society's public service announcements that one in eight women will develop breast cancer, many younger women opt for mammograms. While the percentage of women over fifty-nine having mammograms has declined since 1985, the numbers are growing for both women under fifty and women under forty. Nearly 85 percent of breast cancers, however, strike women over fifty.[17]

Should a forty-year-old woman at average risk have a mammogram? To help decide, consider the following numbers derived from a recent editorial in the *New England Journal of Medicine:*[18]

Thirteen out of every 1,000 women will develop breast cancer between the ages of forty and fifty.

Five of those thirteen cancers will be so slow-growing that the women will survive even if they aren't screened with breast exams and mammograms.

Another 5.7 of those thirteen cancers will be so aggressive that screening will not improve the cure rate.

Another 2.3 of those thirteen cancers will be cured due

to early detection, 1.5 detected via the breast exam, and 0.8 detected via the mammogram.

Of 1,000 women screened with mammograms every year, 345 between the ages of forty and fifty, will receive false positive results—resulting in anxiety, repeat mammograms, and such further testing as biopsies.

For women aged forty to fifty, adding yearly mammograms onto breast exams will save one woman in 1,250, but at considerable hassle and expense. It may be worth it to some women but not to others. It's a decision that each woman should make for herself.

- *Some screening tests not recommended for the general public may be worthwhile for individuals at increased risk of particular conditions.* The recommendations from the U.S. Preventive Services Task Force and from the American Cancer Society shown above are for the general public. People at greater-than-average risk may benefit from additional tests. Consider AIDS tests. The U.S. Preventive Services Task Force found routine HIV tests for the general public unwarranted but recommended them for people whose behavior puts them at increased risk for AIDS.

- *Some tests that are not useful in screening have value in diagnosing people with symptoms.* This chapter only discusses their usefulness to screen for disease in people with no symptoms. Many of the principles that we discussed in the chapter on tests, however, apply to screening tests. They can be falsely positive or falsely negative; they cost money, cause side effects, and may be ordered inappropriately or not ordered when they ought to be.

Prevention Principle 4.
Weigh the Risks and Benefits

For any preventive measure you are considering, from vaccines to mammograms, you should carefully weigh the risks and the benefits before making your decision. Preventive tests and treatments cost money and often have side effects. You have to decide whether the expected benefit justifies the expense, hassle, and risk. Even a simple screening test, if abnormal, can initiate a cascade of events that may not be to your benefit.

Screening for Prostate Cancer

In the past few years there has been a great ballyhoo about the prostate specific antigen (PSA) test. Reports in medical journals, in newspapers, and on TV have heralded this new "breakthrough" in the early detection of prostate cancer. Despite all the enthusiasm, many doctors are not yet convinced the PSA is a useful screening test. Consider the following:

- *The PSA test is far from perfect.* The test is normal in 25 to 45 percent of men with localized prostate cancer and moderately elevated in up to half of men with benign enlargement of the prostate, an extremely common condition of older men.[19] The higher the PSA level, however, the greater the likelihood of prostate cancer. The traditional rectal exam is also an imperfect way to detect prostate cancer. Up to 60 percent of men with prostate cancer have tumors that cannot be felt. By the time many tumors can be felt, they have already spread beyond the prostate.[20]
- *Despite the lack of proof of its usefulness, PSA testing is already in wide use.* Because of all the attention in the press and the recommendation of the American Cancer Society, millions of PSA tests are being done every year. One of the most common questions I get from my male patients is whether they should have "the prostate test."
- *Only a small minority of those screened for prostate cancer will benefit.* The risk of widespread screening programs for prostate cancer is that many men who would have never developed symptoms will be subjected to the expense and inconvenience of further testing, the worry and anxiety of a cancer diagnosis, and the sometimes debilitating side effects and risk of death associated with major prostate surgery.
 Even if treatment for prostate cancer is effective—which

is still unproven—many men with less aggressive forms of prostate cancer will need to be treated to benefit the minority with more aggressive tumors. As we've seen, many men with prostate cancer do not benefit from aggressive treatment and are best treated with watchful waiting.

- *Being labeled with a cancer diagnosis can itself cause harm.* Once a man has been diagnosed with prostate cancer, even if he is one of the majority who will never get symptoms from it, his life will never be the same again. The psychological effects of knowing you have cancer can be profound. Depression and anger are common. This fate seems especially tragic for those men who would have lived out the remainder of their lives not knowing they had cancer. The diagnosis of cancer in your medical records may also make it impossible for you to obtain life insurance or decent medical coverage. Job discrimination also becomes a concern.

- *There is controversy in the medical community about whether we should be screening for prostate cancer at all.* Studies have shown that the incidence of asymptomatic prostate cancer is huge: most men who have prostate cancer never develop symptoms, and many of those who do die from other causes.

The High Incidence of Undiagnosed Prostate Cancer

Men who die from conditions other than prostate cancer are commonly found to have small areas of prostate cancer when autopsies are performed. Almost 30 percent of men aged fifty to fifty-nine, 40 percent of men aged seventy to seventy-nine, and 67 percent of men over eighty were found to have prostate cancer on autopsy, even though it had never caused symptoms and had never been recognized during their lifetimes.[21]

Considering the overall frequency of prostate cancer, even though most men never become symptomatic, prostate cancer is still one of the leading causes of cancer deaths. The problem is that prostate cancer is highly variable. In many men it sits there for decades without causing any problems. In others it is rapidly fatal. Unfortunately, the PSA can't reliably differentiate aggressive prostate cancer from the more common slow-growing forms.

Given these concerns and the lack of evidence that early treatment of prostate cancer improves the outcome, the U.S. Preventive Services Task Force has recommended against routine use of PSA tests. The task force felt there was insufficient evidence to recommend either for or against routine rectal exams. The American Cancer Society, on the other hand, recommends yearly rectal exams starting at forty and PSA tests for all men over fifty.

Routine rectal exams and PSA tests are imperfect methods to screen for prostate cancer, but at this point they are the best imperfect methods we have. You may opt for these tests, but be advised that we don't yet know whether these tests will help lengthen your life or improve its quality. They could do the opposite.

Unfortunately, you have to make your decisions about prevention based on less-than-complete information. All you can do is make an informed judgment and hope for the best. As more information comes in, you can modify your strategy as seems appropriate.

Hormone Treatment at Menopause

At menopause the ovaries stop producing the female hormone estrogen, causing a number of changes in the body. Hot flashes, the best-known symptom of menopause, are due to sudden fluctuations in estrogen levels. Some women barely seem to notice menopause, while others find the symptoms debilitating.

When contemplating estrogen therapy, consider the following issues:

- *Hormone replacement therapy was first introduced to fight the symptoms of menopause but in recent years has been increasingly prescribed for another reason: life extension.* Experts now believe that estrogen therapy lowers the risk of heart disease—the number-one killer of elderly women— and of osteoporosis. Osteoporosis thins bones and leads to fractures of the hips, arms, and spine. Osteoporosis also kills: between 15 and 20 percent of the 250,000 hip fractures per year in the United States are fatal.[22] If an elderly woman breaks her hip and ends up bed-bound, then months later dies of pneumonia, it's fair to say that osteoporosis killed her.

- *The studies reporting the beneficial effects of estrogen are all flawed.* The main problem is that women who choose to take estrogen may have healthier habits and may be at lower risk for various medical conditions than women who don't. Despite the uncertainty, Premarin, one brand of estrogen, is the number-one prescribed drug in the United States.[23]

- *Estrogen therapy is not without risk.* Estrogen increases the risk of cancer of the lining of the uterus, known as endometrial cancer. Endometrial cancer is rarely fatal among women taking estrogens, although the treatment, hysterectomy, like any major surgery, entails some risk. Study results are conflicting, but it appears that estrogen may also increase the risk of breast cancer slightly.

Advantages and Disadvantages of Estrogen Treatment at Menopause

Disadvantages	Advantages
increased risk of endometrial cancer	longer life expectancy
slightly increased risk of breast cancer	lower risk of heart attacks
side effects, including bloating, breast tenderness, vaginal bleeding	lower risk of osteoporosis
increased need for screening tests for endometrial cancer	reduction in menopausal symptoms
increased risk of hysterectomy	fewer urinary problems
need to take medicine daily	better sex

- *Adding another hormone, progestin, to estrogen appears to eliminate the risk of endometrial cancer.* Women who take both hormones together don't need more screening tests for endometrial cancer and should not be at increased risk of hysterectomy. Progestin may increase the risk of breast cancer even further, although the experts aren't sure yet. Progestin's effects on heart disease aren't yet known either. Because doctors have only recently started using estrogen and progestin together, and good studies have not yet been done, all doctors can do is give you their best guess.

  As you'd expect, adding a second drug, progestin, increases the risk of side effects. The majority of women taking both drugs experience vaginal bleeding. Other possible side effects include breast tenderness and depression. Some studies suggest that progestin decreases estrogen's positive effects on sex.

- *Women opting for long-term estrogen therapy to prevent osteoporosis should make the decision right around the time of menopause.* Even before a woman's periods have completely stopped, bone loss is already occurring. If you wait several months or longer to start estrogen, some of the potential benefit in preventing osteoporosis is lost. The risks stay the same, but the benefit declines. I therefore encourage women to think about the issue of estrogen therapy before they hit menopause. Consider too that women who stop taking estrogen quickly lose much of the bone the drug was helping preserve. If you're on it to prevent osteoporosis, you need to stay on it.

- *Women whose primary goal is to alleviate hot flashes and other menopausal symptoms may only need to take hormones for a few months or a few years.* The cancer risk from short-term use is probably small. Most experts recommend hormone therapy to women with severe symptoms. Whether to continue that therapy long-term is a separate question.

- *Different women will look at the advantages and disadvantages of long-term hormone therapy and make different decisions.* Some women will fear the increased risk of cancer and decide against treatment. Some people just don't like the idea of taking a pill every day for the rest of their lives. Others view the prospect of increased life expectancy as worth the effort. Some women consider reducing menopausal symptoms, lowering the risk of urinary infections, and improving sex as motivating factors in their decision for hormone therapy. The point is that the decision to take hormone therapy at menopause is a highly personal one, fraught with uncertainty. It may be decades before scientists sort out all the risks and benefits of therapy. In the meantime I believe the decision is best made by a woman herself and not by her doctor acting in a paternalistic fashion.

As we'll discuss in the following section, the decision on hormone therapy should also be influenced by a women's personal risk for the medical conditions that are affected by treatment. Risk factors for heart disease, osteoporosis, or breast cancer could tip the scales either for or against therapy.

- *Drug therapy is not the only option.* Women at risk for osteoporosis or heart disease can improve their chances considerably by quitting smoking, eating better, and exercising more. Unlike those of drugs, the side effects of these interventions are generally beneficial.

Prevention Principle 5. Personalize Prevention According to Your Risks

Because every person presents a unique constellation of risks, prevention must be personalized. Which preventive measures make sense depends on your age, sex, race, habits, and your family's history of medical problems. Osteoporosis is much more common in women than men and almost never occurs in blacks. Blacks are much more likely to be blinded by glaucoma. Women suffer heart attacks but usually years later than men. As we've seen, dietary, exercise, and smoking habits profoundly affect your risk for cancer, heart attacks, and many other problems.

Which preventive tests are done should also reflect your overall level of health. If you are a sixty-five-year-old man with severe emphysema, screening for elevated cholesterol or colon cancer probably doesn't make sense since you are unlikely to live long enough to benefit from the screening. If you are an active seventy-five-year-old woman, your life expectancy is ten more years, and continued screening for breast cancer may be reasonable.

Let's return to the example of hormone therapy at menopause to explore how your personal risk affects which preventive measures make the most sense.

Individual Factors in Deciding on Hormone Therapy at Menopause

Estrogen therapy lowers the risks of some medical conditions and increases the risk of others. Your decision may depend in large measure on what conditions you're at risk for. Women whose mothers or sisters had breast cancer may be reluctant to take a drug that may even slightly increase their already high risk. Women who have already had a hysterectomy are at no risk of endometrial cancer and experts recommend almost all of them take estrogen. There is no reason, however, to take progestin along with it.

Hormone Therapy and Life Expectancy in Different Women

Researchers from several San Francisco hospitals calculated the effects of hormone therapy at menopause in women at risk for various medical conditions. The table below lists the medical conditions a hypothetical fifty-year-old white woman is at risk for, her life expectancy in years, and the expected change in life expectancy from hormone treatment. The researchers arrived at an optimistic and a pessimistic appraisal of the effects of combined estrogen-progestin therapy on life expectancy, since the therapy has not been studied well enough to provide definitive answers.

Change in Life Expectancy in Years on:

Medical Condition Woman at Risk for	Life Expectancy Without Hormones (in Years)	Estrogen Only	Estrogen-Progestin (Optimistic)	Extrogen-Progestin (Pessimistic)
heart disease	79.6	+1.5	+1.6	+0.6
hip fracture	82.4	+1.0	+1.1	+0.2
breast cancer	82.3	+0.7	+0.8	−0.5

The researchers further calculated that women who have already had a hysterectomy on average gain 1.1 years of life expectancy on estrogen. Women who already have heart disease stand to gain the most from hormone replacement, over two years. Although black women are at markedly lower risk of hip fracture than white women, they are also at somewhat lower risk of breast cancer and endometrial cancer. Their rates of heart disease are similar to those of whites. Weighing all these factors, the authors calculated that black women should achieve about the same gain in life expectancy from hormone therapy as white women. The authors recommend that all women with hysterectomies and all women at risk for heart disease consider hormone therapy. They believe that for other women the best course of action is not yet clear.[24]

The right choice is more than a matter of just looking at the numbers for life expectancy. Taking estrogen may raise the *average* life expectancy, but if a women develops breast cancer who otherwise wouldn't have, she is harmed by the therapy. Breast cancer also tends to strike women younger than those who suffer heart attacks or hip fractures. Women may therefore be trading an increased risk of cancer in the short-term for a lower risk of heart disease and osteoporosis in the long-term.[25] Remember too that the estimates of the improved life expectancy with hormone treatment are based on flawed studies. The real benefit may be less than the experts currently estimate.

Besides looking at your personal risk, you need to consider your personal values. You have to with choose your poison. Would you rather live longer if by doing so you increase your risk of dying of cancer? Some people would rather go sooner of a heart attack. Once again there is no right answer, only the answer that makes the most sense to you.

Should You Take Medication to Lower Your Cholesterol?

The country's current preoccupation with lowering cholesterol is another example of how preventive measures that make sense for one person may be ill-advised in another. Many doctors have a threshold for prescribing cholesterol-lowering drugs: anybody whose level climbs above, say, 240 gets a prescription. The decision to start medication, however, should not be so simple.

Case History: Worried Sick About Her Cholesterol

Margaret DeIulio was crestfallen when she got back her most recent cholesterol level. It had risen from 232 to 254 despite her best efforts to lower the fat in her diet. As a nurse Margaret was aware of the recommendation to "know your number" and has followed her cholesterol closely for years. Now she was worried sick about her risk of suffering a heart attack. I work with Margaret and have seen her study the nutrition labels on boxes of crackers to determine the fat content and have watched her munch carrot sticks and nonfat rice cakes with her lunch.

Despite her elevated cholesterol, Margaret's risk for heart attack is actually lower than most people's. There is no history of premature heart disease in her family. Margaret's mother, a one-time heavy smoker, died in her late eighties of emphysema. Margaret doesn't smoke. She walks regularly, isn't overweight, and doesn't have high blood pressure or diabetes. Her sole risk factor for heart attack is her high cholesterol level.

Because of the synergy between risk factors for heart attack— that is the multiplying effect of multiple risk factors—when you've only got one, your risk isn't very great. That's why I have a problem with the simplistic recommendation of well-intentioned public health experts to "know your number." A more sensible recommendation is to view your cholesterol in context. If it's 250 and if, as in Margaret case, it's your only risk factor, I wouldn't be overly concerned. If your father had a heart attack at the age of forty, I'd worry about a reading of 215.

When I reassured Margaret about her low risk for a heart attack, the furrows in her brow disappeared. I advised her to continue her low-fat diet and her walking program—sensible advice for everyone—but to try not to worry about it all. One thing is for sure: I'd wouldn't recommend she take drugs to lower her cholesterol level.

When contemplating cholesterol-lowering medication, consider the following:

- *The decision on cholesterol-lowering medication should reflect your overall constellation of risk factors for heart attack.* The following appear to increase the risk of a heart attack:
    - —a family history of premature heart disease
      being a male
    - —elevated cholesterol
    - —low HDL "good cholesterol"
    - —elevated triglycerides (another form of fat in the blood)
    - —smoking
    - —diabetes
    - —high blood pressure
      a lack of exercise
    - —being overweight (probably only a mild risk factor)

  Because of the multiplying effect on risk, the presence of several risk factors is of much more concern than just one or two.

- *The total cholesterol number gives only part of the picture.* High levels of LDL "bad cholesterol" and low levels of HDL "good cholesterol" are more strongly correlated with heart attacks than elevations of total cholesterol. Some people have high total cholesterols but low overall risk because their HDL levels are so high. At the time of her cholesterol reading of 258, Margaret's HDL was 52, which is not bad, and her LDL level was only in the borderline elevated range. Margaret's cholesterol problem, like Wagner's music (according to Mark Twain), is not as bad as it sounds.

- *Many labs, particularly labs in doctors' offices, do a poor job of measuring cholesterol.* Before starting on cholesterol-lowering medication, be sure your cholesterol test result is accurate. Finger-stick cholesterol levels, such as those offered at health fairs or in shopping malls, are so inaccurate that they are worthless. Actually, they are probably worse than worthless. By misleading some people into thinking they have high cholesterol, they cause anxiety and lead to unnecessary visits to doctor. More commonly, people are mistakenly informed that their cholesterol is fine and may delay getting rechecked, thereby missing an opportunity for valuable preventive measures.

- *Cholesterol levels vary depending on the time of year and on stress levels.* Because of the natural variation in cholesterol levels and on the lack of accuracy of some cholesterol tests, no one should be placed on cholesterol-lowering medicine on the basis of a single reading. Cholesterol wreaks its damage over decades. A few weeks' delay in starting even needed medication makes little difference in the long run. If you are contemplating treatment, it's best to make the decision based on the average of two or more readings done at a reliable lab. It's also advisable to give diet and exercise six months or more to work before resorting to drugs.

- *It is not proven that drugs that lower cholesterol increase your odds of living longer.* Three large studies have shown that middle aged men given different cholesterol-lowering drugs had fewer fatal heart attacks. The results were mixed, however, on whether the overall death rate was lowered, possibly because of side effects of the drugs. So far there are no good studies demonstrating that cholesterol-lowering drugs improve life expectancy of women, younger men, or the elderly, although doctors aren't waiting for proof.

- *The benefits of drug therapy tend to be framed in a misleading fashion.* One major study reported that the drug Lopid (gemfibrozil) lowered the risk of heart disease by 34 percent in men who took it for five years.[26] The *Boston Globe* ran a front-page headline touting the better than one-third reduction in heart attacks. What those statistics didn't tell was that for every 1,000 men in the study who took Lopid, 973 did not have a heart attack, compared with 959 out of every 1,000 who took a placebo. Stated differently, each man had to take the medicine for five years to improve his chances of not having a heart attack from 96 to 97 percent.

The study's authors also downplayed the fact that taking the drug didn't lower the overall death rate.[27]

This is not to say that cholesterol drugs may not benefit some people. It's just that many people need to take expensive drugs, some of unknown long-term safety, for a few people to benefit. When the results of studies are presented as percentage differences, you tend to come away with an overly optimistic view of a drug's effectiveness. Researchers looking to advance their careers, the media looking for a good story, and the drug companies looking to boost sales all tend to present data in this misleading fashion.

- *The safety and effectiveness of the most prescribed drugs for high cholesterol are unknown.* These days the drug American doctors are most likely to prescribe for high cholesterol is Mevacor (lovastatin). Mevacor is relatively new, so by definition its long-term safety is unknown. Within one year of its introduction on the market it was the number one prescribed drug for elevated cholesterol. It is extremely effective in lowering cholesterol and has few short-term side effects, but there is no evidence it improves life expectancy. The drug is also incredibly expensive. At my local discount pharmacy, a one-month supply of the lowest recommended daily dose of Mevacor costs over $57—almost two bucks a pill. Most people who take it are expected to need it for the rest of their lives.

Since the long-term risks and benefits of most cholesterol-lowering drugs are not yet known, at this point you've got to make your decision based on incomplete information. The higher your risk of a heart attack, the more risk you can justify in trying to prevent it. Even given the uncertainty, I recommend cholesterol-lowering drugs to some people with markedly elevated readings and other risk factors for a heart attack, if changes in diet and exercise haven't sufficed to lower their level. Given the new evidence of the effectiveness of simvastatin, those at very high risk for heart attacks should consider the drug. Keep in mind, however, that like its chemical cousin lovastatin, simastatin is new, expensive, and while it appears relatively safe in the short term, its long-term safety is unknown. Those at lower risk may want to try out non-drug therapies like oat bran or garlic which lower cholesterol moderately with very little risk.

Should You Have Your Home Tested for Radon?

Radon is an odorless and colorless gas that is thought to contaminate one in fifteen homes in the United States. This naturally occurring radioactive gas is believed to cause thousands of lung cancers deaths every year, second only to smoking; the higher the radon level in your home, the greater the risk. Primary care doctors should therefore be asking their patients if they've had their homes tested.

Not everyone needs to test their homes, though. Since radon seeps up from the soil, levels are generally highest in the basement and on the ground floor. People who live above the second floor are not considered to be at risk.

Several factors increase your risk of lung cancer from radon. If you smoke, your risk is multiplied. Your risk also depends on the amount of time you spend at home—particularly on the lower floors—and on the length of time you live in homes with high levels. If you smoke, are at home at lot, or plan to live in your home for many years, it's especially prudent to have your home tested.

Do-it-yourself radon testing kits are inexpensive and available at most hardware stores. Be sure to look for one that says it meets Environmental Protection Agency (EPA) requirements. If high levels are found in your home, effective measures can be taken to lower them. The average fix costs a little over a thousand dollars. For more information, call your state's radon office or the National Radon Hotline at (800) SOS-RADON. For written material, call the Indoor Air Quality Information Clearinghouse at (800) 438-4318.

Prevention Principle 6. Prevent Injuries

Has your doctor ever asked you if you wear your seat belt every time you get into a car? Has the doctor asked you if you ever drive after having a few drinks? If your hobby is mountain biking, has the doctor asked if you wear a helmet? If not, your doctor isn't doing a great job at preventive medicine. You may not feel that injury prevention fits into a doctor's traditional duties. Many doctors feel the same way. When you consider how many routine blood tests and physical exams a doctor must do to save one life, however, it becomes clear why devoting a minute or two to preventing some of the leading causes of death and disability makes sense.

For people under forty-five in the United States, car accidents are the number-one cause of death. While your chance of getting in an accident any one time you drive is low, most of us drive so much that the average American has a one-in-three lifetime risk of getting in a disabling accident. Some of the risk from car accidents is uncontrollable, but one action—buckling up—can make a huge difference. Seat belts cut the risk of death or serious injury in a car accident in half. Working in emergency rooms, I felt I could take one look at the people being wheeled in and guess whether they'd been wearing their seat belts or not. The people with the more serious injuries almost invariably hadn't been. Even so, one-third of Americans don't wear their seat belts.

Most preventable deaths from car accidents happen at low speeds. In many high-speed accidents, the g forces are simply too great for a seat belt or airbag to save you. Even low-speed accidents generate tremendous force. A sudden stop from thirty miles per hour is the equivalent of falling from a three-story building.[29] This is precisely the kind of accident where a seat belt is most likely to make a difference. While airbags lower your risk of death or injury in a head-on accident, they are no substitute for seat belts. Early evidence suggests that an airbag alone may be less effective than a lap and shoulder belt alone. The combination of seat belts and airbags offers the best protection.

Since forty percent of people killed in car accidents are intoxicated by alcohol, doctors ought to advise their patients who drink alcohol to avoid drinking and driving. The message should be *not even one*. Drugs other than alcohol are implicated in 10–20 percent of crashes, so doctors should be talking about them too.

Unintentional injuries are the leading cause of death in young people and still rank number six in people over sixty-five. The largest cause of injuries in the elderly is falling. One of their main risks from a fall is a broken hip. Besides the risk of death, hip fractures also threaten an elderly person's independence. The loss of functioning after a hip fracture is a common reason for admission to a nursing home. A doctor's efforts to prevent osteoporosis by prescribing calcium and hormone treatment can reduce the risk of a hip fracture.

Preventing the fall that causes the hip fracture can be even more effective. A doctor can do several things to try to lessen an elderly patient's risk of falling. First, the doctor should routinely ask if the person has had any falls. Unless they are injured, many people will not mention falls to their doctor.

The doctor should be sure the vision of elderly patients is routinely checked, since failing vision contributes to many falls. Many medicines, including blood pressure pills, sleeping pills, and over-the-counter remedies, can contribute to falls. Sedatives and tranquilizers, in particular, should be avoided. Since different drugs can interact in unexpected ways, the elderly should take as few medications as possible and at the lowest effective dose. The doctor should encourage exercise, since it helps improve strength, balance, and mobility.

In people who have already had falls or who seem at risk for falls, the doctor should ask several questions about the home environment. Is there adequate lighting in the stairways and halls? Are there throw rugs or electrical cords in the house they could trip on? The doctor can make other suggestions: in the bathroom, grab rails, rubber mats, and friction treads in the tub all lessen the risk of falls. Colored tape on stairs and proper handrails can help as well.

There are several other worthwhile measures to prevent accidental injury or death that doctors usually don't have time to mention. Here are a few:

Install smoke detectors in your house.

Wear bicycle and motorcycle helmets.

Don't smoke in bed or near upholstery.

Turn hot water temperature down to 120°F.

Don't keep a gun in the house. If you feel you must, keep it unloaded and lock it up.

Prevention Principle 7. Avoid Ineffective Preventive Measures

If you're spending your time getting routine physical exams instead of Pap smears and flu shots, your preventive efforts may be misdirected. Chest X-rays and routine blood tests have become mainstays of many doctors' preventive efforts, even though they are just about worthless in people with no symptoms. It may seem harmless to have a preventive test you don't really need. Maybe you and your doctor just want to be sure. There are three main drawbacks, though, to using ineffective preventive measures:

- *They cost money.* Billions of dollars every year are wasted on screening tests of no value.

- *They produce of false positives.* When the likelihood of your having a problem is small, an abnormal test result is much more likely to be a false positive than to truly reflect a medical problem. Abnormal test results, even if there's nothing wrong with you, can be alarming and can lead to further unnecessary tests and office visits, with their attendant trouble, risk, and expense.

- *The doctors' time for prevention is limited.* Ineffective preventive efforts in effect steal the opportunity for more effective prevention. When the leading killers of adults under forty are car accidents, murder, suicide, and AIDS, routine EKGs and batteries of blood tests waste more than time and money.

Routine Physical Exams

Routine yearly physicals were once recommended for everybody. There is very little evidence that most of what a doctor does during a routine exam is of value in detecting unsuspected illness. In people who have no symptoms, listening to the lungs, tapping on the knees, and prodding the abdomen—

mainstays of the routine physical—almost never lead to unexpected findings. Only the few preventive tests mentioned in this chapter, like blood pressure screening and breast exams, are useful for most people. Remember, we're talking about the physical exam as it applies to prevention; the exam remains an essential tool in evaluating people with symptoms.

Time saved by eliminating inessential elements of the routine physical exam can be dedicated to talking about personal habits and their relationship to various diseases. Five minutes spent advising you on how to lower your risk for a heart attack or teaching someone how to modify dangerous sexual behavior is much more likely to be of benefit.

The few preventive tests that are of value can usually be incorporated into routine medical care without the need specifically to schedule a complete physical exam. Most people who ought to have preventive tests visit a doctor once or twice a year for other reasons. A doctor can advise a man who comes in with knee pain that he ought to have his cholesterol checked. A woman with a sore throat can be asked how long it's been since she's had a Pap smear. Blood pressure should be checked every time a patient visits a medical clinic or doctor's office. Doctors should routinely inquire if you smoke. As discussed, if preventive care isn't incorporated into routine medical care, it may never happen.

Some doctors persist in ordering screening tests which none of the authorities, including the American Cancer Society, thinks are valuable. Take the case of chest X-rays. Lung cancer is the number-one cancer killer in the United States. Over 140,000 Americans die each year from it. It would make sense to screen for lung cancer if early detection improved outcome. Unfortunately, by the time a chest X-ray can pick up a lung cancer, it has usually spread beyond the lungs. Studies have shown that people whose lung cancer is detected by routine chest X-rays fare no better than those who first go to the doctor when they develop symptoms. Either way, five years later only about 13 percent are alive.

Given these grim statistics, doctors shouldn't be wasting time on routine chest X-rays. It would be better to invest time in counseling their patients to quit smoking, since 90 percent of lung cancer is caused by cigarettes. This country spends $1.5 billion each year on 30 million screening chest X-rays. How much more good could be done if that money were directed toward preventive measures that actually made a difference in people's health?

Putting it Together

Doctors often fail to practice preventive medicine effectively. They may neglect to counsel patients to improve their habits; they may forgo screening tests of proven value, obtain preventive tests of dubious value, or order useful preventive tests more often than can be justified. Consider the following study from one of the nation's most prestigious hospitals.

Too Little and Too Much Prevention

Researchers from Harvard's Brigham and Women's Hospital in Boston compared published guidelines on preventive tests with how often doctors in their medical clinic did the recommended tests. The following table lists the number of times each of various tests should have been performed, if the guidelines had been followed, and the number of times the tests were actually done.

Preventive Test	Number Recommended	Number Done
blood sugar	14	181
blood count	44	181
EKG	0	3
chest X-ray	0	4
glaucoma test	22	148
mammogram	185	9
rectal exam	272	124
stool test for hidden blood	207	100
sigmoidoscopy	44	6
Pap smear	56	98
breast exam	276	209

The authors concluded that doctors failed to live up to both the published guidelines and their own beliefs about the proper number of preventive tests.[30]

What determines whether a doctor practices good preventive medicine? Does the doctor's specialty matter?

Which Doctors Practice Good Preventive Medicine?

Doctors from Stanford University compared twenty specialists and twenty primary care doctors, such as family practitioners and internists, to see if there were differences in how often they performed seven recommended preventive services. Overall, the doctors performed less than half the recommended services. They were particularly unlikely to comply with recommendations for tetanus shots, mammograms, and flu shots. The researchers found no significant differences between specialists and primary care doctors in their compliance rates, but within each group there were huge differences. Some specialists and some primary care doctors practiced excellent prevention, while others largely ignored it. The doctor's age, specialty, and whether he or she was board-certified made little difference in the quality of preventive medicine. The individual doctor's belief that a preventive service was important most strongly correlated with actually providing the service.[31]

Seven Principles of Preventive Medicine

1. Focus on personal health habits.
2. Prevent disease with vaccines.
3. Detect treatable diseases early with screening tests.
4. Weigh the risks and benefits.
5. Personalize prevention according to your risk.
6. Prevent accidents.
7. Avoid ineffective preventive measures.

Once again, it appears that the doctor's values and biases are the biggest determinant of how that doctor practices. Some doctors believe in prevention, some don't. Using the seven principles of preventive medicine outlined in this chapter, you should be able to tell how well your doctor is doing. Even some doctors who are otherwise quite good neglect prevention. With a little prodding, however, you may be able to get the few preventive tests you need.

7

TAKING CONTROL OF YOUR MEDICAL CARE

IF YOU WANT TO AVOID BAD MEDICAL CARE, YOU'VE GOT TO TAKE control of your encounters with doctors. You need to continually scrutinize a doctor's performance, ask questions, and get involved in the decision-making process. Physicians vary so greatly—in their competence, philosophies of practice, and agendas—that to simply accept a doctor's recommendations on faith is a risky proposition. It's your body, after all, and you're the one who'll have to live with the results.

Active involvement in your medical care is a radical concept. Historically, patients have been the passive recipients of medical care, asking few questions and making few attempts to influence their physicians' behavior. Physicians, in turn, have acted as benevolent—and sometimes not so benevolent—dictators. In fact, until recently even the phrase "patient involvement" usually meant either the presence of a nonmedical person on the board of trustees of a hospital or instructions from the doctor about what you could do about your medical problems once you got home.[1]

Being assertive is sometimes the only way to avoid a disaster. Consider the following case.

Case History: Could I Please See the Real Doctor?

Ray Hargrove is always in a hurry. Wonderfully creative and hopelessly disorganized, his life springs from one crisis to the

275

next. If a project is due at 5 P.M. on Thursday, he's likely to be up most of Wednesday night working and to be scrambling at ten to five Thursday afternoon to apply the final touches. He was in his usual predicament a few years ago when his haste led to an unusual injury.

Trying to fit in a quick shower before a date, he took off his shirt and trousers in his bedroom. While rushing into the bathroom, lowering his briefs en route to save time, he caught the tip of his ring finger in the groove of the door frame into which the latchbolt fits. He heard a pop like the uncorking of a bottle of champagne. He screamed in pain, but after ten minutes his finger no longer hurt. Even so, he couldn't straighten it, so he went to the emergency room of a renowned university hospital near where he lived.

The doctor—who later turned out to be only an intern— listened to Ray's story, examined his finger, and left the room without a word. Ten minutes later he returned, assuring Ray that he'd simply sprained his finger and would be fine. He started to apply a bandage.

"Wait a minute," Ray protested. "Why can't I move the end of my finger?" He held up his hand palm down and showed the doctor how the end of his ring finger drooped from the last knuckle. "I can bend it down but I can't straighten it. Could I have torn the tendon?"

"No, no, no," the doctor assured him. He grabbed Ray's finger near the nail, and moved the last knuckle up and down. "You see?" he said. "It hurts you when I do this." This was the first time he'd examined Ray's finger in this fashion.

"No," Ray said, "it doesn't."

"But it hurts when I do this," the doctor repeated, again bending the knuckle up and down.

"No, it doesn't."

The doctor's expression changed from confident to worried. "Oh. Uh...I'll be right back."

He returned a half hour later with another doctor, a specialist, whom Ray affectionately refers to as "the real doctor." The real doctor examined his finger and said, "Yup, you got the tendon all right." He recognized that Ray had an injury commonly referred to as mallet finger. He prescribed a special splint and told Ray how to protect the finger. He told Ray that if Ray hadn't got the splint within the first week of the injury, the tendon might have shrunk. Ray might never have regained full function of the finger, even with surgery.

Ray has no medical training; he's a designer and an amateur musician. He knew enough, however, to suspect that the doctor was missing something and to assert himself when he needed to. If he'd been intimidated by the first doctor's overconfident assurances and walked out with only a bandage, he might not still be playing the piano and guitar.

One of Ray's coworkers was not so fortunate. He'd sustained the identical injury playing volleyball. His doctor had failed to offer the proper treatment and only bandaged the finger, resulting in a permanent loss of function.

SEVEN PRINCIPLES FOR TAKING CONTROL OF YOUR MEDICAL CARE

Taking Control Principle 1. Be Assertive

The days of the passive "you're the doctor" mentality are over, or at least they ought to be. Earlier this century, when doctors had little to offer patients, it may not have been as risky to follow a physician's dictates blindly. With advances in our understanding of various diseases and with increasingly effective—and increasingly dangerous—interventions to diagnose and treat disease, you need to get actively involved.

Assertive Patients Get Better Care

Researchers from the New England Medical Center in Boston trained a group of patients to ask questions, express their feelings, and assert control of the doctor-patient interaction. They discovered that the assertive patients stayed healthier than similar patients who weren't taught to be assertive. Assertive patients with hypertension had lower blood pressure readings; assertive diabetics had lower blood sugars. The patients taught to be assertive reported that they functioned better, had fewer health problems, and lost fewer days from work.[2]

Your Rights as a Patient

You have a right to expect your doctor to explain every-thing that's done to you. If a test or a therapy is planned, its risks and benefits should be reviewed. If you're given a drug, you should be told what it is, why you need it, how long you'll have to take it, and what its side effects are. For each diagnosis made, the doctor should explain what the condition is, how you got it, and what needs to be done. If a test or procedure is done, its results should be discussed with you. Don't assume every-thing is fine just because you haven't heard anything from the doctor. There are tragic cases in which nobody bothered to inform a patient that her Pap smear was abnormal or that a biopsy showed cancer. If your doctor doesn't volunteer the information, ask. If you don't hear anything, call the doctor's office.

The American Hospital Association publishes what they call the Patient's Bill of Rights, a copy of which should be given to all patients on admission to the hospital and which hospitals should also post in conspicuous locations. According to the association, you have the right to:

- receive complete information about your diagnosis, treat-ment, and prognosis in language you can understand.
- be informed about the nature, risks, and benefits of any proposed test or treatment and be asked for your consent to proceed.
- refuse any tests or treatment.
- refuse to participate in medical research.
- have your privacy respected to the extent possible while getting medical care.
- have your medical records remain private and confidential.
- receive emergency care.
- know the name of the physician in charge of your case.
- know the name and function of any person providing treatment.
- receive an explanation of your bill.

- express complaints about your care and have those complaints investigated.

Getting What's Coming to You in an HMO

To get good care in the traditional fee-for-service system, you need to be aware that the doctors are paid for every service they provide. The situation in HMOs is reversed. To keep costs down, HMOs try to restrict members from using unnecessary, and sometimes necessary, services. **How successful you are in getting services in an HMO is often a function of how effective and how persistent you are in asking for them.** Some basic HMO survival tactics include the following:

- *Learn the system.* Different HMOs have different rules and regulations, different services they will pay for, different services they deny. People who know the services they're entitled to are more likely to get them. Study the brochures before you join, remembering that advertisements only stress a plan's advantages. After you join, read the member handbook to get to know the ins and outs of your plan. Glance through the newsletters and other material they mail out for updates and changes in their policies. When you go for visits, ask the nurses and doctors or other members you bump into in the waiting room how to work the system to your benefit.

- *Find out how the doctors are paid.* HMOs pay some doctors a salary, some a monthly fee per patient, and some by fee-for-service. Many use a combination of all three methods. Within the same HMO, for example, a primary care doctor may be paid a salary, while a specialist gets a fee for every service. Most plans pay bonuses to primary care doctors who keep expenses down or penalize ones who spend too much on patient care, but a few do not. Some bonus plans are tied to the use of expensive services like hospitalization and referrals to specialists. The different incentive systems affect how doctors order tests and allocate other services. It's much easier to evaluate a doctor's suggestions if you know where the incentives lie.

- *Get a good primary care doctor.* Since primary care doctors act as gatekeepers in HMOs, getting a good doctor is one key to success in a plan. Part of what defines a good doctor in an HMO is a willingness to go to bat for you when a test or treatment that is not usually covered is necessary. You may be able to learn through the grapevine who the good doctors are, but since word-of-mouth is not completely reliable, ultimately you'll have to depend on your experience. If after several visits you're dissatisfied, consider switching to another doctor.

  Remember too that choosing a good primary care doctor is only half the battle. Next you need to be able to get an appointment. Often the schedules of good primary care doctors fill up quickly, and the HMO will attempt to shunt you to a nurse practitioner or to a physician assistant, not coincidentally saving them money. For some problems seeing a nonphysician may be fine with you. For others you may prefer to see your regular doctor.

  There are sometimes tricks to getting appointments that you can learn from receptionists or from other members. Some plans, for example, will only book appointments for a given month starting on a particular day. If you can find out when that day is, you may have no problem getting an appointment with the doctor of your choice.

- *Complain, complain, complain.* The squeaky wheel gets the grease is the number-one survival rule in an HMO. If there is a service that you feel you are being unjustly denied, tell your primary care doctor. Doctors in HMOs often have a hard time denying services to well-informed patients who can make a good case for why something is necessary. If you get no satisfaction from your doctor, turn to the plan's administrators. With a single phone call, a sympathetic administrator can knock down barriers that previously seemed impenetrable. Remember, HMOs are businesses. Ultimately their survival depends on satisfying their customers. Administrators or people in the member services departments may be more in touch with this fact than the doctors who feel pressured to keep expenses down or who are required to live by rules that powerful administrators can sometimes simply waive. If you still have no luck, all HMOs have formal grievance procedures.

When appealing a decision, remember that HMOs are set up to make doctors appear to be the bad guys. The administrators make the decisions about what will be covered, but it's usually the doctors who inform you of the policy. One particularly pernicious practice in some HMOs is to force physicians to misrepresent why something is not being done. The doctor may feel a test or therapy is advisable but is supposed to tell you that it's not medically necessary rather than that the HMO won't cover it. Doctors who object to this policy or who are truthful with their patients have been threatened with dismissal.

- *Don't be deflected on the telephone.* HMOs may discourage "excessive" doctors' visits by making appointments, especially specialist appointments, difficult to obtain. When you call you may be told the first opening is months down the road. If the first appointment you're offered seems too distant, ask if they haven't got anything sooner. Could they call you if they get a cancellation? Sometimes if you have your primary care doctor make an appointment with a specialist for you, you can be seen more quickly. For routine checkups or for nonurgent problems, you may simply have to wait a while to be seen, so make your appointment as soon as you think of it. **If your HMO doesn't have walk-in services and you're truly sick, don't let them tell you that you can't be seen that day. Instead, simply announce that you're coming in and expect to be seen.**

- *Vote with your feet.* If your HMO fails to meet your expectations because it's poorly organized, isn't responsive to your needs, or doesn't have quality doctors, switch plans when your period of obligation is up. And write a letter to the administration telling them why you switched. If enough people do likewise, they'll get the message.

Taking Control Principle 2. Grade Your Doctor

After you have worked with a doctor for a while, you can begin to assess the doctor's abilities. By looking at a doctor's overall pattern of strengths and weaknesses—and even the very best doctors have weaknesses—you can form a composite profile of that doctor. One doctor, working in private practice, might be affable, good at explaining things, not bad about obtaining recommended preventive tests, but a little out of date and too disposed to prescribing new, heavily promoted drugs. Another doctor, working in a university hospital, might be knowledge-able, up-to-date, well versed in the latest high technology, but not so good at bedside manner and neglectful of prevention.

Using the relevant sections of this book as a guide, try to evaluate your doctor in the following ten categories:

1. *Knowledge.* How well informed is your doctor? How up-to-date? Does your doctor's knowledge extend beyond his or her specialty?

2. *Technical Skills.* If you're thinking of having a procedure or operation done, how many has the doctor done? If the procedure is new, what training does your doctor have in it? What's the doctor's track record? Complication rate?

3. *Agenda.* Does your doctor seem overly interested in making money? Is he or she swayed by monetary incentives to provide more or fewer services than advisable? Worried about getting sued? Primarily interested in research? Try-ing to satisfy the customer, even if it's not good medical practice?

4. *Communication Skills.* Does your doctor spend enough time with you to do a good job? Perform an in-depth interview? Explain things? Speak in a language you can understand?

5. *Examination Skills.* Does your doctor perform a thorough physical exam? Examine you before ordering tests? Wash his or her hands?

6. *Test Ordering.* Does your doctor order tests prudently? Start with less-invasive tests? Miss the obvious? Waste time and money by looking for zebras instead of horses at the sound of hoofbeats? Is your doctor overly enamored of high technology?

7. *Drug Prescribing.* Does your doctor prescribe drugs spar-ingly? Use generics? Favor older, safer drugs? Personalize

the prescription? Is the office filled with notepads, pens, and other assorted freebies from the drug companies?

8. *Preventive Medicine.* Does your doctor counsel you about a healthy lifestyle? Recommend vaccines? Perform tests like Pap smears and breast exams to detect treatable diseases early?

9. *Judgment.* Does your doctor display common sense? Can he or she tell the difference between something trivial and something serious? Does your doctor know when *not* to order tests, prescribe drugs, or otherwise intervene?

10. *Patient Involvement.* Does your doctor involve you in decisions? Give you the facts you need to decide? Talk with you while you're well about your preferences for resuscitation and other interventions if you become irreversibly ill? Encourage you to learn more about your medical conditions? Grant you access to your medical records?

You may want to write out a report card on your doctor, assigning a letter grade in each category, A for excellent, B for good, C for fair, D for poor, and F for failing. As you work with a doctor longer and learn more about his or her practice style, you may modify some of the grades. With a little encouragement and hard work, maybe your doctor can even improve some of his or her poorer grades.

By grading your doctor, you begin to understand the ways you may need to compensate to get the quality care you want. Knowing, for example, that your doctor seems to order a lot of tests "just in case" can help you decide to forgo some of them. If your doctor is generally good but is perhaps a few years out of date, you may be tempted to get frequent second opinions. If your doctor consistently neglects to recommend preventive measures like flu shots or Pap smears, you can suggest them.

Similarly, if you understand how doctors are affected by financial incentives and by the setting in which they practice, you can strategize to get better care. If you belong to an HMO and have symptoms your doctor can't explain, you may insist on seeing a specialist even though your doctor recommends against it. In a walk-in clinic you may refuse tests that seem superfluous if the doctor can't give an adequate explanation of why they're necessary.

Taking Control Principle 3. Get Smart

A few years ago a listener to the nationally syndicated public radio program *Car Talk* called in to ask how she should go about finding a good mechanic. The host answered that the first step was to "know your make." Only if you have an understanding of your car, he asserted, can you assess a mechanic's competence. The same principle applies to finding a good doctor: The better you understand your body and your medical problems, the better you'll be able to judge the quality of your doctor and know what to make of that doctor's advice.

By making a habit of learning about every disorder you develop, every drug that's prescribed, and every major intervention that's proposed, you get, in effect, a low-cost second opinion. Say you ask your doctor about the side effects of a particular drug. If you go home and look the drug up, you'll be able to assess how accurate your doctor's information was. If what you read seems to contradict what your doctor told you, or if your doctor has made important omissions, you may have cause for concern.

I'm continually amazed at how little many otherwise well informed people know about their medical care. They've had surgery, they tell me, but they're not sure what for. They've been taking pills for high blood pressure for several years, but they don't know the name or the dose. They know they're allergic to some antibiotic, but they're not sure which one.

At a minimum, anyone who wants to be involved in their medical care should keep a record of the following:

- *Major diagnoses.* Include when the diagnosis was made and, if possible, how the diagnosis was made. Know *both* the medical terminology and what it means in plain English. If you only know your diagnosis in layman's terms, another doctor may not be able to figure out exactly what you have.
- *Major test results.* Write down the name and date of any major test and why it was done. Also list tests with normal

results. You may want to keep a photocopy of your last EKG in your records.

- *Medications.* Include a mention of what each drug is for, when it was first prescribed, what the dose is, and how often you're supposed to take it.
- *Surgery or other procedures.*
- *Drug allergies.*

If you visit a new doctor, bring this information with you. One of the most difficult problems facing doctors seeing a patient for the first time is to reconstruct what has happened to the patient before. Medical records may not be available, and if you're unable to inform the doctor about your history, the quality of the care that doctor gives you may be compromised. The doctor may have to make an educated guess about your diagnoses and medications or to repeat tests needlessly.

Knowing your medical history will help you get better care from your own doctor and will protect you when your doctor is unavailable. If you have a problem in the middle of the night or while your doctor is on vacation, the covering doctor won't know your history. Your chart may not be immediately accessible. If you need emergency care while you're traveling away from home, the doctors may need to rely entirely on the information you provide.

Educating Yourself About Medicine

It's good to have access to a few books on medical care. You may want to purchase an inexpensive manual on drugs and their side effects and a general medical guide. CompuServe and other on-line computer services offer information on drugs and medical problems that is updated regularly. The internet is becoming an excellent source of medical information. It is also home to hundreds of medically-related discussion groups with topics ranging from AIDS to Lyme disease to women's health.

The U.S. government offers many health-related brochures free of charge. The American Cancer Society, the American Diabetes Association, the Arthritis Foundation, and dozens of other groups offer free information on specific diseases. Many of these organizations run toll-free hotlines. The National Cancer Institute, for example, answers questions and offers publications at (800) 4-CANCER. For the addresses and phone numbers of organizations offering medical information, see Appendices 2–4.

Public libraries are often good sources of medical information. In addition to carrying health-related books and magazines, many libraries also subscribe to such medical journals as the *New England Journal of Medicine* and the *Journal of the American Medical Association*. A librarian can help you to find recent articles on the topic of your choice in both the general and medical press.

For people who want to do more detailed research and are willing to wade through more technical material, medical libraries carry the most information; unfortunately, they sometimes restrict access to the general public. If there is a medical school in your area, call and ask what their policy is. Another possibility for the particularly motivated is to search the medical databases of the National Library of Medicine on-line. Their databases summarize information from thousands of medical journals from all over the world and are the best place to locate the latest research findings. Inexpensive software called Grateful Med (believe it or not) is available from the National Library of Medicine. For information, call (800) 638-8480.

Motivated patients can sometimes even figure things out that mystify their doctors. The movie, *Lorenzo's Oil*, you may recall, portrayed the efforts of concerned parents who researched possible treatments for their son's fatal disease.

Case History: Teaching the Doctor a Lesson

Martin Palmer had just moved to Boston's North End, a neighborhood known for its fine Italian restaurants, when he noticed his taste in food was changing. He decided he didn't like Italian food anymore; he thought the tomato sauce was giving him indigestion and diarrhea. He stopped liking Wheaties too, his cereal of choice as a kid, because they seemed to cause flatulence. Cheerios weren't any better. He never thought to mention any of this to his doctor. He just couldn't understand how people could eat those things.

Several years later, as a graduate student in architecture, he developed an itchy rash on his knees, elbows, and upper back. He consulted a dermatologist, but Martin found it difficult to talk with the guy. Even though the doctor couldn't make a diagnosis, he always acted supremely confident. He was really pushy too. Martin told him the rash itched like "all get out." The doctor responded, "Is it really itchy or just a little itchy?" Martin felt the doctor wanted him to say just a little itchy because that's what fit with what he thought Martin had. "Just a little itchy," Martin answered but thought to himself, I'm just scratching it all the time, that's all.

Half out of pique at the doctor's imperious manner, Martin went to the health sciences library at his university to see what he could find out. He consulted a number of dermatology textbooks. At first he leafed through the three-inch-thick ones but found them too daunting. Finally he settled on a thin picture book of clinical dermatology. He paged through looking at the photographs, stopping a few times to read the accompanying write-ups. He'd been at it about a half hour when he saw something that looked just like what he had. It was called dermatitis herpetiformis, or DH for short.

The book described an intensely itchy rash made up of small blisters that usually appeared on the elbows and knees. Men got it more often than women but not usually until after the age of twenty. It occurred primarily in people of European extraction. All the pieces seemed to fit his case. DH was caused, he read, by an allergy to gluten, a protein found in wheat. Many people with DH also have intestinal symptoms due to gluten sensitivity. That's got to be it, *he thought. Martin went back to several of the bigger books and read everything he could find on it.*

Martin set up another appointment with the dermatologist to discuss his discovery. Before he could say much, though, the doctor told him to "drop your drawers and get up on the table." Martin later told me, "I knew the guy would start running me through the drill. But by then I was pretty sure of myself. I gritted my teeth, set myself, and said, 'I've been doing some research. I think you ought to listen.'"

The doctor looked annoyed. Martin figured he was thinking, Who does this jerk think he is? *but he let Martin speak. After a couple of minutes it finally hit the doctor that Martin might know what he was talking about. He asked Martin if he'd noticed any connection with his diet.* Yes! *he responded. Pretty soon the doctor was acting all proud of himself. He even called in some other doctors to have them look at the great case he'd diagnosed.*

By the time of their next appointment, the doctor must have done his homework, because he seemed to know a lot more about DH. He told Martin a number of things that by that time Martin already knew. He referred Martin to a nutritionist. Martin ended up teaching her about hidden sources of dietary gluten, such as beer and Chinese food made with MSG.

Within twenty-four hours of restricting the gluten in his diet, Martin noticed an improvement in his bowel symptoms. Within weeks his rash was better. Buoyed by his discovery and his improved health, Martin enthusiastically began to look for alternatives to wheat in his diet. He started baking bread at home, for example, substituting rice flour for wheat. He found a group that published a newsletter containing dietary tips and recipes as well as the latest research findings on DH and a related gluten allergy problem called celiac sprue. Five years later Martin is symptom-free. He even gets away with an occasional beer.

Get Your Medical Records

In many states you have a right to have a copy of all your medical records. You can find out your rights by contacting your state's department of health. Even if your state does not grant you the right to your records, some doctors will still provide them if you ask. Once you request your records, expect to wait several weeks to get them (unless it's an emergency) and to pay for photocopying. Because of a lack of responsiveness on the part of some doctors and hospitals, you may have to request your records more than once.

Your medical records should contain the results of any tests you've had and all your doctors' notes. Since doctors aren't always as communicative as they should be, you can often learn a lot by reviewing your medical records. You may also be able to catch errors which otherwise might be perpetuated. Insurance companies sometimes reject applicants for a policy based on erroneous information in their charts.

Because of all the abbreviations, medical jargon, and illegible handwriting, you may need help deciphering your records. Ask your doctor to spend a few minutes going over things with you, or if you happen to have a friend in medicine or nursing, you might ask him or her. Since hospital records are often bulky, rather than request your entire chart, you might simply ask for a copy of the discharge summary for each hospitalization, which provides a synopsis of what happened during your stay and which lists all your diagnoses and medications on discharge. Discharge summaries, by the way, are usually typed and contain few abbreviations.

Even if you won't use them yourself, it's not a bad idea to have a copy of your records for future reference. If you move or change doctors, having a copy assures more ready access. Since files can be lost and buildings can burn, it's advisable to have a fail-safe.

Some doctors may resist giving you a copy of your records. This is a bad sign. **Doctors who don't want you to have access to your records may either feel they have something to hide or are resistant to the idea of your active participation in your medical care.** When interviewing a new doctor, ask what his or her policy is toward medical records before you sign on. If your current doctor puts up serious roadblocks to your obtaining your records, that may be a reason to consider switching.

Making Sense of Media Reports

Although newspapers, magazines, and TV frequently report on medical topics, I encourage you to be skeptical of reports of medical advances. Be particularly wary of the "good news for [fill in the blank] sufferers" stories, which often hype new drugs or surgical techniques, the effectiveness and long-term safety of which are usually not yet known.

When evaluating medical reports, ask yourself:

- *What's the source?* Health reporters vary enormously in their scientific training and in their ability to separate what's important from what's not. Some are interested in getting at the truth; some are interested in providing "info-tainment." Some stories are based on press conferences given by scientists or by "news releases" from drug com-panies. Be more impressed if the information comes from studies in reputable medical journals and is reported in detail.

In an egregious example of advertising disguised as news, ex–New York Yankee great Mickey Mantle appeared in August 1988 on the *Today* show. The NBC interview began with these words: "The most famous knees in sports history are back, thanks in part to some exciting new arthritis therapy." Mantle described how his knees had forced his retirement from baseball, even prevented him from playing golf. He talked about how the drug Voltaren had changed his life and joked that it was even good for hangovers. (Since then Mantle has sought treatment for alcoholism.) An ar-thritis specialist appeared on the show with Mantle and was enthusiastic in his praise of the drug. What the millions of viewers were not told was that both Mantle and the arthritis doctor were paid spokesmen of the Swiss pharmaceutical giant Ciba-Geigy. Mantle had, in fact, tried Voltaren at the company's suggestion before signing on. Patients reportedly flocked to their doctors asking for "Mickey Mantle's wonder drug."[3] Voltaren, by the way, is a classic me-too drug, with little advantage over ibuprofen and other previously avail-able drugs but with a much higher price tag.

• *Whom do they interview?* A scientist who has just discovered something new is usually very optimistic about its signifi-cance. Careers and future funding for studies can be made or wiped out by the success or failure of a new development. Many scientists receive funding for their studies from drug companies or medical device manufacturers. Some also serve as paid consultants to the companies or even hold equity interest in them. Their conclusions may be biased, whether consciously or not. Reputable medical journals now require researchers to reveal possible conflicts of interest, but media reports on these studies may not mention them. Be more impressed when the experts interviewed are neu-tral observers, rather than the study's authors.

- *Is the finding preliminary or confirmed?* An exciting "break-through" makes for better copy than an interesting prelimi-nary finding of unclear significance, even if the latter is a much more realistic assessment of the new discovery. Re-member all the hoopla a few years back about interferon being a cure for cancer? The drug has turned out to be useful for a few conditions but nothing like what you would have thought from the initial reports. If the news story ends with something like, "Doctors don't expect it to be available for several more years," you can usually just forget it.

- *Was the group studied like me?* Until recently, almost all major studies of heart disease were done on men, even though heart disease is the number-one killer of women too. Drug studies are usually not performed on the elderly, even though they are precisely the group most likely to take medications. If the group studied is different from you, the results may not apply.

In January of 1990 a study in the *New England Journal of Medicine* made headline news all over the country. Contrary to earlier reports, the study suggested that oat bran didn't lower cholesterol levels.[4] Millions of Americans had been supplementing their diets with this cheap, safe, natural source of fiber, and when the reports aired, many of them stopped. Oats sales plummeted.

What the media reports neglected to mention was that dozens of prior studies had shown that oat bran led to significant reductions in elevated cholesterol levels.[5] Few reporters had the savvy to place the new study in its proper historical context. The beneficial effects of oat bran on hemorrhoids, constipation, diverticulitis, and even possibly on preventing colon cancer were also neglected in the reports.

Most of the reports also failed to mention something possibly even more significant: who the participants in the study were. If you had read the study itself, you'd have learned that the participants were healthy young women, most of whom worked in hospitals as dietitians. They were already eating low-fat diets, weren't overweight, didn't smoke, and had normal blood pressures and normal cholesterol levels. This highly select group supplemented their already healthy diets with oat bran, and lo and behold, their already desirable cholesterol levels only went down a little.

What does this finding mean for overweight, middle-aged men with high cholesterol levels who consume the typical American high-fat diet? As one doctor put it in a rebuttal to the study published by the *New England Journal,* "Nothing!"[6] In fact, most of the published letters were highly critical of the study's design and conclusions. These criticisms were published five months after the original study and were essentially ignored by the press.

Given the uncertain significance of media reports, it's probably best to speak with your doctor before making any changes in your treatment plan based on what you read or hear.

Taking Control Principle 4. Decide What's Right for You

When it comes to medical decisions, I believe it's healthiest to think of your doctor in the same way you might think of an accountant, that is, as someone who works for you, makes recommendations, but doesn't dictate what you do. You depend on an accountant's expertise, especially when your situation is complex, but only you know your values and priorities, and many decisions will hinge on these. There's one more similarity: if an accountant fails to live up to your expectations, you hire a replacement.

Many patients agree to tests and therapies they don't want. Some people find it difficult to go against the doctor's advice, perhaps out of their desire to please the doctor or out of their respect for authority. As a competent adult, you have the legal right to refuse any therapy a doctor recommends, no matter how advisable the doctor or anyone else feels it is or how irrational they feel you're being. You should only consent to intervention when you favor it, not when you perceive your doctor favors it. Telling the doctor that you're not sure and need time to think the decision over can be a nonthreatening way to assert your preference.

Differences of opinion between doctors and patients often

revolve around value differences. Competent physicians whose values differ from yours may make "medically correct" decisions that may nonetheless be wrong for you. If an operation offers you a chance at a few extra months of life, but you don't think it's worth it, it is not the doctor's prerogative to overrule your decision. A doctor may place more value on giving you a chance at a longer life and give less weight to your short-term risk of death or complications or to your comfort. You may not feel the same way. You may opt for a treatment that minimizes your pain, anxiety, and inconvenience even if it's not the "medically correct" choice.

There are times when because of illness you may feel you can't shoulder the burden of decision making alone. Try to anticipate this possibility and find someone who knows you well who can help you make decisions. If you are more gravely ill and completely unable to make decisions, having filled out a living will or appointed a health care proxy makes it more likely your wishes will be respected. If you return to better health, you can resume control of decisions.

Informed Consent

Traditionally, physicians simply made decisions for patients based on their expertise. Doctors did not necessarily even inform patients of their diagnoses, much less involve them in medical decisions. A woman I know in New Orleans who had breast cancer many years ago was in the hospital recovering from her mastectomy when she learned by chance that she was being given chemotherapy. A nurse had come into her room to change her IV and casually mentioned it was for the chemotherapy. The woman didn't object—at that time it was rare for a patient to do so—she just found it strange that her doctor hadn't even mentioned it.

These days **doctors are required by law to inform you of your options before performing tests or instituting treatment.** They are required to lay out in plain language

- what they think you have
- what they propose doing

- the potential risks
- what stands to be gained
- alternatives approaches, including doing nothing
- the risks and benefits of the alternatives

For major procedures doctors will ask you to sign a form acknowledging your understanding and agreement. These forms are, unfortunately, often a poor substitute for real informed consent. They may be written in medical jargon and may only be presented to you minutes before you are scheduled to undergo a procedure. Many informed consent forms are more designed to protect doctors from malpractice suits than truly to involve you in decision making.

Case History: Uninformed Consent

Elizabeth Burch's husband was in the end stages of Alzheimer's disease when he was brought to the hospital for fever and dehydration. A fiercely independent woman, Elizabeth felt uneasy about much of what had been done to her husband during past hospitalizations. Just a few weeks earlier a nurse had cut her husband's beard off against his will, apparently because the beard made it more difficult to feed him. Elizabeth had arrived for a visit and discovered him clean-shaven, only to be told by the man in the next bed how her husband had screamed and resisted the whole time the nurse had been snipping it off.

This time Elizabeth was told the doctor wanted to perform a spinal tap on her husband, a procedure in which a small needle is inserted in the lower back to remove fluid from the spinal canal. The doctor, a heavy-set man in his sixties, wanted to be sure her husband didn't have meningitis—although he never told her that—and had already positioned her husband curled up on his side to do the test.

"Do you know what a spinal tap is?" he asked her.

"Yes," she said.

The nurse handed her a form and said, "Sign this." No further explanation was given.

"I just want to read it first," Elizabeth said, adding that she

was going to take the form out into the hall where the light was better.

The nurse followed her to the hall. "Well, are you going to sign it or not?"

"It's a rather broad statement," Elizabeth said. The form stated among other things that "all consequences have been explained to you."

At that point the doctor started picking up his things, loudly announcing, "I'm getting out of here."

As he walked out the door, he scowled at Elizabeth. "He's not getting any antibiotics until the spinal tap's done."

"Well, he needs them," she said, "so I'll sign."

A spinal tap is not a particularly risky procedure and in this instance was appropriate. When meningitis is a possibility, there is a need to act quickly, but a couple of quick sentences of explanation were all that would have been necessary to assuage Elizabeth's doubts. The attitude of this doctor and nurse was that informed consent is a bothersome formality and that patients, and in this case family members, should just do as they're told.

Too many physicians remain reluctant to inform patients fully or to involve them in decisions. Some believe adequately informing patients to make decisions is too time-consuming. Some think, often incorrectly, that they already know what their patients want. Some may simply have a hard time putting themselves in their patients' shoes. If the decision of what to do seems obvious to the doctor, he or she may have a hard time understanding why you want more information. For other doctors, it's a power trip: they've got it and they don't want to give it up. And as usual, money can play a role: fee-for-service doctors are accustomed to regulating the demand for their services. They recommend a profitable test and the patient agrees. Giving up control over decisions could cost them.[7]

My advice is to not agree to anything if you don't feel things have been explained adequately or if you have lingering doubts. In a nonemergency situation, a cooling off period to think over the decision is often an excellent idea. Go home, talk with your family, do a little reading, then make your decision. You can even ask the doctor, "Will anything be lost if I wait a few days to have this done?"

Taking Control Principle 5. Work With Your Doctor as a Team

The best doctor-patient relationships are cooperative, not adversarial. You supply information about your symptoms and agree to be examined and tested; the doctor provides expertise and makes recommendations. Once you get home, you try to follow the agreed-on plan. If you have complications or further problems, the doctor attempts to handle them. There are several secrets to fostering a good relationship with a doctor. They include the following:

- *Prepare for your visits.* Try to be organized for your visits to the doctor. It's often a good idea *before* your appointment to prepare a brief list of questions and problems you'd like to see addressed. That way, you'll be less likely to forget things in the office. Be realistic, though. The doctor's time is limited, so try to concentrate on the matters of greatest concern to you.

  If you're taking medicines, either prescription or over-the-counter, bring them in so the doctor can see exactly what you're taking. Because of faulty record keeping or miscommunication, doctors don't always know what their patients are taking. If you're new to a doctor, either know your medical history or arrange to have past medical records forwarded to the doctor *before* your visit.

  Studies show that patients forget about half of what they're told by doctors almost immediately. The more emotionally charged the information, the harder it can be to recall. After the doctor utters the word *cancer,* for example, some patients won't hear a word for the next several minutes. If you're worried that you may forget things or become intimidated in the presence of the doctor, ask if you can bring a friend or family member along for the visit. But don't bring someone whose presence will stop you from mentioning important but embarrassing problems. It's also useful to take notes during your visit, so you can remember what the doctor says.

- *Be honest and forthcoming.* People sometimes neglect to tell their doctors information that can be vital to their medical care. If you're gay, use drugs, drink twelve pots of coffee a day, or are having problems at work or home, be honest about it. Don't let embarrassment stop you from mentioning sexual difficulties, bad breath, or bowel problems. If there is some information that you'd like to share but that you don't want to appear in your medical record, ask the doctor to not write it down.

  If you're not taking medicines the doctor has prescribed, say so. Maybe the doctor didn't realize your concern about their expense or side effects. Tell the doctor if you have no intention of filling a prescription or showing up for a scheduled test. If your doctor knows what you're willing to do and what you're not willing to do, you may be able to reach a mutually satisfactory solution. If you're dissatisfied with the care you're receiving or with a bill, tell the doctor. If you can't do it in person, write a letter. Many differences can be resolved if they're openly aired.

  Try to avoid having a hidden agenda for your visit. If you're worried that your symptoms might be caused by cancer, say so. The doctor may not be able to allay your fears if the doctor doesn't know what your fears are. Try to mention your major concerns as early as possible in the visit. Many patients let the doctor spend 90% of the allotted time on trivial matters, then spring their real concern in the last minute, almost assuring that it can't be done justice.

- *Carefully describe your symptoms.* In general doctors prefer you to describe your symptoms rather than outline your theory about what's causing them. Say "I've been getting this gnawing stomach pain" rather than "My ulcer's been acting up." Something else could be causing your symptoms, after all. It's the doctor's job to sort things out and to make diagnoses. Good doctors, however, will also be interested in your opinions about the cause of your symptoms.

  Try to describe your symptoms as precisely as possible.

How long have you had the symptom? Do you have it all the time, or does it come and go? What makes it better? What makes it worse? Have you ever had it before? Do any other symptoms accompany it? If your problem is pain, where is it exactly? Is it dull? Throbbing? Stabbing?

- *Keep up your end of the bargain.* Show up for your appointments or try to cancel them in a timely fashion. Don't call your doctor in the middle of the night for a problem you've had for weeks, unless it's suddenly much worse. If you do need to call the doctor, either at work or at home, try to get to the point quickly. If the bill is reasonable, pay it. If you can't afford to, see if you can make arrangements. Perhaps it seems silly to mention personal hygiene, but if the doctor may be examining you, bathe before your visit. I can tell you from painful personal experience that many patients don't.

- *Take as much autonomy as you can handle.* Some people are willing and able to take on more responsibility for their medical problems than others. Some very motivated diabetics check their own blood sugars at home and adjust their insulin doses accordingly. Asthmatics can tell when their breathing is becoming more labored, and as they've previously worked out with their doctors, will add extra medicines. Women with recurrent bladder infections may recognize the early symptoms and start themselves on antibiotics, prescribed for just such a situation, before the infection gets bad, avoiding the wait for an appointment or a late-night trip to an emergency room. People with high blood pressure can measure it themselves at home, record the numbers, and bring them in with them to their appointments, allowing their doctors to gauge better how well their medication is working. Of course people with hypertension can also work on lowering their blood pressure by exercising, losing weight, quitting smoking, cutting back on alcohol, limiting salt, and lowering their stress levels.

- *Be respectful.* You catch more flies with honey than with vinegar, goes the old saying. There is a way of being assertive that can rankle some doctors. Try not to seem hostile or antagonistic. Your goal should not be to try to show your physician up but rather to do what you can to get your questions answered and to get good care. Usually you'll get the best results if you're assertive and persistent while remaining polite and respectful. Some doctors, however, object to any meaningful participation of patients in medical care, no matter how diplomatically it's broached. If you find yourself in a medical dictatorship, try to switch to a democracy.

- *Try to negotiate differences.* It's inevitable that doctors and patients with their different values and different life experiences are at times going to disagree about the best course of action. Reasonable people can usually negotiate their differences, find a consensus, or at the very least respectfully agree to disagree. Confrontation seldom helps, but there are times when physicians and patients who cannot see eye to eye need to part company. Even in these instances, vitriol serves little purpose.

Taking Control Principle 6. Trust But Verify

When Ronald Reagan began negotiating with Mikhail Gorbachev to limit the number of nuclear weapons in each of their country's arsenals, he frequently quoted a Russian proverb, Trust but verify. A similarly cautious stance is appropriate when dealing with physicians.

It's reasonable to expect doctors to be competent and caring but unreasonable to expect them to be perfect. Doctors are human beings. Even the best ones make mistakes. They forget things. They sometimes fail to recognize conditions that should be obvious. With the boom in medical knowledge, there is simply more information out there than any doctor can master and what is out there is constantly changing. Even an otherwise well informed doctor may not know some fact that might be helpful in your case.

Second Opinions

Second opinions are usually done before elective surgery, but there are other times when they can be useful. If your primary care doctor can't figure out what's wrong with you, it may be time to get another doctor's input. This is true even if you're generally satisfied with your doctor and don't intend on changing. If there is some doubt about the interpretation of a biopsy, you might have a pathologist from another hospital look at the slides under the microscope. If there is a questionable area on a mammogram, you might ask for a second radiologist to have a look. If your doctor proposes a major intervention, be it a test, an invasive procedure or a drug with serious side effects, consider getting another point of view. If your doctor is a little behind-the-times, you may want to check with a specialist every now and again to make sure that your condition is being well-managed. In fact, **anytime you have doubts about the way your care is being managed, consider getting a second opinion. If you have the feeling your doctor may be missing something, you may be right.**

In order to increase your likelihood of benefiting from a second opinion, keep the following tips in mind:

- *Tell your primary care doctor you want a second opinion.* Even though it may be difficult for you to do so, it's best to inform your doctor of your desire for a second opinion. That way copies of all relevant medical records and test results can be forwarded to the second doctor. Even if your doctor doesn't agree with the need for a second opinion, he or she should respect your wish for more information and cooperate with the process. If a doctor is so insecure as to resist or object to a second opinion, you need to ask yourself if you're seeing the right doctor. Good doctors realize they have little to lose and might even learn something by hearing the opinion of a colleague.

- *Try to get your second opinion from a doctor unaffiliated with the first, preferably one practicing at another institution.* Doctors with close affiliations may share biases and you may simply end up hearing the same opinion twice, even though other doctors might disagree about the best way to manage your case. Many people rely on their physicians to provide the name of doctor to provide a second opinion. I'd advise against this practice, as doctors are more likely to recommend colleagues with whom they share biases. There are other ways to find doctors for second opinions. Some consumer groups will provide names of specialists in your area. If there is a medical school nearby, you can call up and ask for the name of a specialist in the relevant area.

- *If you are seeking a second opinion on surgery, consider seeing a nonsurgeon.* Surgeons tend to be more convinced than other doctors of the power of the scalpel, particularly of *their* scalpel. It is sometimes joked that if you ask a surgeon to name the three greatest surgeons in the world, he or she will be hard-pressed to come up with the other two. One study showed that surgeons were much more likely to recommend ulcer surgery than medical specialists were.[8] If you have hip or knee surgery recommended, consider a second opinion from a joint and arthritis specialist, a rheumatologist, rather than from another orthopedic surgeon. For intestinal surgery, try a gastroenterologist, a medical specialist in the stomach and intestines. For back surgery, see a neurologist; for heart surgery, a cardiologist. These nonsurgeons will understand the problems but may have a less rosy view of the effectiveness of surgery.

- *Expect the second doctor to thoroughly review your records, interview you, and perform a physical examination.* If the consultation is about the need for surgery, the doctor should comment not only on whether the operation is necessary but on whether you've been adequately diagnosed. The doctor might think that more tests are required before a definitive recommendation can be made. If the doctor providing the second opinion agrees with your diagnosis, that doctor should give you his or her take on alternative treatments and their relative risk and benefits and make specific recommendations.

- *When the opinions of two physicians greatly differ, your preferences should guide your decision.* Considering the frequency of unnecessary surgery, when one doctor recommends an operation that another considers inadvisable, the odds are that you don't need it. Keep in mind that medicine is an inexact science. Given the lack of proof of the effectiveness of many interventions, particularly surgery, different doctors of equal competence may look at the same information and come to different conclusions.

When opinions differ and you're unsure what to do, it's reasonable to discuss the situation with your primary care physician. If necessary, you can get a third or even a fourth opinion, if you can afford it. Many insurance companies will pay for a second opinion before a proposed operation and sometimes for a third opinion when the first two differ.

Remember, though, that just because two opinions differ, one isn't necessarily wrong. The two doctors may be proposing similarly effective alternative approaches. Of course, even when both doctors agree, the advice can turn out to be wrong. If you had breast cancer not so many years ago, most surgeons would have recommended a radical mastectomy, a disfiguring operation we now know was unnecessarily harsh.

Remember, too, that even when both doctors agree that you need an operation or other intervention, you can still decide against it. Ultimately, it's your body, and your values count most.

Taking Control Principle 7. Cultivate an Attitude of Healthy Skepticism

We know from history that much of what doctors do at any particular time is ineffective or even dangerous when viewed in retrospect. Years ago a famous professor warned his graduating medical students that half of what he'd taught them was wrong, but the trouble was he didn't know which half. Medical practice has evolved significantly since then, but the principle still applies: we don't know which of the well-intentioned therapies of the present will end up looking like the leeches and bloodletting of ancient time or like the thalidomide, Dalkon shields, and routine tonsillectomies of a more recent era gone by. Accordingly, the pronouncements of doctors should be viewed with healthy skepticism.

The Limits of Medicine

Despite all the PR to the contrary, modern medicine can't alter the outcome of most diseases. The vast majority of problems that lead people to doctors either go away on their own or aren't affected much by medical therapy. Although advances have been made, the "war on cancer" is far from won. The reduction in the threat of many infectious diseases, such as cholera and rheumatic fever, had a lot more to do with improvements in living conditions than with magic bullets from the medical profession. The recent decline in the rate of heart disease in this country is mostly attributable to improvements in diet, exercise, and smoking habits, not to drugs or bypass surgery. Huge gaps still exist in what we know. Even today many of our most trusted remedies are unproved.

Nonetheless, many doctors and many patients have the attitude that modern medicine, particularly in its more high-tech manifestations, is all-powerful. Doctors who are uncritical believers in modern medicine are much more likely to intervene, even in cases where the likelihood of benefit is small and the risk is great. Others doctors, much less sanguine about the powers of modern medicine, realize that high-tech solutions when appropriately marshaled can work wonders but that they also have the power to cause great harm.

The Seven Principles for Taking Control of Your Medical Care

1. Be assertive.
2. Grade your doctor.
3. Get smart.
4. Decide what's right for you
5. Work with your doctor as a team.
6. Trust but verify.
7. Cultivate an attitude of healthy skepticism

Putting It Together

It's no coincidence that I've chosen to end the book with a chapter on taking control of your medical care. Better informed patients force their doctors to stay on their toes. Only by getting involved in medical decisions can you be sure that what's done reflects *your* values and goals. Assertive patients also get better care and end up more satisfied with the results. With practice, you should be able to assume more responsibility for your medical care and become less dependent on doctors.

Remember, all doctors have weaknesses. Even the very best ones make mistakes. Since no doctor can know it all, none should be trusted blindly. If you understand your doctor's limitations, scrutinize his or her advice, and play an active role in decision making, you can enjoy excellent medical care from less-than-perfect physicians.

A Final Word

If by reading this book, you've started to view your doctor in a more questioning light, you're already on the road to better medical care. To benefit fully from the book, however, you need to continue to invest time and energy. When contemplating a doctor's recommendation for a test or for surgery, for example, you may need to take a trip to the library to do some research or to reread sections from the relevant chapters in this book.

This book has not attempted to be encyclopedic in the medical conditions it discusses or to cover every possible scenario. Instead it provides a conceptual framework to help you understand your medical care and give you the tools to analyze situations as they arise. More than anything, this book aims to teach you how to think about doctors and the practice of medicine.

In the years ahead much in medical practice will change. New drugs will come on the market, and new uses for old ones will be discovered. New diseases will appear. New technologies for diagnosis and treatment will be invented. New studies will alter some of our present thinking about which treatments work and which ones don't. Whatever changes occur, though, the principles of how medicine should and should not be practiced will endure.

Our system for delivering health care is also changing. More and more patients are moving to managed care plans. Giant insurance companies are buying HMOs or starting their own. Hospitals are gobbling each other up. Even without health care reform, the landscape of American medicine has been altered dramatically in the last few years, and more changes, from the government on down, are coming.

But even a revolution in health care won't take away the need to be an informed and assertive medical consumer. No matter what shape future developments take, one fact will remain: the primary determinant of the quality of your medical care is what happens one-on-one between you and your doctor. You can make it better.

APPENDIX I

NOTES

CHAPTER ONE: Are You Seeing the Right Doctor?

1. "Prevalence of Substance Use Among U.S. Physicians," P. H. Hughes, et al., *Journal of the American Medical Association*, May 6, 1992, pp. 2333–39.

2. "The Medical Association of Georgia's Impaired Physicians Program: Review of the First 1000 Physicians: Analysis of Specialty," G. D. Talbott, et al., *Journal of the American Medical Association*, June 5, 1987, pp. 2927–30.

3. "Preventable Deaths: Who, How Often and Why?" R. W. Dubois, et al., *Annals of Internal Medicine*, October 1, 1988, pp. 582–89.

4. "Incidence of Adverse Events and Negligence in Hospitalized Patients: Results of the Harvard Medical Practice Study I," T. A. Brennan, et al., *New England Journal of Medicine*, February 7, 1991, pp. 370–76.

5. "Relation Between Malpractice Claims and Adverse Events Due to Negligence: Results of the Harvard Medical Practice Study III," A. R. Localio, et al., *New England Journal of Medicine*, February 7, 1991, pp. 245–51.

6. "Malpractice in Massachusetts: Regulatory System in Shambles; Negligent Doctors Stay on the Job," B. Butterfield, et al., *Boston Globe*, October 1, 1994, p. 1.

7. "Specialty Distribution of U.S. Physicians—The Invisible Driver of Health Care Costs," S. A. Schroeder, et al., *New England Journal of Medicine*, April 1, 1993, pp. 961–63.

8. "Variations in Resource Utilization Among Medical Specialties and Systems of Care: Results from the Medical Outcomes Study," S. Greenfield, et al., *Journal of the American Medical Association*, March 25, 1992, pp. 1624–30.

9. "What Role for Nurse Practitioners in Primary Care?" J. P. Kassirer, *New England Journal of Medicine*, January 20, 1994, pp. 204–205.

10. " "Physician Assistants and Health System Reform: Clinical Capabilities, Practice Activities, and Potential Roles," P. E. Jones, et al., *Journal of the American Medical Association*, April 27, 1994, pp. 1266–72.

11. "M.D. Specialty Listings: Let Your Fingers Do the Walking," L. Page, *American Medical News*, September 8, 1989, p. 71.

12. "Pride and Prejudice: Can M.D.s and D.O.s Heal the Rift Between Them?" J. Berlfein, *New Physician*, October 1989, pp. 17–21.

13. "Board-Certified Physicians in the United States, 1971–86," D. G. Langley, *New England Journal of Medicine*, July 4, 1991, p. 67.

14. "Quality of Care in Episodes of Respiratory Illness Among Medicaid Patients in New Mexico," K. N. Lohr, et al., *Annals of Internal Medicine*, January 1980, pp. 99–106.

15. "Access to Information—Physicians' Credentials and Where You Can't Find Them," J. M. Reade, et al., *New England Journal of Medicine*, August 17, 1989, pp. 466–68.

16. "Yellow Professionalism: Advertising by Physicians in the Yellow Pages," J. M. Reade, et al., *New England Journal of Medicine*, May 21, 1987, pp. 1315–19.

17. "10,289 Questionable Doctors," *Health Letter*, Public Citizen Health Research Group, November 1993, pp. 4–7.

18. "The Use of Ambulatory Testing in Prepaid and Fee-for-Service Group Practices: Relation to Perceived Profitability," A. M. Epstein, et al., *New England Journal of Medicine*, April 24, 1986, pp. 1089–93.

19. "Physician's Responses to Financial Incentives: Evidence From a For-Profit Ambulatory Care Center," D. Hemenway, et al., *New England Journal of Medicine*, April 12, 1990, pp. 1059–63.

20. "Health Maintenance Organizations, Financial Incentives and Physicians' Judgments," A. L. Hillman, *Annals of Internal Medicine*, June 15, 1990, pp. 891–93.

21. "Patients' Ratings of Outpatient Visits in Different Practice Settings: Results From the Medical Outcomes Study," H. R. Rubin, et al., *Journal of the American Medical Association*, August 18, 1993, pp. 835–40.

22. "AMA Study Says Group Practices Pay More but Make Patients Wait," M. Mitka, *American Medical News*, March 7, 1994, p. 4.

23. "Are HMOs the Answer?" *Consumer Reports*, August 1992, pp. 519–31.

24. "Use of the Hospital in a Randomized Trial of Prepaid Care," A. L. Siu, et al., *Journal of the American Medical Association*, March 4, 1988, pp. 1343–46.

25. "Managed Care Plan Performance Since 1980: A Literature Analysis," R. H. Miller, et al., *Journal of the American Medical Association*, May 18, 1994, pp. 1512–19.

26. "Primary Care Performance in Fee-for-Service and Prepaid Health Care Systems: Results from the Medical Outcomes Study," D. G. Safran, et al., *Journal of the American Medical Association*, May 25, 1994, pp. 1579–86.

27. "The Pressure to Keep Prices High at a Walk-In Clinic," R. S. Bock, *New England Journal of Medicine*, September 22, 1988, pp. 785–87.

28. "The Nature of Adverse Events in Hospitalized Patients: Results of the Harvard Medical Practice Study II," L. L. Leape, et al., *New England Journal of Medicine*, February 7, 1991, pp. 377–84.

29. "The Relation Between Hospital Experience and Mortality for Patients with AIDS," V. E. Stone, et al., *Journal of the American Medical Association*, November 18, 1992, pp. 2655–61.

30. "Hospital Characteristics and Quality of Care," E. B. Keeler, et al., *Journal of the American Medical Association*, October 7, 1992, pp. 1709–14.

31. "Investigation of the Relationship Between Volume and Mortality for Surgical Procedures Performed in New York State Hospitals," E. L. Hannan, et al., *Journal of the American Medical Association*, July 28, 1989, pp. 503–10.

CHAPTER TWO: Is Your Doctor Taking the Time to Do the Job Right?

1. "Diagnosis and Treatment of Congenital Dislocation of the Hip," C. A. Churgay, et al., *American Family Physician*, March 1992, pp. 1217–28.

2. "Contributions of the History, Physical Examination and Laboratory Investigation in Making Medical Diagnoses," M. C. Peterson, et al., *Western Journal of Medicine*, February 1992, pp. 163–65.

3. "The Impact of Long Working Hours on Resident Physicians," T. B. McCall, *New England Journal of Medicine*, March 24, 1988, pp. 775–78.

4. "The Effect of Physician Behavior on the Collection of Data," H. B. Beckman, et al., *Annals of Internal Medicine*, November 1984, pp. 692–96.

5. "Making Good Interview Skills Better," E. J. Cassell, et al., *Patient Care*, March 30, 1989, pp. 145–65.

6. "Psychological Stress and Susceptibility to the Common

Cold," S. Cohen, et al., *New England Journal of Medicine*, August 29, 1991, pp. 606–11.

7. "The Relationship Between 'Job Strain,' Workplace Diastolic Blood Pressure and Left Ventricular Mass Index: Results of a Case-Control Study," P. L. Schanall, et al., *Journal of the American Medical Association*, April 11, 1990, pp. 1929–35.

8. "Self-Perceived Psychological Stress and Incidence of Coronary Artery Disease in Middle-Aged Men," A. Rosengren, et al., *American Journal of Cardiology*, November 1, 1991, pp. 1171–75.

9. "Stress and Relapse of Breast Cancer," A. J. Ramirez, et al., *British Medical Journal*, April 8, 1989, pp. 291–93.

10. "Emotional Support and Survival After Myocardial Infarction: A Prospective, Population-Based Study of the Elderly," L. F. Berkman, et al., *Annals of Internal Medicine*, December 15, 1992, pp. 692–96.

11. "Postponement of Death Until Symbolically Meaningful Occasions," D. P. Phillips, et al., *Journal of the American Medical Association*, April 11, 1990, pp. 1947–54.

12. "Treating Depression and Anxiety in Primary Care: Closing the Gap Between Knowledge and Practice," L. Eisenberg, *New England Journal of Medicine*, April 16, 1992, pp. 1080–83.

13. "Recognition and Management of Benzodiezepine Dependence," J. J. Gonzales, et al., *American Family Physician*, May 1992, pp. 2269–76.

14. "The Recognition and Control of Occupational Disease," P. J. Landrigan , et al., *Journal of the American Medical Association*, August 7, 1991, pp. 676–80.

15. "The Teaching of Occupational Health in United States Medical Schools: Five-Year Follow-up of an Initial Survey," B. S. Levy, *American Journal of Public Health*, January 1985, pp. 79–80.

16. "The Sexual History in General Medicine Practice," J. Ende, et al., *Archives of Internal Medicine*, March 1984, pp. 558–61.

17. "Effects of Antihypertensive Agents on Sexual Function," R. J. Weiss, *American Family Physician*, December 1991, pp. 2075–82.

18. "Health Risk Behaviors and Medical Sequelae of Childhood Sexual Abuse," F. E. Springs, et al., *Mayo Clinic Proceedings*, June 1992, pp. 527–32.

19. "Choices About Cardiopulmonary Resuscitation in the Hospital: When Do Physicians Talk With Patients?" S. E. Bedell, et al., *New England Journal of Medicine*, April 26, 1984, 1089–93.

20. "Assessing Housestaff Diagnostic Skills Using a Cardiology Patient Simulator," E. W. St. Clair, et al., *Annals of Internal Medicine*, November 1, 1992, pp. 751–56.

21. "Hand-Washing Patterns in Medical Intensive-Care Units," R. K. Albert, et al., *New England Journal of Medicine*, June 11, 1981, pp. 1465–66.

22. "Patient-to-Patient Transmission of Hepatitis B in a Dermatology Practice," W. G. Hlady, et al., *American Journal of Public Health*, December 1993, pp. 1689–93.

23. "Examination Gloves as Barriers to Hand Contamination in Clinical Practice," R. J. Olsen, et al., *Journal of the American Medical Association*, July 21, 1993, pp. 350–53.

24. "Preventive Care for Women: Does the Sex of the Physician Matter?" N. Lurie, et al., *New England Journal of Medicine*, August 12, 1993, pp. 478–82.

25. "Avoidable Errors in Emergency Practice," S. Jacobson, ed., *Emergency Medicine*, February 28, 1990, p. 94.

26. "Health Science Information Management and Continuing Education of Physicians: A Survey of U.S. Primary Care Practitioners and Their Opinion Leaders," J. W. Williamson, et al., *Annals of Internal Medicine*, January 15, 1989, pp. 151–60.

27. "Changes Over Time in the Knowledge Base of Practicing Internists," P. G. Ramsey, et al., *Journal of the American Medical Association*, August 28, 1991, pp. 1103–07.

28. "Some Older Doctors Run Afoul of Law," L. Tye, *Boston Globe*, July 7, 1987, p. 1.

29. "Patient, Provider and Hospital Characteristics Associated with Inappropriate Hospitalization," A. L. Siu, et al., *American Journal of Public Health*, October 1990, pp. 1253–56.

30. "Changes Over Time," Ramsey, et al.

31. "Withdrawal of Digoxin From Patients With Chronic Heart Failure Treated With Angiotensin-Converting-Enzyme Inhibitors," M. Packer, et al., *New England Journal of Medicine*, July 1, 1993, pp. 1–7.

CHAPTER THREE: Is Your Doctor Ordering the Right Tests?

1. "The Use and Misuse of Upper Gastrointestinal Endoscopy," K. L. Kahn, et al., *Annals of Internal Medicine*, October 15, 1988, pp. 664–70.

2. "Physicians' Perceptions of the Risk of Being Sued," A. G. Lawthers, et al., *Journal of Health Politics, Policy and Law*, Fall 1992, pp. 463–82.

3. "Biochemical Profiles," R. D. Cebul, et al., *Annals of Internal Medicine*, March 1987, pp. 403–13.

4. "Usefulness of Complete Blood Counts as a Case-Finding Tool in Medical Outpatients," S. Ruttimann, et al., *Annals of Internal Medicine*, January 1, 1992, pp. 44–50.

5. "Utility of the Routine Electrocardiogram Before Surgery and on General Hospital Admission: Critical Review and New Guidelines," A. L. Goldberger, et al., *Annals of Internal Medicine*, October 1986, pp. 552–57.

6. "The Utility of Routine Chest Radiographs," T. G. Tape, et al., *Annals of Internal Medicine*, May 1986, pp. 663–70.

7. "Routine Use of the Prothrombin and Partial Thromboplastin Times," S. B. Erban, et al., *Journal of the American Medical Association*, November 3, 1989, pp. 2428–32.

8. "Commercial Laboratory Testing for Chronic Fatigue Syndrome," D. P. Dooley, *Journal of the American Medical Association*, August 19, 1992, p. 873–74.

9. "The Psychological Consequences of Predictive Testing for Huntington's Disease," S. Wiggins, et al., *New England Journal of Medicine*, November 12, 1992, pp. 1401–05.

10. "Detection of Breast Cancer in Young Women," G. J. Lesnick, *Journal of the American Medical Association*, March 7, 1977, pp. 967–69.

11. "Evaluation of a Palpable Breast Mass," W. L. Donegan, *New England Journal of Medicine*, September 24, 1992, pp. 937–42.

12. "Maternal Serum Alpha-Fetoprotein Screening," F. G. Cunningham, et al., *New England Journal of Medicine*, July 4, 1991, pp. 55–57.

13. "Interpretation by Physicians of Clinical Laboratory Results," W. *Casscells*, et al., *New England Journal of Medicine*, November 2, 1978, pp. 999–1001.

14. "The Overdiagnosis of Lyme Disease," A. C. Steere, et al., *Journal of the American Medical Association*, April 14, 1993, pp. 1812–16.

15. "A Comparison of Ambulatory Test Ordering for Hypertensive Patients in the United States and England," A. M. Epstein, et al., *Journal of the American Medical Association*, October 5, 1984, pp. 1723–26.

16. "Frequency and Costs of Diagnostic Imaging in Office Practice—a Comparison of Self-Referring and Radiologist-Referring Physicians," B. J. Hillman, et al., *New England Journal of Medicine*, December 6, 1990, pp. 1604–08.

17. "The Overutilization of X-rays," H. L. Abrams, *New England Journal of Medicine*, May 24, 1979, pp. 1213–16.

18. "Quality of MD Labs Questioned," D. M. Gianelli, *American Medical News*, May 13, 1988, p. 1.

19. "CAP Moves to Improve Lipid Tests," P. Cotton, *Medical World News*, June 13, 1988, p. 55.

20. "Searching for Inaccuracy in Clinical Laboratory Testing Using Medicare Data: Evidence for Prothrombin Time," S. T. Mennemeyer, et al., *Journal of the American Medical Association*, February 24, 1993, pp. 1030–33.

21. "M.D.s' Investments Reap Controversial Profits," B. Bradley, et al., *Christian Science Monitor*, December 8, 1988, p. 1.

22. "New Evidence of the Prevalence and Scope of Physician Joint Ventures," J. M. Mitchell, et al., *Journal of the American Medical Association*, July 1, 1992, pp. 80–84.

23. "Conflicts of Interest: Physician Ownership of Medical Facilities," American Medical Association's Council on Ethical and Judicial Affairs, *Journal of the American Medical Association*, May 6, 1992, pp. 2366–69.

CHAPTER FOUR: Is Your Doctor Prescribing the Right Drugs?

1. "Mr. Rehnquist's Painful Episode," *Newsweek*, January 11, 1982, p. 20.

2. "Bad Medical Advice for Rehnquist," C. O'Connor, et al., *Newsweek*, August 25, 1986, p. 32.

3. "The Medication Errors That Get Doctors Sued," M. Crane, *Medical Economics*, November 22, 1993, pp. 36–41.

4. "Internists and Nicotine Gum," S. R. Cummings, et al., *Journal of the American Medical Association*, September 16, 1988, pp. 1565–69.

5. "Cimetidine Use in Nursing Homes: Prolonged Therapy and Excessive Doses," D. S. Sherman, et al., *Journal of the American Geriatrics Society*, November 1987, pp. 1023–27.

6. "From the Agency for Health Care Policy and Research: Acute Pain Management Can Be Improved," J. J. Clinton, *Journal of the American Medical Association*, May 20, 1992, p. 2580.

7. "The Neglected Medical History and Therapeutic Choices for Abdominal Pain: A Nationwide Study of 799 Physicians and Nurses," J. Avorn, et al., *Archives of Internal Medicine*, April 1991, pp. 694–98.

8. "How Common is White Coat Hypertension?" T. G. Pickering, et al., *Journal of the American Medical Association*, January 8, 1988, pp. 225–58.

9. "Drug-Induced Illness Leading to Hospitalization," G. J. Car-

anasos, et al., *Journal of the American Medical Association*, May 6, 1974, pp. 713–17.

10. "Adverse Drug Reactions During Hospitalization," R. I. Ogilvie, et al., *Canadian Medical Association Journal*, December 9, 1967, pp. 1450–57.

11. "Scientific Versus Commercial Sources of Influence on the Prescribing Behavior of Physicians," J. Avorn, et al., *American Journal of Medicine*, July 1982, pp. 4–8.

12. "Frequent-Flyer Programs for Drug Prescribing," J. Graves, *New England Journal of Medicine*, July 23, 1987, p. 252.

13. "Pharmaceutical Promotions—A Free Lunch?" D. R. Waud, *New England Journal of Medicine*, July 30, 1992, pp. 351–53.

14. "Final Report on the Aspirin Component of the Ongoing Physicians' Health Study," Steering Committee of the Physicians' Health Research Group, *New England Journal of Medicine*, July 20, 1989, pp. 129–35.

15. "Cost-Conscious Prescribing of Nonsteroidal Anti-inflammatory Drugs for Adults With Arthritis: A Review and Suggestions," J. M. Greene, et al., *Archives of Internal Medicine*, October 1992, pp. 1995–2002.

16. "Adverse Drug Reaction Processing in the United States and Its Dependence on Physician Reporting: Zomepirac (Zomax) as a Case in Point," K. A. Corre, et al., *Annals of Emergency Medicine*, February 1988, pp. 65–69.

17. "Comparison of an Anti-inflammatory Dose of Ibuprofen, an Analgesic Dose of Ibuprofen and Acetaminophen in the Treatment of Patients With Osteoarthritis of the Knee," J. D. Bradley, et al., *New England Journal of Medicine*, July 11, 1991, pp. 87–91.

18. "The Case for Low Dose Diuretics in Hypertension: Comparison of Low and Conventional Doses of Cyclopenthiazide," G. McVeigh, et al., *British Medical Journal*, July 9, 1988, pp. 95–98.

19. "Short-Term Treatment of Uncomplicated Lower Urinary Tract Infections in Women," S. R. Norrby, *Reviews of Infectious Diseases*, December 1990, pp. 458–67.

20. "Torsades de Pointes Occurring in Association with Terfenadine Use," B. P. Monahan, et al., *Journal of the American Medical Association*, December 5, 1990, pp. 2788–90.

21. "Examining Product Risk in Context: Market Withdrawal of Zomepirac as a Case Study," D. Ross-Degnan, et al., *Journal of the American Medical Association*, October 17, 1993, pp. 1937–42.

22. AMA Drug Evaluations, 4th ed., (Chicago: American Medical Association, 1980), pp. 80–81.

23. "Adverse Drug Reaction Processing," Corre, et al.

24. "The Pharmaceutical Tango," K. Franklin, *New Physician,* July–August 1989, pp. 24–28.

25. "Cost and Price of Comparable Branded and Generic Pharmaceuticals," B. S. Bloom, et al., *Journal of the American Medical Association,* November 14, 1986, pp. 2523–30.

26. "Overmedication of the Low-Weight Elderly," E. W. Campion, et al., *Archives of Internal Medicine,* May 1987, pp. 945–47.

27. "Initial Therapy for Hypertension—Individualizing Care," G. L. Schwartz, *Mayo Clinic Proceedings,* January 1990, pp. 73–87.

28. "Communicating With Patients About Their Medication," D. A. Kessler, *New England Journal of Medicine,* December 5, 1991, pp. 1650–52.

29. "Who Provides Patients With Drug Information?" T. McMahon, et al., *British Medical Journal,* February 7, 1987, pp. 355–56.

30. "How Often is Medication Taken as Prescribed? A Novel Assessment Technique," J. A. Cramer, et al., *Journal of the American Medical Association,* June 9, 1989, pp. 3273–77.

31. "Medication Use and Misuse: Physician-Patient Discrepancies," B. S. Hulka, et al., *Journal of Chronic Disease,* January 1975, pp. 7–21.

32. "Benzodiezapines of Long and Short Elimination Half-Life and the Risk of Hip Fracture," W. A. Ray, et al., *Journal of the American Medical Association,* December 15, 1989, pp. 3303–07.

33. "High Anxiety," *Consumer Reports,* January 1993, pp. 19–24.

34. "Quality of Care in Episodes of Respiratory Illness Among Medicaid Patients in New Mexico," K. N. Lohr, et al., *Annals of Internal Medicine,* January 1980, pp. 99–106.

35. "Initiation of Antihypertensive Treatment During Nonsteroidal Anti-Inflammatory Drug Therapy," J. H. Gurwitz, et al., *Journal of the American Medical Association,* September 14, 1994, pp. 781–86.

36. "Withdrawing Payment for Nonscientific Drug Therapy: Intended and Unexpected Effects of a Large-Scale Natural Experiment," S. B. Soumerai, et al., *Journal of the American Medical Association,* February 9, 1990, pp. 831–39.

CHAPTER FIVE: Does Your Doctor Know When to Intervene (and When Not to)?

1. "Arrogance," F. J. Ingelfinger, *New England Journal of Medicine,* December 25, 1980, pp. 1507–11.

2. "The Rational Management of Labor," M. A. Smith, et al., *American Family Physician,* May 1, 1993, pp. 1471–81.

3. "The Rational Management of Labor," Smith, et al.

4. "Effects of Electronic Fetal-Heart-Rate Monitoring, as Compared With Periodic Auscultation, on the Neurologic Development of Premature Infants," K. K. Shy, et al., *New England Journal of Medicine*, March 1, 1990, pp. 588–93.

5. "The Cascade Effect in the Clinical Care of Patients," J. W. Mold, et al., *New England Journal of Medicine*, February 20, 1986, pp. 512–14.

6. "Variations in the Use of Medical and Surgical Services by the Medicare Population," M. R. Chassin, et al., *New England Journal of Medicine*, January 30, 1986, pp. 285–90.

7. "The Physician Factor in Cesarean Birth Rates," G. L. Goyert, et al., *New England Journal of Medicine*, March 16, 1989, pp. 706–709.

8. "The Cesarean Section Rate," P. R. Overhulse, *Journal of the American Medical Association*, August 22/29, 1990, p. 971.

9. "Results of a Second-Opinion Trial Among Patients Recommended for Coronary Angiography," T. B. Graboys, et al., *Journal of the American Medical Association*, November 11, 1992, pp. 2537–40.

10. "The Physician-Patient as an Informed Consumer of Surgical Services," J. P. Bunker, et al., *New England Journal of Medicine*, May 9, 1974, pp. 1051–55.

11. "Patient-Reported Complications and Follow-Up Treatment After Radical Prostatectomy: The National Medicare Experience: 1988–1990 (Updated June 1993)," F. J. Fowler, et al., *Urology*, December 1993, pp. 622–29.

12. "Racial Differences in the Elderly's Use of Medical Procedures and Diagnostic Tests," J. J. Escarce, et al., *American Journal of Public Health*, July 1993, pp. 948–54.

13. "Racial Variation in Cardiac Procedure Use and Survival Following Acute Myocardial Infarction in the Department of Veterans Affairs," E. D. Peterson, et al., *Journal of the American Medical Association*, April 20, 1994, pp. 1175–80.

14. "Patterns of Care Related to Age of Breast Cancer Patients," S. Greenfield, et al., *Journal of the American Medical Association*, May 22/29, 1987, pp. 2766–70.

15. "Gender Disparities in Clinical Decision Making," American Medical Association's Council on Ethical and Judicial Affairs, *Journal of the American Medical Association*, July 24/31, 1991, pp. 559–62.

16. "Cesarean Section Use and Source of Payment: An Analysis of California Hospital Discharge Abstracts," R. S. Stafford, *American Journal of Public Health*, March 1990, pp. 313–15.

17. "The Association Between On-Site Cardiac Catheterization Facilities and the Use of Coronary Angiography After Acute Myocar-

dial Infarction," N. R. Every, *New England Journal of Medicine*, August 19, 1993, pp. 546–51.

18. "Effects of Electronic Fetal-Heart-Rate Monitoring," Shy, et al.

19. "Patterns of Obstetric Procedures Use in Maternity Care," G. Baruffi, et al., *Obstetrics & Gynecology*, October 1984, pp. 493–98.

20. "Continuous Emotional Support During Labor in a U.S. Hospital: A Randomized Controlled Trial," J. Kennell, et al., *Journal of the American Medical Association*, May 1, 1991, pp. 2197–2201.

21. "Fallacy of the Five-Year Survival in Lung Cancer," B. J. McNeil, et al., *New England Journal of Medicine*, December 21, 1978, pp. 1397–1401.

22. "Treating the Patient, Not Just the Cancer," I. F. Tannock, *New England Journal of Medicine*, December 10, 1987, pp. 1534–35.

23. "Latent Carcinoma of the Prostate," L. M. Franks, *Journal of Pathology and Bacteriology*, 1954, pp. 603–16.

24. "A Decision Analysis of Alternative Treatment Strategies for Clinically Localized Prostate Cancer," C. Fleming, et al., *Journal of the American Medical Association*, May 26, 1993, pp. 2650–58.

25. "A Decision Analysis," Fleming, et al.

26. "Patient-Reported Complications," Fowler, et al.

27. "An Assessment of Radical Prostatectomy: Time Trends, Geographic Variation and Outcomes," G. L. Lu-Yao, et al., *Journal of the American Medical Association*, May 26, 1993, pp. 2633–36.

28. "A Decision Analysis," Fleming, et al.

29. "An Assessment of Radical Prostatectomy," Lu-Yao, et al.

30. "Clinical Policies and the Quality of Clinical Practice," D. M. Eddy, *New England Journal of Medicine*, August 5, 1982, pp. 343–47.

31. "Technology Follies: The Uncritical Acceptance of Medical Innovation," D. A. Grimes, *Journal of the American Medical Association*, June 16, 1993, pp. 3030–33.

32. "A Prospective Cohort Study of Vasectomy and Prostate Cancer in U.S. Men," E. Giovannucci, et al., *Journal of the American Medical Association*, February 17, 1993, pp. 873–77.

33. "A Regional Prospective Study of In-Hospital Mortality Associated With Coronary Artery Bypass Grafting," G. T. O'Connor, et al., *Journal of the American Medical Association*, August 14, 1991, pp. 803–809.

34. "The Learning Curve," B. Gaster, *Journal of the American Medical Association*, September 15, 1993, p. 1280.

35. "Surgical Injuries Lead to New Rule: New York Assails the Training for a Popular Technique," L. K. Altman, *New York Times*, June 14, 1992, p. 1.

36. "Predictors of Laparoscopic Complications After Formal Training in Laparoscopic Surgery," W. A. See, et al., *Journal of the American Medical Association*, December 8, 1993, pp. 2689–92.

37. "Should Operations Be Regionalized? The Empirical Relation Between Surgical Volume and Mortality," H. S. Luft, et al., *New England Journal of Medicine*, December 20, 1979, pp. 1364–69.

38. "A Successful Program to Lower Cesarean-Section Rates," S. A. Myers, et al., *New England Journal of Medicine*, December 8, 1988, pp. 1511–16.

39. "Impact of a Mandatory Second-Opinion Program on Medicaid Surgery Rates," S. G. Martin, et al., *Medical Care*, January 1982, pp. 21–45.

40. "A Leap of Faith: What Can We Do to Curtail Intrainstitutional Transmission of Tuberculosis?" M. C. Iseman, *Annals of Internal Medicine*, August 1, 1992, pp. 251–53.

41. "The Outcome of Hospitalization for Acute Illness in the Elderly," C. T. Lamont, et al., *Journal of the American Geriatrics Society*, May 1983, pp. 282–88.

42. "The Idle Intravenous Catheter," F. A. Lederle, et al., *Annals of Internal Medicine*, May 1, 1992, pp. 737–38.

43. "Hazards of Hospitalization of the Elderly," M. C. Creditor, *Annals of Internal Medicine*, February 1, 1993, pp. 219–23.

44. "Inappropriate Use of Hospitals in a Randomized Trial of Health Insurance Plans," A. L. Siu, et al., *New England Journal of Medicine*, November 13, 1986, pp. 1259–66. "Patient, Provider and Hospital Characteristics Associated with Inappropriate Hospitalization," A. L Siu, et al., *American Journal of Public Health*, October 1990, pp. 1253–56.

45. "Just How Short Can Hospital Stays Be? With Third Parties Demanding Earlier and Earlier Discharges, Doctors' Concern Over Their Patients' Welfare Is Growing," L. M. Walker *Medical Economics*, September 26, 1994, pp. 38–47.

46. "R.I. Doctors Face 'Absurd' Inpatient Limits," G. Borzo, *American Medical News*, March 21, 1994, p. 1.

47. "The Variability of Transfusion Practice in Coronary Artery Bypass Surgery," L. T. Goodnough, et al., *Journal of the American Medical Association*, January 2, 1991, pp. 86–90.

48. "Transfusion Medicine Faces Time of Major 'Challenges and Changes,'" A. A. Skolnick, *Journal of the American Medical Association*, August 12, 1992, p. 697.

49. "Transfusion Practice in Medical Patients," S. Saxena, et al., *Archives of Internal Medicine*, November 22, 1993, pp. 2575–80.

50. "Influence of Clinical Knowledge, Organizational Context and Practice Style on Transfusion Decision Making," S. R. Salem-Schatz,

et al., *Journal of the American Medical Association*, July 25, 1990, pp. 476–83.

51. "Prudent Strategies for Elective Red Blood Cell Transfusion," H. G. Welch, et al., *Annals of Internal Medicine*, March 1, 1992, pp. 393–402.

52. "Indications for Hysterectomy," K. J. Carlson, et al., *New England Journal of Medicine*, March 25, 1993, pp. 856–60.

53. "Comparison of Medical and Surgical Treatment for Unstable Angina Pectoris: Results of a Veterans Administration Cooperative Study," R. J. Luchi, et al., *New England Journal of Medicine*, April 16, 1987, pp. 977–84.

54. "The Appropriateness of Performing Coronary Artery Bypass Surgery," C. M. Winslow, et al., *Journal of the American Medical Association*, July 22/29, 1988, pp. 505–509.

55. "Risk of Carotid Endarterectomy in the Elderly," E. S. Fisher, et al., *American Journal of Public Health*, December 1989, pp. 1617–20.

56. "Predicting the Appropriate Use of Carotid Endarterectomy, Upper Gastrointestinal Endoscopy and Coronary Angiography," R. H. Brook, et al., *New England Journal of Medicine*, October 25, 1990, pp. 1173–77.

57. "Incidence of Unwarranted Implantation of Permanent Cardiac Pacemakers in a Large Medical Population," A. M. Greenspan, et al., *New England Journal of Medicine*, January 21, 1988, pp. 158–63.

58. "Complications of Permanent Transvenous Pacing," B. Phibbs, et al., *New England Journal of Medicine*, May 30, 1985, pp. 1428–32.

59. "Complications of Permanent Transvenous Pacing," B. Phibbs, et al.

60. "CPR in Hospitalized Patients: When Is It Futile?" C. F. Von Gunten, *American Family Physician*, December 1991, pp. 2130–34.

61. "Do Physicians' Own Preferences for Life-Sustaining Treatment Influence Their Perceptions of Patients' Preferences?" L. J. Schneiderman, et al., *Journal of Clinical Ethics*, Spring 1993, pp. 28–33.

62. "Limitations of Listing Specific Medical Interventions in Advance Directives," A. S. Brett, *Journal of the American Medical Association*, August 14, 1991, pp. 825–28.

CHAPTER SIX: Is Your Doctor Practicing Good Preventive Medicine?

1. "Advance Report of Final Mortality Statistics, 1990," National Center for Health Statistics, U.S. Department of Health and Human Services, 1993.

2. "Actual Causes of Death in the United States," J. M. McGinnis,

et al., *Journal of the American Medical Association*, November 10, 1993, pp. 2207–12.

3. "Odds and Ends," *Wall Street Journal*, June 9, 1993, p. B1.

4. "Are Physicians Advising Smokers to Quit? The Patient's Perspective," R. F. Anda, et al., *Journal of the American Medical Association*, April 10, 1987, pp. 1916–19.

5. "Actual Causes of Death in the United States," McGinnis, et al.

6. *Guide to Clinical Preventive Services: An Assessment of the Effectiveness of 169 Interventions*, U.S. Preventive Services Task Force, (Baltimore: Williams and Wilkins, 1989).

7. "The Need for Adult Immunizations," P. Gardner, *Infectious Diseases Clinical Updates*, December 1993, pp. 1–4.

8. "Clinical Effectiveness of Influenza Vaccination in Manitoba," D. S. Fedson, et al., *Journal of the American Medical Association*, October 27, 1993, pp. 1956–61.

9. "Frequency of Adverse Reactions to Influenza Vaccine in the Elderly: A Randomized, Placebo-Controlled Trial," K. L. Margolis, et al., *Journal of the American Medical Association*, September 5, 1990, pp. 1139–41.

10. "Sexual Transmission Efficiency of Hepatitis B Virus and Human Immunodeficiency Virus Among Homosexual Men," L. A. Kingsley, et al., *Journal of the American Medical Association*, July 11, 1990. pp. 230–34.

11. "Quality Assurance in Cervical Cytology: The Papanicolaou Smear," the American Medical Association's Council on Scientific Affairs, *Journal of the American Medical Association*, September 22/29, 1989, pp. 1672–79.

12. "Quality Assurance in Cervical Cytology," American Medical Association's Council on Scientific Affairs.

13. "Screening for Cervical Cancer," D. M. Eddy, *Annals of Internal Medicine*, August 1, 1990, pp. 214–26.

14. "Screening for Cervical Cancer," Eddy.

15. *Guide to Clinical Preventive Services*, U.S. Preventive Services Task Force.

16. "Cancer-Related Checkups," American Cancer Society, rev. February 1993.

17. "Mammographic Screening," D. Lee Davis, et al., *Journal of the American Medical Association*, January 12, 1994, pp. 152–53.

18. "Screening and Informed Consent," J. M. Lee, *New England Journal of Medicine*, February 11, 1993, pp. 438–40.

19. "Prostate Cancer: Screening, Diagnosis, and Management," M. B. Garnick, *Annals of Internal Medicine*, May 15, 1993, pp. 804–18.

20. "The Prostate Puzzle," *Consumers Reports*, July 1993, pp. 459–65.

21. "Latent Carcinoma of the Prostate," L. M. Franks, *Journal of Pathology and Bacteriology*, 1954, pp. 603–16.

22. "Falls in the Elderly," T. M. Cutson, *American Family Physician*, January 1994, pp. 149–56.

23. "Top 200 Drugs of 1992: What Are Pharmacists Dispensing Most Often?" L. La Piana Simonsen, *Pharmacy Times*, April 1993, pp. 29–44.

24. "Hormone Therapy to Prevent Disease and Prolong Life in Postmenopusal Women," D. Grady, et al., *Annals of Internal Medicine*, December 15, 1992, pp. 1016–37.

25. "Hormone Replacement Therapy: The Need for Reconsideration," Lynn Rosenberg, *American Journal of Public Health*, December 1993, pp. 1670–73.

26. "Randomised Trial of Cholesterol Lowering in 4444 Patients With Coronary Heart Disease: The Scandinavian Simvastatin Survival Study," Scandinavian Simvastatin Survival Study Group, *Lancet*, November 19, 1994, pp. 1383–89.

27. "Helinski Heart Study: Primary-Prevention Trial With Gemfibrozil in Middle-Aged Men With Dyslipidemia: Safety of Treatment, Changes in Risk Factors, and Incidence of Coronary Heart Disease," M. H. Frick, et al., *New England Journal of Medicine*, November 12, 1987, pp. 1237–45.

28. "Treating Hypercholesterolemia: How Should Practicing Physicians Interpret the Published Data for Patients?" A. S. Brett, *New England Journal of Medicine*, September 7, 1989, pp. 676–80.

29. "Motor Vehicle Crash Injury: Mechanisms and Prevention," T. D. Peterson, et al., *American Family Physician*, October 1991, pp. 1307–14.

30. "Screening Procedures in the Asymptomatic Adult: Comparison of Physicians' Recommendations, Patients' Desires, Published Guidelines, and Actual Practice," B. Woo, et al., *Journal of the American Medical Association*, September 20, 1985, pp. 1480–84.

31. "Preventive Content of Adult Primary Care: Do Generalists and Subspecialists Differ?" A. J. Dietrich, et al., *American Journal of Public Health*, March 1984, pp. 223–27.

CHAPTER SEVEN: Taking Control of Your Medical Care

1. "Expanding Patient Involvement in Care: Effects on Patient Outcomes," S. Greenfield, et al., *Annals of Internal Medicine*, April 1985, pp. 520–28.

2. "Assessing the Effects of Physician-Patient Interactions on the Outcomes of Chronic Disease," S. H. Kaplan, et al., *Medical Care*, March 1989, pp. S110–27.

3. "How Drug Firms Romance Doctors: Junkets, Favors Influence Prescriptions," J. Rosenbloom 3rd, *Boston Globe*, March 26, 1989, pp. A25–26.

4. "Comparison of the Effects of Oat Bran and Low-Fiber Wheat on Serum Lipoprotein Levels and Blood Pressure," J. F. Swain, et al., *New England Journal of Medicine*, January 18, 1990, pp. 147–52.

5. "Oat Products and Lipid Lowering: A Meta-analysis," C. M. Ripsin, et al., *Journal of the American Medical Association*, June 24, 1992, pp. 3317–25.

6. "Oat Bran and Serum Cholesterol," J. F. Burris, *New England Journal of Medicine*, June 14, 1990, p. 1748.

7. "The Patient's Role in Clinical Decision-Making," D. S. Brody, *Annals of Internal Medicine*, November 1980, pp. 718–22.

8. "Physician Recommendations of Elective Surgery for Duodenal Ulcer Patients: A Comparison of Surgeons and Medical Specialists," J. D. Elashoff, et al., *Gastroenterology*, October 1980, pp. 750–53.

When consulting the information sources listed in the pages that follow, keep in mind that there is no such thing as unbiased information. Everybody has a point of view. Some of the organizations listed present mainstream points of view; others have more alternative slants. Some present both sides of various controversies; some offer only their preferred dogma. I have included some organizations whose positions I don't always agree with. My advice is to obtain as broad a range of opinion as possible, including that of your doctor, and to make up your own mind.

Because of frequent address and phone number changes, some listings may not remain accurate.

APPENDIX 2

SOURCES OF INFORMATION ON SPECIFIC MEDICAL CONDITIONS

The following is a list of organizations providing information on a variety of medical conditions. If you can't find information in the area you're seeking, there are two resources you might try. The U.S. government runs a service that refers callers to some twelve hundred organizations that may be able to provide information:

National Health Information Center
P.O. Box 1133
Washington, DC 20013
(800) 336-4797

Another possiblity is to contact the group that acts as a clearinghouse for information on various rare medical problems:

National Organization for Rare Disorders
P.O. Box 8923
New Fairfield, CT 06812
(800) 999-NORD

Finally, two organizations act as clearinghouses for hundreds of national and local self-help groups:

The American Self-Help Clearinghouse
St. Clares–Riverside Medical Center
25 Pocono Road
Denville, NJ 07834
(201) 625-7101
(201) 625-9053 (TDD)
(800) 367-6274 New Jersey only

National Self-Help Clearinghouse
Graduate School and University Center of the City University
of New York
25 West Forty-third Street, Room 6
New York, NY 10036
(212) 642-2944

Acquired Immunodeficiency Syndrome (AIDS)

CDC National AIDS Clearinghouse
P.O. Box 6003
Rockville, MD 20849
(800) 458-5231
(800) 243-7012 (TTY/TDD)

Gay Men's Health Crisis
129 West Twentieth Street
New York, NY 10011
(212) 807-6664
AIDS hotline (212) 807-6655

American Social Health Association
P.O. Box 13827
Research Triangle Park, NC 27709
AIDS hotline (800) 342-2437
AIDS hotline in Spanish (800) 344-7432

Addison's Disease

National Adrenal Disease Foundation
505 Northern Boulevard, Suite 200
Great Neck, NY 11021
(516) 487-4992

Alcohol and Other Drug Abuse

Alcoholics Anonymous
P.O. Box 459
Grand Central Station
New York, NY 10163
(212) 870-3400
(212) 870-3199 (TDD)

National Council of Alcoholism and Drug Dependence
12 West Twenty-first Street
New York, NY 10010
(800) 622-2255

National Clearinghouse for Alcohol and Drug Information
P.O. Box 2345
Rockville, MD 20847
(800) SAYNOTO
(800) 487-4889 (TDD)

Center for Substance Abuse Treatment Information and Treatment
  Referral Hotline
11426-28 Rockville Pike, Suite 410
Rockville, MD 20852
(800) 662-HELP

Narcotics Anonymous
P.O. Box 9999
Van Nuys, CA 91409
(818) 780-3951

Alzheimer's Disease

Alzheimer's Association
919 Michigan Avenue, Suite 1000
Chicago, IL 60611
(800) 272-3900

Allergies

Asthma and Allergy Foundation of America
1125 Fifteenth Street NW, Suite 502
Washington, DC 20005
(800) 7-ASTHMA

National Institute of Allergy and Infectious Diseases
9000 Rockville Pike, Building 31, Room 7A-50
Bethesda, MD 20892
(301) 496-5717

Amyotrophic Lateral Sclerosis (Lou Gehrig's Disease)

Amyotrophic Lateral Sclerosis Association
21021 Ventura Boulevard, Suite 321
Woodland Hills, CA 91364
(800) 782-4747

Arthritis and Other Joint Problems

Arthritis Foundation
1314 Spring Street NW
Atlanta, GA 30309
(800) 283-7800

National Arthritis and Musculoskeletal and Skin Diseases Information Clearinghouse
Box AMS
9000 Rockville Pike
Bethesda, MD 20892
(301) 495-4484

Spondylitis Association of America
P.O. Box 5872
Sherman Oaks, CA 91413
(800) 777-8189

Asbestos (see also *Lung Problems*)

Asbestos Victims of America
P.O. Box 559
Capitola, CA 95010
(408) 476-3646

White Lung Association
P.O. Box 1483
Baltimore, MD 21203
(410) 243-5864

Asthma

American Lung Association
1740 Broadway
New York, NY 10019-4374
(800) 586-4872

Asthma and Allergy Foundation of America
1125 Fifteenth Street NW, Suite 502
Washington, DC 20005
(800) 7-ASTHMA

Ataxia

National Ataxia Foundation
750 Oaks Center
15500 Wayzata Boulevard
Wayzata, MN 55391
(612) 473-7666

Attention Deficit Disorder

National Attention-Deficit Disorder Association
P.O. Box 488
West Newbury, MA 01985
(800) 487-2282

Bechet's Syndrome

American Bechet's Association
P.O. Box 54063
Minneapolis, MN 55454-0063
(800) 7BECHETS

Blood Conditions

Aplastic Anemia Foundation
P.O. Box 22689
Baltimore, MD 21203
(800) 747-2820

Cooley's Anemia Foundation (Thalassemia)
105 East Twenty-second Street, Suite 911
New York, NY 10010
(800) 221-3571
(800) 522-7222 New York only

Leukemia Society of America
600 Third Avenue
New York, NY 10016
(800) 955-4LSA

National Association for Sickle Cell Disease
3345 Wilshire Boulevard, Suite 1106
Los Angeles, CA 90010
(800) 421-8453

National Hemophilia Foundation
110 Greene Street, Suite 303
New York, NY 10012
(212) 219-8180

Burn Injuries

Phoenix Society for Burn Survivors
11 Rust Hill Road, Suite 146
Levittown, PA 19056
(800) 888-BURN

Cancer

American Brain Tumor Association
2720 River Road, Suite 146
Des Plaines, IL 60018
(800) 886-2282

American Cancer Society
1599 Clifton Road NE
Atlanta, GA 30329
(800) ACS-2345

Cancer Information Service
Office of Cancer Communication
NCI/NIH, Building 31, 10A24
9000 Rockville Pike
Bethesda, MD 20892
(800) 4-CANCER

Leukemia Society of America
600 Third Avenue, 4th Floor
New York, NY 10016
(800) 955-4LSA

Skin Cancer Foundation
245 Fifth Avenue, Suite 2402
New York, NY 10016
(212) 725-5751

United Ostomy Association
36 Executive Park, Suite 120
Irvine, CA 92714
(800) 826-0826

Carpal Tunnel Syndrome/Repetitive Motion Injuries

American Carpal Tunnel Syndrome Association
P.O. Box 6730
Saginaw, MI 48608

National Institute for Occupational Safety and Health (NIOSH)
4676 Columbia Parkway
Cincinnati, OH 45226
(800) 35-NIOSH

Celiac Disease (see also *Intestinal Problems)*

American Celiac Society/Dietary Support Coalition
58 Musano Court
West Orange, NJ 07052
(201) 325-8837

Celiac Disease Foundation
13251 Ventura Boulevard, Suite 3
Studio City, CA 91604
(818) 990-2354

Celiac Spruce Association/USA
P.O. Box 31700
Omaha, NE 68131
(402) 558-0600

Cerebral Palsy

> United Cerebral Palsy Associations
> 1522 K Street, Suite 1112
> Washington, DC 20005
> (800) USA-5UCP

Chronic Fatigue Syndrome

> CFIDS Association
> P.O. Box 220398
> Charlotte, NC 28222-0398
> (800) 442-3437

> National Chronic Fatigue Syndrome Association
> 3521 Broadway, Suite 222
> Kansas City, MO 64111
> (816) 931-4777

Cleft Palate

> American Cleft Palate–Craniofacial Association
> 1218 Grandview Avenue
> Pittsburgh, PA 15211
> (800) 242-5338

Crohn's Disease/Ulcerative Colitis (see also *Intestinal Problems*)

> Crohn's and Colitis Foundation of America
> 386 Park Avenue South
> New York, NY 10016-7374
> (800) 932-2423

Cystic Fibrosis

> Cystic Fibrosis Foundation
> 6931 Arlington Road, No. 200
> Bethesda, MD 20814
> (800) 344-4823

Depression (see also Mental Health)

National Depressive and Manic Depressive Association
730 N. Franklin, Suite 501
Chicago, IL 60610
(800) 82-NDMDA

National Foundation for Depressive Illnesses
P.O. Box 2257
New York, NY 10016
(800) 248-4344

DES (Diethylstilbestrol) Exposure

DES Action, USA
1615 Broadway, Suite 510
Oakland, CA 94612
(510) 465-4011

Diabetes

American Diabetes Association
P.O. Box 25757
1660 Duke Street
Alexandria, VA 22314
(800) ADA-DISC

National Diabetes Information Clearinghouse
P.O. Box NDIC
9000 Rockville Pike
Bethesda, MD 20892
(301) 468-2162

Down's Syndrome

National Down's Syndrome Congress
1605 Chantilly Drive, Suite 250
Atlanta, GA 30324
(800) 232-NDSC

National Down's Syndrome Society
666 Broadway
New York, NY 10012
(800) 221-4602

Ear Problems

Acoustic Neuroma Association
P.O. Box 12402
Atlanta, GA 30355
(404) 237-8023

American Tinnitis Association
P.O. Box 5
Portland, OR 97207
(503) 248-9985

Better Hearing Institute
P.O. Box 1840
Washington, DC 20013
(800) EAR-WELL

Meniere's Network
Ear Foundation
2000 Church Street
P.O. Box 111
Nashville, TN 37236
(800) 545-HEAR

National Hearing Aid Society
20361 Middlebelt Road
Livonia, MI 48152
Hearing Aid Helpline
(800) 521-5247

National Institute on Deafness and Other Communication Disorders Information Clearinghouse
P.O. Box 37777
Washington, DC 20013
(800) 241-1044
(800) 241-1055 (TDD)

Vestibular Disorders Association
P.O. Box 4467
Portland, OR 97208
(503) 229-7705

Eating Disorders

Anorexia Nervosa and Related Eating Disorders
P.O. Box 5102
Eugene, OR 97405
(503) 344-1144

National Association of Anorexia Nervosa and Associated
Disorders
Box 7
Highland Park, IL 60035
(708) 831-3438

Obesity Foundation
5600 South Quebec, Suite 109-A
Englewood, CO 80111
(303) 850-0328

Overeaters Anonymous
383 Van Ness Avenue, Suite 1601
Torrance, CA 90501
(310) 618-8835

Take Off Pounds Sensibly (TOPS)
c/o Susan Trones
4575 South Fifth Street
P.O. Box 07360
Milwaukee, WI 53207
(800) 932-8677

Endometriosis

Endometriosis Association
8585 North Seventy-sixth Place
Milwaukee, WI 53223
(800) 992-3636

Epilepsy

Epilepsy Foundation of America
4531 Garden City Drive
Landover, MD 20785
(800) EFA-1000

Eye Problems

American Council of the Blind
1155 Fifteenth Street NW, Suite 720
Washington, DC 20005
(800) 424-8666

Association for Macular Disorders
210 East Sixty-fourth Street
New York, NY 10021
(212) 605-3719

National Eye Institute
National Institutes of Health
Building 31, Room 6A-32
9000 Rockville Pike
Bethesda, MD 20892
(301) 496-5248

National Federation of the Blind
1800 Johnson Street
Baltimore, MD 21230
(800) 638-5555

National Society to Prevent Blindness
500 East Remington Road
Schaumberg, IL 60173
(800) 331-2020

Foundation for Glaucoma Research
490 Post Street, Suite 830
San Francisco, CA 94102
(800) 826-6694

RP (Retinitis Pigmentosa) Foundation Fighting Blindness
1401 Mount Royal Avenue, 4th Floor
Baltimore, MD 21217
(800) 638-5555

Fibromyalgia

Fibromyalgia Association of Central Ohio
3545 Olentangy River Road, Suite 8
Columbus, OH 43214
(614) 262-2000

Fibromyalgia Association of Texas
5650 Forest Lane
Dallas, TX 75230
(214) 363-2473

Gaucher's Disease

National Gaucher's Foundation
19241 Montgomery Village Avenue, Suite E-21
Gaithersburg, MD 20879
(800) 925-8885

Genetic Disorders

Alliance of Genetic Support Groups
35 Wisconsin Circle, Suite 440
Chevy Chase, MD 20815
(800) 336-4363

March of Dimes Birth Defects Foundation
1275 Mamaroneck Avenue
White Plains, NY 10605
(914) 428-7100

National Maternal and Child Health Clearinghouse
8201 Greensboro Drive, Suite 600
McLean, VA 22102
(703) 821-2098

Guillain-Barre Syndrome

Guillain-Barre Syndrome Foundation
P.O. Box 262
Wynnewood, PA 19096
(215) 667-0131

Hair Loss

American Hair Loss Council
100 Independence Place, Suite 207
Tyler, TX 75703
(800) 274-8717

Headache

National Headache Foundation
5252 North Western Avenue
Chicago, IL 60625
(800) 843-2256

Head Injury

National Head Injury Foundation
1776 Massachusetts Avenue NW, Suite 100
Washington, DC 20036
(800) 444-6443

Heart Disease

American Heart Association
7272 Greenville Avenue
Dallas, TX 75231-4596
(800) 242-8721

National Heart, Lung, and Blood Institute Information Center
P.O. Box 30105
Bethesda, MD 20824
(301) 251-1222

Hemochromatosis

Hemochromatosis Foundation
P.O. Box 8569
Albany, NY 12208
(518) 489-0972

Iron Overload Diseases Association
433 Westwind Drive
North Palm Beach, FL 33408
(407) 840-8512

Hemophilia

National Hemophilia Foundation
110 Greene Street, Suite 303
New York, NY 10012
(212) 219-8180

High Blood Pressure (see also *Heart Disease*)

High Blood Pressure Information Center
4733 Bethesda Avenue, Suite 530
Bethesda, MD 20814-4820
(301) 951-3260

Huntington's Disease

Huntington's Disease Society of America
140 West Twenty-second Street, 6th Floor
New York, NY 10011
(800) 345-HDSA
(212) 242-1968 New York only

Hypoglycemia

Adrenal Metabolic Research Society of the Hypoglycemia
Foundation
153 Pawling Avenue
Troy, NY 12180
(518) 272-7154

Immune Deficiency (primary, as opposed to acquire, as with AIDS)

Immune Deficiency Foundation
25 Chesapeake Avenue, Suite 206
Towson, MD 21204
(800) 296-4433

Impotence

Geddings Osbon Sr. Foundation
1246 Jones Street
P.O. Drawer 1593
Augusta, GA 30903–1593
(800) 433-4215

Impotence Institute of America/Impotents Anonymous
119 South Ruth Street
Maryville, TN 37801
(615) 983-6064

Recovery of Male Potency
27211 Lahser Road, No. 208
Southfield, MI 48034
(800) TEL-ROMP

Incontinence

Help for Incontinent People
P.O. Box 544
Union, SC 29379
(800) BLADDER

Simon Foundation for Continence
Box 815
Wilmette, IL 60091
(800) 23-SIMON

Infertility

Resolve, Inc.
1310 Broadway
Somerville, MA 02144
(617) 623-1156

Intestinal Problems

Crohn's and Colitis Foundation of America
386 Park Avenue South
New York, NY 10016-7374
(800) 932-2423

Intestinal Disease Foundation
1323 Forbes Avenue, Suite 200
Pittsburgh, PA 15219
(412) 261-5888

National Digestive Diseases Information Clearinghouse
Box NDDIC
9000 Rockville Pike
Bethesda, MD 20892
(301) 468-6344

United Ostomy Association
36 Executive Park, Suite 120
Irvine, CA 92714
(800) 826-0826

Kidney and Urinary Problems

American Association of Kidney Patients
111 South Parker Street, Suite 405
Tampa, FL 33606
(800) 749-2257

American Kidney Fund
6110 Executive Boulevard, Suite 1010
Rockville, MD 20852
(800) 638-8299

National Kidney and Urological Diseases Information
   Clearinghouse
Box NKUDIC
9000 Rockville Pike
Bethesda, MD 20892
(301) 468-6345

National Kidney Foundation
30 East Thirty-third Street, Suite 1100
New York, NY 10016
(800) 622-9010

Polycystic Kidney Research Foundation
922 Walnut Street, Suite 411
Kansas City, MO 64106
(800) PKD-CURE

Leprosy (Hansen's Disease)

American Leprosy Mission
1 ALM Way
Greenville, SC 29601
(800) 543-3131

Leukodystrophy

United Leukodystrophy Foundation
2304 Highland Drive
Sycamore, IL 60178
(800) 728-5483

Liver Problems

American Liver Foundation
1425 Pompton Avenue, Suite 1-3
Cedar Grove, NJ 07009
(800) 223-0179

National Digestive Diseases Information Clearinghouse
Box NDDIC
9000 Rockville Pike
Bethesda, MD 20892
(301) 654-3810

Lung Problems (see also *Asthma*)

American Lung Association
1470 Broadway
New York, NY 10019
(800) 586-4872

Black Lung Association (Coal Miners)
P.O. Box 872
Crab Orchard, WV 25827
(304) 252-9654

Brown Lung Association (Cotton Mill Workers)
P.O. Box 7583
Greenville, SC 29610
(803) 269-8048

White Lung Association (Asbestos)
P.O. Box 1483
Baltimore, MD 21203
(410) 243-5864

Lupus

American Lupus Society
3914 Del Amo Boulevard, Suite 922
Torrance, CA 90503
(800) 331-1802

Lupus Foundation of America
4 Research Place, Suite 180
Rockville, MD 20850-3326
(800) 558-0121

Lyme Disease

Lyme Disease Foundation
One Financial Plaza, 18th Floor
Hartford, CT 06103
(800) 886-LYME

Lymphedema

National Lymphedema Network
2111 Post Street, Suite 404
San Francisco, CA 94115
(800) 541-3259

Marfan Syndrome

National Marfan Foundation
382 Main Street
Port Washington, NY 11050
(800) 862-7326

Mental Health (see also *Depression*)

Information Resources and Inquiries Branch
National Institute of Mental Health
5600 Fishers Lane, Room 7-99
Rockville, MD 20857
(301) 443-4513

National Alliance for the Mentally Ill
2101 Wilson Boulevard, Suite 302
Arlington, VA 22201
(703) 524-7600

National Mental Health Association
1021 Prince Street
Alexandria, VA 22314
(800) 969-NMHA

National Mental Health Consumer Self-Help Clearinghouse
311 South Juniper Street, Room 1000
Philadelphia, PA 19107
(800) 553-4539

Obsessive Compulsive Foundation
P.O. Box 70
Milford, CT 06460
(203) 878-5669

President's Committee on Mental Retardation
U.S. Department of Health and Human Services
William J. Cohen Building, Room 5325
330 Independence Avenue SW
Washington, DC 20201
(202) 619-0634

Multiple Sclerosis

Multiple Sclerosis Foundation
6350 North Andrews Avenue
Fort Lauderdale, FL 33309
(800) 441-7055

National Multiple Sclerosis Society
733 Third Avenue
New York, NY 10017
(800) 624-8236

Muscular Dystrophy

Muscular Dystrophy Association
3300 East Sunrise Drive
Tucson, AZ 85718
(800) 572-1717

Myasthenia Gravis

Myasthenia Gravis Foundation
53 West Jackson Boulevard, Suite 1352
Chicago, IL 60604
(800) 541-5454

Neurofibromatosis

National Neurofibromatosis Foundation
141 Fifth Avenue, Suite 7-S
New York, NY 10010
(800) 323-7398

Neurofibromatosis, Inc.
8855 Annapolis Road, Suite 110
Lanham, MD 20706
(800) 942-6825

Osteoporosis

National Osteoporosis Foundation
1150 Seventeenth Street NW, Suite 500
Washington, DC 20037
(202) 223-2226

Paget's Disease

Paget Foundation for Paget's Disease of Bone and Related
Disorders
200 Varick Street, Suite 1004
New York, NY 10014
(800) 23-PAGET

Pain

American Chronic Pain Association
P.O. Box 850
Rocklin, CA 95677
(916) 632-0922

National Chronic Pain Outreach Association
7979 Old Georgetown Road, Suite 100
Bethesda, MD 20814
(301) 652-4948

Panic Disorder

Panic Disorder Education Program
National Institute of Mental Health
National Institutes of Health
5600 Fishers Lane, Room 7-99
Rockville, MD 20857
(800) 64-PANIC

Parkinson's Disease

American Parkinson Disease Association
60 Bay Street, Suite 401
Staten Island, NY 10301
(800) 223-APDA

Parkinson's Disease Foundation
William Black Medical Research Building
Columbia Presbyterian Medical Center
650 West 168th Street
New York, NY 10032
(800) 457-6676

Parkinson's Educational Program/USA
3900 Birch Street, No. 105
Newport Beach, CA 92660
(800) 344-7872

Polio

Polio Society
P.O. Box 106273
Washington, DC 20016
(301) 897-8180

Porphyria

American Porphyria Foundation
P.O. Box 22712
Houston, TX 77227
(713) 266-9617

Premenstrual Syndrome

PMS Access
P.O. Box 9326
Madison, WI 53715
(800) 222-4PMS

PMS Research Foundation
P.O. Box 14574
Las Vegas, NV 89114
(702) 369-9248

Prostate Problems

American Prostate Society
1340 Charwood Road, Suite F
Hanover, MD 21076
(800) 678-1238

National Kidney and Urological Diseases Information
Clearinghouse
9000 Rockville Pike
Box NKUDIC
Bethesda, MD 20892
(301) 654-4415

Reflex Sympathetic Dystrophy

Reflex Sympathetic Dystrophy Association
P.O. Box 821
Haddenfield, NJ 08033
(609) 795-8845

Sarcoidosis

National Sarcoidosis Family Aid and Research Foundation
P.O. Box 22868
Newark, NJ 07101
(800) 223-6429

Scoliosis

Scoliosis Association
P.O. Box 811705
Boca Raton, FL 33481
(800) 800-0669

Sexually Transmitted Diseases (STDs) (see also *AIDS*)

American Social Health Association
P.O. Box 13827
Research Triangle Park, NC 27709
AIDS hotline (800) 342-2437
AIDS hotline in Spanish (800) 344-7432
AIDS hotline (TTY) (800) 243-7889
National STD hotline (800) 227-8922
Herpes Resource Center hotline (800) 230-6039

Sjogren's Syndrome

National Sjogren's Syndrome Association
3201 West Evans Drive
Phoenix, AZ 85023
(800) 395-6772

Sjogren's Syndrome Foundation
382 Main Street
Port Washington, NY 11050
(516) 767-2866

Skin Conditions

FIRST—Foundation for Ichthyosis and Related Skin Types
P.O. Box 20921
Raleigh, NC 27619
(800) 545-3286

National Arthritis and Musculoskeletal and Skin Diseases Information Clearinghouse
P.O. Box AMS
Bethesda, MD 20892
(301) 468-3235

National Organization for Albinism and Hypopigmentation
1500 Loust Street, Suite 2405
Philadelphia, PA 19102
(800) 473-2310

National Psoriasis Foundation
6600 SW Ninety-second, Suite 300
Portland, OR 97223
(800) 248-0886

National Vitiligo Foundation
P.O. Box 6337
Tyler, TX 75711
(903) 534-2925

Scleroderma Federation
Peabody Office Building
One Newbury Street
Peabody, MA 01960
(800) 422-1113

United Scleroderma Foundation
P.O. Box 399
Watsonville, CA 95077
(800) 722-4673

Sleep Disorders

American Narcolepsy Association
425 California Street, No. 201
San Francisco, CA 94104
(415) 856-7564

American Sleep Apnea Association
2700 East Main Street, Suite 206
Columbus, OH 43209-2536
(614) 239-4200

National Sleep Foundation
122 South Robertson Boulevard, 3rd Floor
Los Angeles, CA 90048
(310) 288-0466

Smoking

American Cancer Society
1599 Clifton Road NE
Atlanta, GA 30329
(800) ACS-2345

American Lung Association
1740 Broadway
New York, NY 10019-4374
(800) 586-4872

National Clearinghouse for Smoking and Health
Office on Smoking and Health

Centers for Disease Control and Prevention
4770 Buford Highway NE
Mailstop K50
Atlanta, GA 30341
(404) 488-5708

Spina Bifida

Spina Bifida Association of America
4590 MacArthur Boulevard NW, Suite 250
Washington, DC 20007
(800) 621-3141

Spinal Cord Injury/Paralysis

American Paralysis Association
500 Morris Avenue
Springfield, NJ 07081
(800) 225-0292
Spinal Cord Injury Hotline (800) 526-3456

National Spinal Cord Injury Association
600 West Cummings Park, Suite 2000
Woburn, MA 01801
(800) 962-9629

Stress

American Institute of Stress
124 Park Avenue
Yonkers, NY 10703
(800) 24-RELAX

Stroke

National Stroke Association
8480 East Orchard Road, Suite 1000
Englewood, CO 80111-5015
(800) STROKES

Stroke Clubs, International
805 Twelfth Street
Galveston, TX 77550
(409) 762-1022

Sturge-Weber Disease

Sturge-Weber Foundation
P.O. Box 460931
Aurora, CO 80046
(800) 627-5482

Stuttering

National Center for Stuttering
200 East Thirty-third Street
New York, NY 10016
(800) 221-2483

Thyroid Problems

Thyroid Foundation of America
Massachusetts General Hospital
Ruth Sleeper Hall 350
Boston, MA 02114
(617) 726-8500

Torticollis

National Spasmodic Torticollis Association
P.O. Box 476
Elm Grove, WI 53122
(800) HURTFUL

Tourette's Syndrome

Tourette's Syndrome Association
42-40 Bell Boulevard
Bayside, NY 11361
(800) 237-0717

Transplants

Organ Transplant Fund
1027 South Yates Road
Memphis, TN 38119
(800) 489-3863

Transplant Recipients International Organization
244 North Bellfield Avenue
Pittsburgh, PA 15213
(412) 687-2210

Tuberous Sclerosis

National Tuberous Sclerosis Association
8000 Corporate Drive, Suite 120
Landover, MD 20785
(800) 225-6872

Wilson's Disease

Wilson's Disease Association
P.O. Box 75324
Washington, DC 20013
(703) 636-3014

Besides the information sources listed above, a few governmental agencies not cited also provide information on various medical conditions. These include the Agency for Health Care Policy and Research. This agency provides "Clinical Practice Guidelines," reviewing for physicians' expert recommendations on the best way to treat various conditions, for instance, heart failure and cancer pain. "Patient Guides" summarizing the guidelines in plain English are also available.

Agency for Health Care Policy and Research
Publications Clearinghouse
P.O. Box 8547
Silver Spring, MD 20907
(800) 358-9295

Another source of written material on a wide variety of subjects, medical and otherwise, is the

Consumer Information Center
Pueblo, CO 81009
(719) 948-4000

Finally, a section of the National Institutes of Health holds Consensus Development Conferences on various subjects, including the treatment of sleep disorders in older people and the diagnosis and treatment of melanoma:

> Office of Medical Applications of Research
> National Institutes of Health
> Federal Office Building, Room 618
> Bethesda, MD 20892

"Consensus Statement" brochures are excellent summaries of current thinking but are written in technical medical language.

APPENDIX 3

Sources of Other Medical Information

The following is a list of various organizations that provide information on a wide variety of health-related subjects from board certification of doctors to women's health issues.

Board Certification for D.O.'s

Two competing organizations certify doctors of osteopathy. You may have to call both to find out if a doctor is certified.

American Association of Osteopathic Specialists
804 Main Street, Suite D
Forest Park, GA 30050
(800) 447-9397

American Osteopathic Association
142 East Ontario Street
Chicago, IL 60610
(800) 621-1773

Board Certification for M.D.'s

American Board of Medical Specialties
1007 Church Street, Suite 404
Evanston, IL 60201-5913
(800) 776-CERT

Childbirth

American College of Nurse-Midwives
818 Connecticut Avenue NW, Suite 900
Washington, DC 20006
(202) 728-9860

American Society for Psychoprophylaxis in Obstetrics (Lamaze
  Method)
1101 Connecticut Avenue NW, Suite 700
Washington, DC 20036
(800) 368-4404

Association for Childbirth at Home, International
P.O. Box 430
Glendale, CA 91205
(213) 667-0839

Cesareans: Support Education and Concern
22 Forest Road
Framingham, MA 01701
(508) 877-8266

Informed Homebirth: Informed Birth and Parenting
P.O. Box 3675
Ann Arbor, MI 48106
(313) 662-6857

International Cesarean Awareness Network
P.O. Box 152
Syracuse, NY 13210
(315) 424-1942

International Childbirth Education Association
P.O. Box 20048
Minneapolis, MN 55420
(800) 624-4934

Midwives Alliance of North America
P.O. Box 175
Newton, KS 67114
(316) 283-4543

Consumer Groups

Center for Medical Consumers and Health Care Information
237 Thompson Street
New York, NY 10012
(212) 674-7105

People's Medical Society
462 Walnut Street
Allentown, PA 18102
(215) 770-1670

Public Citizen Health Research Group
2000 P Street NW, 6th Floor
Washington, DC 20036
(202) 833-3000

Disabilities

American Coalition of Citizens With Disabilities
1012 Fourteenth Street NW, Suite 901
Washington, DC 20005
(202) 628-3470

Clearinghouse of Disability Information
Office of Special Education and Rehabilitative Services
Switzer Building, Room 3132
330 C Street SW
Washington, DC 20202
(202) 205-8241

National Easter Seal Society
70 East Lake Street
Chicago, IL 60601
(312) 726-6200

National Information Clearinghouse for Infants With Disabilities
    and Life-Threatening Conditions
Benson Building, 1st Floor
University of South Carolina, Center for Developmental
    Disabilities
Columbia, SC 29208
(800) 922-9234 x 201
(800) 922-1107 South Carolina only

National Rehabilitation Information Center
8455 Colesville Road, Suite 935
Silver Spring, MD 20910
(800) 34-NARIC

Domestic Abuse

Clearinghouse on Family Violence Information
P.O. Box 1182
Washington, DC 20013
(703) 385-7565

National Coalition Against Domestic Violence
P.O. Box 18749
Denver, CO 80218
(303) 839-1852

National Council on Child Abuse and Family Violence
1155 Connecticut Avenue NW, Suite 400
Washington, DC 20036
(800) 222-2000

National Gay and Lesbian Domestic Violence Victims' Network
3506 South Ouray Circle
Aurora, CO 80013
(303) 266-3477

Drug Information, Prescription and Nonprescription

Food and Drug Administration
Office of Consumer Affairs
5600 Fishers Lane, HFE-50
Rockville, MD 20857
(301) 443-3170

Elder Health Issues

American Association of Retired Persons (AARP)
601 E Street NW
Washington, DC 20049
(800) 424-3410

Gray Panthers
2025 Pennyslvania Avenue NW, Suite 821
Washington, DC 20006
(202) 466-3132

Mature Outlook
6001 North Clark Street
Chicago, IL 60660
(800) 336-6330

National Citizens' Coalition for Nursing Home Reform
1424 Sixteenth Street NW, Suite 202
Washington, DC 20036-2211
(202) 332-2275

National Clearinghouse on Aging
Administration on Aging
330 Independence Avenue SW
Washington, DC 20201
(202) 619-0441

National Institute on Aging Information Office
National Institutes of Health
Building 31, Room 5C35
9000 Rockville Pike
Bethesda, MD 20892
(301) 496-1752

Older Women's League
666 Eleventh Street NW, Suite 700
Washington, DC 20001
(202) 783-6686

Environmental and Job-Related Problems

American Lung Association
1740 Broadway
New York, NY 10019-4374
(800) 586-4872

Center for Environmental Health and Injury Control
Centers for Disease Control and Prevention (CDC)
Building 1, Room 2047
1600 Clifton Road NE
Atlanta, GA 30333
(404) 639-3286

Citizens' Clearinghouse for Hazardous Waste
P.O. Box 6806
Falls Church, VA 22040
(703) 237-2249

Environmental Protection Agency (EPA)
Public Information Center, PM-211B
401 M Street SW
Washington, DC 20460
(202) 260-2080

Indoor Air Quality Information Clearinghouse
P.O. Box 37133
Washington, DC 20013
(800) 438-4318

National Institute for Occupational Safety and Health (NIOSH)
4676 Columbia Parkway
Cincinnati, OH 45226
(800) 35-NIOSH

National Safety Council
1121 Spring Lake Drive
Itasca, IL 60143
(800) 621-7615

Occupational Safety and Health Administration (OSHA)
U.S. Department of Labor
Room N-3647
Washington, DC 20210
(202) 219-8148

Family Planning

Office of Family Planning
U.S. Department of Health and Human Services
P.O. Box 37299
Washington, DC 20013
(301) 585-6636

Planned Parenthood Federation of America
810 Seventh Avenue
New York, NY 10019
(212) 541-7800

Fitness

Aerobics and Fitness Association of America
15250 Ventura Boulevard, Suite 200
Sherman Oaks, CA 91403
(800) 446-AFAA

National Heart, Lung, and Blood Institute Information Center
P.O. Box 30105
Bethesda, MD 20824
(301) 251-1222

President's Council on Physical Fitness and Sports
450 Fifth Street NW, Suite 7103
Washington, DC 20001
(202) 272-3430

Free Medical Care for Low-Income People

Hill-Burton Program
U.S. Department of Health and Human Services
5600 Fishers Lane, Room 11-25
Rockville, MD 20857
(800) 638-0742
(800) 492-0359

Gay/Lesbian Health Issues

National Lesbian and Gay Health Foundation
P.O. Box 65472
Washington, DC 20035
(202) 797-3708

Hospice and Home Care

Foundation for Hospice and Home Care
519 C Street NE
Stanton Park
Washington, DC 20002
(202) 547-6586

Hospice Education Institute
190 Westbrook Road
Essex, CT 06426
(800) 331-1620

National Hospice Organization
1901 North Moore Street, Suite 901
Arlington, VA 22209
(800) 658-8898

National Institute for Jewish Hospice
8723 Alden Drive, Suite 652
Los Angeles, CA 90048
(800) 446-4448

Hospital Accreditation

Joint Commission on Accreditation of Healthcare Organizations
One Renaissance Boulevard
Oak Brook Terrace, IL 60181
(708) 916-5600

Hysterectomy

Hysterectomy Educational Resources and Services Foundation
422 Bryn Mawr Avenue
Bala Cynwyd, PA 19004

Injury Prevention

National Injury Information Clearinghouse
5401 Westbard Avenue, Room 625
Washington, DC 20207
(301) 504-0424

National Safety Council
1121 Spring Lake Drive
Itasca, IL 60143
(800) 621-7615

International Traveler's Information

Centers for Disease Control and Prevention (CDC)
Atlanta, GA 30333
CDC Automated Traveler's Hotline (404) 332-4559

Living Wills and Health Care Proxies

Choice in Dying
200 Varick Street
New York, NY 10014
(800) 989-WILL

National Library of Medicine

National Library of Medicine
National Institutes of Health
Bethesda, MD 20894
(800) 638-8480

Maternal and Child Health

March of Dimes Birth Defects Foundation
1275 Mamaroneck Avenue
White Plains, NY 10605
(914) 428-7100

National Maternal and Child Health Clearinghouse
8201 Greensboro Drive, Suite 600
McLean, VA 22102
(703) 821-2098

Medicare/Medicaid Information

Health Care Financing Administration, Office of Public Affairs
U.S. Department of Health and Human Services
Hubert H. Humphrey Building, Room 435-H
200 Independence Avenue SW
Washington, DC 20001
(202) 690-6113
Medicare hotline (800) 638-6833

Minority Health Issues

Association of Asian/Pacific Community Health Organizations
1212 Broadway, No. 730
Oakland, CA 94612
(510) 272-9536

National Black Men's Health Network
250 Georgia Avenue, Suite 321
Atlanta, GA 30312
(404) 524-7237

National Black Women's Health Project
1237 Ralph David Abernathy Boulevard SW
Atlanta, GA 30310
(800) ASK-BWHP

National Indian Health Board (Native American)
1385 South Colorado Boulevard, Suite A-708
Denver, CO 80222
(303) 759-3075

Office of Minority Health Resource Center
U.S. Department of Health and Human Services
P.O. Box 37337
Washington, DC 20013
(800) 444-6472 English, Spanish, and Asian languages

Preventive Medicine

American Health Foundation
320 East Forty-third Street
New York, NY 10017
(212) 953-1900

Office of Disease Prevention and Health Promotion
ODPHP National Health Information Center
P.O. Box 1133
Washington, DC 20013
(800) 336-4797

Product Safety

U.S. Consumer Product Safety Commission
Office of Information and Public Affairs
5401 Westbard Avenue, Room 332
Bethesda, MD 20207
(800) 638-CPSC
(800) 638-8270 (TDD/TTY)
(800) 492-8104 (TTY in Maryland)

Radon

American Lung Association
1740 Broadway
New York, NY 10019
(800) 586-4872

Environmental Protection Agency (EPA)
Public Information Center, PM-211B
401 M Street SW
Washington, DC 20460
(202) 260-2080
National Radon Hotline (800) SOS-RADON

National Safety Council's Radon Program
1019 Nineteenth Street NW
Washington, DC 20036
(800) 55-RADON

Indoor Air Quality Information Clearinghouse
P.O. Box 37133
Washington, DC 20013
(800) 438-4318

Sexual Abuse

Survivors of Incest Anonymous
P.O. Box 26870
Baltimore, MD 21212
(410) 433-2365

Women's Health Issues

National Black Women's Health Project
1237 Ralph David Abernathy Boulevard SW
Atlanta, GA 30310
(800) ASK-BWHP

National Women's Health Network
514 Tenth Street NW
Suite 400
Washington, DC 20004
(202) 347-1140

Older Women's League
666 Eleventh Street NW, Suite 700
Washington, DC 20001
(202) 783-6686

APPENDIX 4

Sources of Information on Alternative Medicine

The federal government has recently opened an office to investigate the effectiveness of various forms of alternative medical care:

Office of Alternative Medicine
National Institutes of Health
6120 Executive Boulevard, EPS Suite 450
Rockville, MD 20892
(301) 402-2466

They distribute a directory of alternative health care associations. I'll list only a few below.

American Association of Acupuncture and Oriental Medicine
1400 Sixteenth Street NW, Suite 710
Washington, DC 20036
(202) 265-2287

American Association of Ayurvedic Medicine
c/o Dr. Deepak Chopra
P.O. Box 1382
South Lancaster, MA 01561
(800) 532-8332

American Botanical Council
P.O. Box 201660
Austin, TX 78720
(512) 331-8868

American Center for the Alexander Technique
129 West Sixty-seventh Street
New York, NY 10023
(212) 799-0468

American Chiropractic Association
1701 Clarendon Boulevard
Arlington, VA 22209
(703) 276-8800

American Foundation for Alternative Healthcare, Research and
    Development
25 Landfield Avenue
Monticello, NY 12701
(914) 794-8181

American Foundation of Traditional Chinese Medicine
1280 Columbus Avenue, Suite 302
San Francisco, CA 94133
(415) 776-0502

American Holistic Medical Association
4101 Lake Boone Trail, Suite 201
Raleigh, NC 27607
(919) 787-5146

Association for Applied Psychophysiology and Biofeedback
10200 West Forty-fourth Avenue, Suite 304
Wheatbridge, CO 80033
(800) 477-8892

Committee for Freedom of Choice in Medicine
1180 Walnut Avenue
Chula Vista, CA 92011
(800) 227-4473

Herb Research Foundation
1007 Pearl Street, Suite 200F
Boulder, CO 80302
(303) 449-2265

National Center for Homeopathy
801 Fairfax Street, Suite 306
Alexandria, VA 22314
(703) 548-7790

RECOMMENDED READING

Arnot, Robert, M.D. *The Best Medicine: How to Choose the Top Doctors, the Top Hospitals, and the Top Treatments*, Reading, Mass.: Addison Wesley, 1992.

The Boston Women's Health Book Collective. *The New Our Bodies, Ourselves: A Book by and for Women*. Updated and expanded. New York: Touchstone, 1992.

Bursztajn, Harold, M.D., Richard I. Feinbloom, M.D., Robert M. Hamm, Ph.D., and Archie Brodsky. *Medical Choices, Medical Chances: How Patients, Families, and Physicians Can Cope with Uncertainty*. New York: Routledge, 1990.

Consumer Reports Books. *The New Medicine Show: Consumers Union's New Practical Guide to Some Everyday Health Problems and Health Products*. Mount Vernon, N.Y.: Consumer Reports Books, 1989.

Doress-Worters, Paula B., and Diana Laskin Siegal in cooperation with the Boston Women's Health Book Collective. *The New Ourselves, Growing Older: Women Aging With Knowledge and Power*. New York: Touchstone, 1994.

Feinbloom, Richard I. *Pregnancy, Birth, and the Early Months: A Complete Guide*. 2nd ed. Reading, Mass.: Addison Wesley, 1993.

Graedon, Joe, and Theresa Graedon. *50+: The Graedons' People's Pharmacy for Older Adults*. New York: Bantam Books, 1988.

Inlander, Charles B., and Ed Weiner. *Take This Book to the Hospital With You: A Consumer Guide to Surviving Your Hospital Stay*. Revised and updated. Emmaus, Penn.: Rodale Press, 1993.

_____ , and the staff of the People's Medical Society. *Good Operations, Bad Operations: The People's Medical Society's Guide to Surgery*. New York: Viking, 1993.

Long, James W., M.D., and James J. Rybocki, Pharm. D. *The Essential Guide to Prescription Drugs: Everything You Need to Know for Safe Drug Use*. New York: HarperPerennial, 1994.

Mendelsohn, Robert S., M.D. *Confessions of a Medical Heretic*. Chicago: Contemporary Books, 1979.

Ornish, Dean, M.D. *Eat More, Weigh Less: Dr. Dean Ornish's Life Choice Program for Losing Weight Safely While Eating Abundantly*. New York: HarperCollins, 1993.

———. *Dr. Dean Ornish's Program for Reversing Heart Disease: The Only System Scientifically Proven to Reverse Heart Disease Without Drugs or Surgery.* New York: Ballantine Books, 1990.

Payer, Lynn. *Medicine & Culture: Varieties of Treatment in the United States, England, West Germany, and France.* New York: Henry Holt, 1988.

Robin, Eugene D., M.D. *Matters of Life & Death: Risks vs. Benefits of Medical Care.* New York: W. H. Freeman, 1984.

Scully, Thomas, M.D., and Celia Scully. *Playing God: The New World of Medical Choices.* New York: Simon & Schuster, 1987.

University of California, Berkeley, Wellness Letter. *The Wellness Encyclopedia: The Comprehensive Family Resource for Safeguarding Health and Preventing Illness.* Boston: Houghton Mifflin, 1991.

Vickery, Donald M., M.D., and James F. Fries, M.D. *Take Care of Yourself: The Consumer's Guide to Medical Care.* 5th ed. Reading, Mass.: Addison Wesley, 1993.

Weil, Andrew, M.D. *Health and Healing: Understanding Conventional and Alternative Medicine.* 2nd ed. Boston: Houghton Mifflin, 1988.

———. *Natural Health, Natural Medicine: A Comprehensive Manual for Wellness and Self-Care.* Boston: Houghton Mifflin, 1990.

Wolfe, Sidney, M.D., Phyllis McCarthy, Alana Bame, and Durrie McKnew. *10,289 Questionable Doctors: Disciplined by States or the Federal Government.* Washington, D.C.: Public Citizen Health Research Group, 1993. (state editions also available)

———, Rose-Ellen Hope, R. Ph., and the Public Citizen Health Research Group. *Worst Pills, Best Pills II: The Older Adult's Guide to Avoiding Drug-Induced Death or Illness.* Washington, D.C.: Public Citizen Health Research Group, 1993.

AFTERWORD

In this book I've tried to paint as honest a portrait as I could of the medical profession. I hope you've found it accurate and helpful. You can help me now by providing honest feedback. Please send any comments, corrections, or suggestions for future editions to

Timothy B. McCall, M.D.
PO Box 390945
Cambridge, MA 02139

or send email to

examinedoc@aol.com

Thanks!

INDEX